Cellular and Molecular Aspects of Glucuronidation

Aspects Cellulaires et Moléculaires de la Glucuronoconjugaison

Cellular and Molecular Aspects of Glucuronidation

Aspects Cellulaires et Moléculaires de la Glucuronoconjugaison

Proceedings of the International Congress on Cellular and Molecular Aspects of Glucuronidation
Held in Montpellier (France), 27-29 April 1988

Sponsored by the Institut National de la Santé et de la Recherche Médicale (INSERM)

Edited by

Gérard Siest
Jacques Magdalou
Brian Burchell

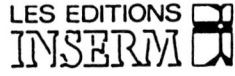

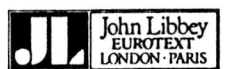

British Library Cataloguing in Publication Data

Cellular and molecular aspects of glucuronidation.
  1. Drugs. Chemical analysis
  I. Burchell, B.   II. Magdalou, J.
  III. Siest, Gerard   IV. Series
  615'.19015

ISBN 0 86196 182 X
ISSN 0768-3154

First published in 1988 by

John Libbey & Company Ltd
80/84 Bondway, London SW8 1SF, England.
(01) 582 5266
John Libbey Eurotext Ltd
6 rue Blanche, 92120 Montrouge, France. (1) 47 35 85 52
ISBN 0 86196 182 X

Institut National de la Santé et de la Recherche Médicale
101 rue de Tolbiac, 75654 Paris Cedex 13, France.
(1) 45 84 14 41
ISBN 2 85598 353 3

ISSN 0768-3154

© 1988 Colloques INSERM/John Libbey Eurotext Ltd,
All rights reserved
Unauthorised publication contravenes applicable laws

Editors/*Responsables éditoriaux*

Gérard Siest
Jacques Magdalou
Brian Burchell

Scientific committee/*Comité scientifique*

K.W. Bock
B. Burchell
J. Caldwell
J. Magdalou
G.J. Mulder
G. Siest

Secretary/*Secrétariat*

C. Thirion
M.A. Pham

Organizing committee/*Comité d'organisation*

Professeur Gérard Siest et Docteur Jacques Magdalou, Centre du Médicament, UA CNRS 597, 30, rue Lionnois, 54000 Nancy, France

Doctor Brian Burchell, Department of Biochemistry, Medical Sciences Institute, The University, Dundee DD1 4HN, UK

Acknowledgements

The organization committee would like to greatly acknowledge the following organizations for their auspices for the symposium « Cellular and molecular aspects of glucuronidation » :

— Société de Chimie Biologique (Groupe Thématique Enzymes du Métabolisme du Médicament)
— European Society of Biochemical Pharmacology
— International Society for the Study of Xenobiotics

The committee is also indebted to the following organizations and industrial firms for providing financial support :

— Ministère de la Recherche et de l'Enseignement Supérieur, Département Agriculture et Industries Agroalimentaires
— Institut National de la Recherche Agronomique
— Université de Nancy I
— Madaus (Koln), Sanofi, Sandoz (Basel), Bayer-Pharma, Duphar, Fabre, Fournier, Lers, Merck, Rhône-Poulenc Santé, Sarget, Servier

The Institut National de la Santé et de la Recherche Médicale has permitted the publication of this volume.

We would like to thank also the local organizing committee in Montpellier, Sanofi Recherche (J-P Cano) and especially Mrs Menu and Soullier.

Remerciements

Le comité d'Organisation exprime ses vifs remerciements aux organismes qui ont apporté leur patronage pour le Symposium « Aspects Cellulaire et Moléculaire de la Glucuronoconjugaison » :

— Société de Chimie Biologique (Groupe Thématique Enzymes du Métabolisme du Médicament)
— Société Européenne de Biochimie Pharmacologique
— Société Internationale pour l'Étude des Xénobiotiques

Ces remerciements s'adressent également aux organismes et aux industries pharmaceutiques qui nous ont apporté leur aide matérielle :

— Ministère de la Recherche et de l'Enseignement supérieur, Département Agriculture et Industries Agroalimentaires
— Institut National de la Recherche Agronomique
— Université de Nancy I
— Madaus (Cologne), Sanofi, Sandoz (Bâle), Bayer-Pharma, Duphar, Fabre, Fournier, Lers, Merck, Rhône-Poulenc Santé, Sarget, Servier

L'Institut National de la Santé et de la Recherche Médicale assure la publication des actes du colloque.

Enfin, nous remercions particulièrement Monsieur J.-P. Cano ainsi que Mesdames Menu et Soullier pour l'organisation locale à la Sanofi Recherche de Montpellier.

Foreword

The Workshop « Cellular and Molecular Aspects of Glucuronidation » took place, from 27 to 29 april 1988 at the Sanofi Recherche Center, in Montpellier, France. The purpose of this event, which attracted together more than 70 specialists coming from 11 countries, including Australia, Japan and United States was to discuss the recent advances in the study of the UDP-glucuronosyltransferases. The Workshop was the fifth devoted UDP-glucuronosyltransferases, after those held in London (1974), Bonn (1977), Göttingen (1981) and Titisee (1984).
This family of enzymes plays an important role in the ultime metabolism of foreign compounds, such as drugs, food additives, pesticides... It is also responsible for transformation of endogenous substances, some of them potentially toxic such as bilirubin.
The first part of the Workshop was devoted to the molecular basis of the existence of multiple enzyme forms in animals and also in man. The staggering success of the techniques in molecular biology will lead in the near future to the determination of the structure of the active sites and to the conception of new effectors and pharmacologically active molecules. Polymorphism and genetic deficiency in glucuronidation have been deeply investigated. The understanding of the molecular origin in the lack of glucuronidation, which can be studied with particular strains of rats and the development of new probes will help us to better detect or even prevent, in the human population, genetic diseases such as Gilbert's or Crigler-Najjar' syndrome.
The second part of the meeting was focused on the opportunity to use and valid new biological tools to characterize this enzyme : hepatoma cell lines, from man hepatocytes, isolated and perfused organs. The study of extrahepatic glucuronidation in brain or skin has begun to expand. However such models need the development of more specific and sensitive analytical methods for the detection and quantitation of glucuronides (HPLC, immunochemistry, monoclonal antibodies, mass spectrometry). Examples of applications and limits of these techniques have been described.
Finally, in the last part of the Workshop, the pharmacological and toxicological aspects of glucuronidation were discussed. Formation of toxic metabolites or influence of inducers was the subject of several oral presentations and posters.
In conclusion, this Workshop was a good opportunity to establish collaboration between researchers. The hectic working atmosphere did not exclude friendly interactions, which will also favour further progress in the field of UDP-glucuronosyltransferase.

The Editors

Avant-propos

Le colloque « Aspects Cellulaire et Moléculaire de la Glucuronoconjugaison » s'est tenu du 27 au 29 Avril 1988 dans les locaux de la Sanofi Recherche à Montpellier.

Cette manifestation, qui a réuni plus de 70 spécialistes venus de 11 pays, dont l'Australie, le Japon et les Etats-Unis, se proposait de faire le point sur les découvertes récentes concernant l'étude des UDP-glucuronosyltransférases. Il s'agissait du 5e colloque européen consacré à cette enzyme, après ceux de Londres (1974), Bonn (1977), Göttingen (1981) et Titisee (1984).

Cette famille d'enzymes joue un rôle primordial dans le métabolisme final des substances étrangères à l'organisme tels les médicaments, additifs alimentaires, pesticides... Elle intervient également dans la transformaion de composés endogènes dont certains sont potentiellement toxiques comme la bilirubine.

La première partie du colloque a été consacrée aux bases moléculaires supportant l'existence d'une multiplicité de formes enzymatiques tant chez l'animal que chez l'homme. Les progrès foudroyants des techniques de biologie moléculaire permettront, dans un avenir proche, d'élucider la séquence primaire de la protéine, la structure des sites actifs, et conduiront à l'élaboration de nouveaux effecteurs et molécules pharmacologiquement actifs.

Le problème du polymorphisme et de la déficience génétique a été approfondi. La compréhension de l'origine moléculaire des lacunes de la glucuronoconjugaison observées chez des souches de rats et le développement de sondes permettront de mieux dépister dans la population humaine les maladies génétiques de type Gilbert ou Crigler-Najjar et peut être un jour de les prévenir.

La seconde partie a fait le point sur l'opportunité d'utiliser et de valider de nouveaux modèles biologiques pour caractériser cette enzyme, comme les cultures de cellules d'hépatomes d'origine humaine, d'hépatocytes ou l'utilisation d'organes isolés perfusés. L'étude de la glucuronoconjugaison dans des organes autres que le foie ou le rein, tels le cerveau ou la peau, commence à se développer.

Cependant l'utilisation de ces modèles exige la mise au point de méthodes analytiques spécifiques et sensibles. Elles permettront la détection de plus en plus performante de glucuronides (HPLC, immunochimie, anticorps monoclonaux, spectrométrie de masse). Des exemples d'applications, mais aussi des limites de ces techniques, ont été présentés.

Enfin, dans une dernière partie, les aspects pharmacologique et toxicologique ont été rassemblés. La formation de métabolites toxiques ou l'influence de l'induction ont souvent été à la base des présentations.

En conclusion, ce colloque a été un lieu privilégié et propice à l'établissement de collaborations entre chercheurs. Son ambiance de travail n'a pas exclu un tissage de relations humaines amicales qui favoriseront sans nul doute de rapides progrès dans le domaine de l'UDP-glucuronosyltransférase.

Les Editeurs

List and Addresses of contributors
Liste et adresses des auteurs

Antoine B., Centre du médicament, UA CNRS 597, 30, rue Lionnois, 54000 Nancy, France.

Armstrong R.N., Dept. Chem and Biochem., University of Maryland, College Park, College Park, MD 20742, USA.

Batt A.M., Centre du Médicament, UA CNRS 597, 30, rue Lionnois, 54000 Nancy, France.

Bock K.W., Institut für Toxikologie, Universität Tübingen, Wilhelmstrasse 56, 7400 Tubingen, Allemagne.

Caldwell J., Dept. Pharmacology, St. Mary's Hospital, Medical School, Norfolk Place, W2 1PG Londres, Angleterre.

Carrera G., INSERM U 87, Groupe de Recherches sur la Toxicologie des Aliments et des Boissons, 2, rue François Magendie, 31400 Toulouse, France.

Celier C., INSERM U 75, Biochimie Pharmacologique et Métabolique, Faculté de Médecine, Necker-Enfants Malades, 156, rue de Vaugirard, 75730 Paris Cedex 15, France.

Coughtrie M.W.H., Biochemistry Department, Medical Sciences Institute, The University, Dundee DD1 4HN Ecosse.

Durand A., L.E.R.S. — Synthelabo, 23-25, avenue Morane Saulnier, 92366 Meudon La Forêt Cedex, France.

Fabre G., Sanofi Recherche Service Métabolisme et Pharmacocinétique, rue du Professeur J. Blayac, 34082 Montpellier Cedex, France.

Fevery J., Hepatology, Dept. of Medical Research, University of Leuven, B 3000 Leuven, Belgique.

Foliot A., Service de Biochimie, Hôpital Saint-Joseph, 7, rue Pierre Larousse, 75674 Paris Cedex 14.

Fournel-Gigleux S., Centre du Médicament, UA CNRS 597, 30, rue Lionnois, 54000 Nancy, France.

Ghersi Egea J.-F., Centre du Médicament, UA CNRS 597, 30, rue Lionnois, 54000 Nancy, France.

Gollan J.-L., Gastroenterology division, Brigham and Women's Hospital, 75 Francis Street, Boston, Mass. 02115, USA.

Goudonnet H., Formation de Biochimie Pharmacologique, Faculté de Pharmacie et Médecine, 7, Bd Jeanne d'Arc, 21033 Dijon Cedex.

Grant M.H., Dept. of Medicine and Therapeutics, Clinical Pharmacology Unit, Polwarth Building, Foresterhill, Aberdeen AB9 2ZD, Angleterre.

Harding D., Biochemistry Department, Medical Sciences Institute, The University, Dundee DD1 4HN, Ecosse.

Iyanagi T., Division of Biochemistry, Institute of Basic Medical Sciences, University of Tsukuba, Ibaraki 305, Japon.

Jayyosi Z., Centre du Médicament, UA CNRS 597, 30, rue Lionnois, 54000 Nancy, France.

Klaassen C.D., Department of Pharmacology, Toxicology and Therapeutics, University of Kansas Medical Center, 39th and Rainbow Blvd, Kansas City, KS 66103, USA.

Koster A.S., Rijksuniversiteit Utrecht, Dept. of Pharmacology and Pharmacotherapy, Catharijnesingel 60, NL — 3511 GH Utrecht, The Netherlands.

Mackenzie P.I., Department of Clinical Pharmacology, Flinders Medical Centre, Bedford Park, South Australia 5042.

Magdalou J., Centre du Médicament, UA CNRS 597, 30, rue Lionnois, 54000 Nancy, France.

Matern H., Abteilung Innere Medizin III der Medizinischen Fakultät der Rheinisch-Westfälischen, Technischen Hochschule Aachen, Pauwelsstrasse, D-5100 Aachen, Allemagne.

Matsui M., Kyoritsu College of Pharmacy, Shibakoen, Minato-ku, Tokyo 105, Japon.

Meyerinck von L., Dept. of Pharmacology, University of Hamburg, Martinistr. 52, D-2000 Hamburg 20, RFA.

Mulder G.J. Dept. of Pharmacology, University of Leiden, Sylvius Laboratories, P.O. Box 9503, 2300 RA Leiden, Pays-Bas.

Nicolas A., Faculté des Sciences Pharmaceutiques et Biologiques, Laboratoire de Chimie Analytique, 5, rue Albert Lebrun, 54001 Nancy Cedex, France.

Pacifici G.M. Instituto di Patologia Generale, Universita di Pisa, Via Roma 55, I — 56100 Pisa, Italie.

Padieu P., Faculté de Médecine, Laboratoire de Biochimie Médicale, 7, Bd Jeanne d'Arc, 21000 Dijon, France.

Rivière J.-L., INRA, Ecole Nationale Vétérinaire, Laboratoire d'Ecotoxicologie, 69752 Charbonnières Cedex.

Roy Chowdhury J., Liver Research Center, Albert Einstein College of Medicine, Bronx, NY 10461, USA.

Spahn H., Dept. of Pharmacy, School of Pharmacy, University of California, San Francisco, CA 94143-0446, USA.

Tephly T.R., The Toxicology Center, Dept. of Pharmacology, The University of Iowa, Iowa City, IA 52242, USA.

Totis M., Centre du Médicament, UA CNRS 597, 30, rue Lionnois, 54000 Nancy, France.

Ury A., ULP, Institut de Botanique, Laboratoire de Biochimie Végétale, et de Chimie Enzymatique, 28, rue Goethe, 67083 Strasbourg Cedex.

Van Breemen R.B., Department of Chemistry, North Carolina State University, Raleigh, North Carolina 27695, USA.

Van Es H.H.G., Academisch Ziekenhuis bij de Universiteit van Amsterdam, Meibergdreef 9, 1105 AZ Amsterdam, NL.

Van Stapel F., Biomedical NMR Unit, Campus Gathuisberg O/N 08, 3000 Leuven, Belgique.

Weil A., Laboratoires Fournier, Dept. Pharmacocinétique et Métabolisme, Route de Dijon, Daix, 21121 Fontaine les Dijon, France.

Williams G.M., American Health Foundation, Dana Road, Valhalla, New-York 10595, USA.

Contents
Sommaire

VII   Acknowledgments
VIII *Remerciements*
IX   Foreword
X   *Avant-propos*
XI   List of Contributors
      Liste des auteurs

MOLECULAR BASIS OF MULTIPLICITY AND REGULATION OF UDP-GLUCURONOSYLTRANSFERASES/*BASES MOLECULAIRES DE LA MULTIPLICITE ET DE LA REGULATION DES UDP-GLUCURO-NOSYLTRANSFERASES*

3   T. Iyanagi
    Cloning and characterization of 3-methylcholanthrene inducible rat liver UDP-glucuronosyltransferase mRNA
    Clonage et caractérisation du mRNA de l'UDP-glucuronosyltransférase hépatique de rat induite par le 3-methylcholanthrène

13 D. Harding, M.R. Jackson, R. Wooster, S. Fournel-Gigleux and B. Burchell
    Cloning of human UDP-glucuronosyltransferase cDNAs
    Clonage des cDNAs d'UDP-glucuronosyltransférases humaines

21 P.I. Mackenzie
    Expression of UDP glucuronosyltransferase cDNA
    Expression du cDNA de l'UDP glucuronosyltransférase

29 J. Roy Chowdhury, P. Lahiri, P.I. Mackenzie, F.F. Becker and N. Roy Chowdhury
    Expression of UDP-glucuronosyltransferase isoforms during development and carcinogen-induced preneoplastic transformation of liver in rats
    Expression des isoformes de l'UDP-glucuronosyltransférase pendant le développement et les transformations préneoplasiques hépatiques de rats

37 T. Tephly, M. Townsend, B. Coffman, J. Puig and M. Green
    Characterization of UDP-glucuronosyltransferases from animal and human liver
    Caractérisation des UDP-glucuronosyltransférases hépatiques animales et humaines

43 S. Fournel-Gigleux, J. Magdalou, G. Siest, M.C. Carré, S.R.P. Shepherd, M.R. Jackson, D. Harding and B. Burchell
Carboxylic acids as inhibitors and substrates of UDP-glucuronosyltransferases
Les acides carboxyliques substrats et inhibiteurs des UDP-glucuronosyltransférases

51 R.N. Armstrong, J.C. André and J.G.M. Bessems
Mechanistic and stereochemical investigations of UDP-glucuronosyltransferases
Aspects mécanistiques et stéréochimiques des UDP-glucuronosyltransférases

59 M. Matsui, F. Nagai and H. Homma
Genetic deficiency of UDP-glucuronosyltransferase in the rat
Déficience génétique de l'UDP-glucuronosyltransférase chez le rat

69 M.W.H. Coughtrie, D. Harding, S. Wilson, M.R. Jackson, S. Fournel-Gigleux, R. Hume and B. Burchell
Genetic deficiency of rat and human UDP-glucuronosyltransferases
Déficience génétique des UDP-glucuronosyltransférases de rat et d'homme

CELLULAR AND SUBCELLULAR BASIS OF GLUCURONIDATION/ *BASES CELLULAIRES ET SUBCELLULAIRES DE LA GLUCURONO-CONJUGAISON*

79 B. Antoine, J.A. Boutin and G. Siest
Investigation of UDP-glucuronosyltransferase isoenzymes restricted-specificity in liver microsomes
Etude de la spécificité restreinte d'isoenzymes d'UDP-glucuronosyltransférase

85 D.I. Whitmer and J.L. Gollan
Modulation of hepatic bilirubin transport and glucuronidation by the lipid microenvironment of substrate
Modulation du transport hépatique de la bilirubine par le microenvironnement lipidique du substrat

93 G.M. Pacifici, M. Franchi and L. Giuliani
Is there cytosolic glucuronyl transferase in human liver?
Existe-t-il une glucuronyltransférase cytosolique dans le foie humain?

103 F. Van Stapel and N. Blanckaert
Evidence that bilirubin UDP-glucuronosyltransferase faces the lumen of the endoplasmic reticulum in rat liver
Evidence de la présence de la bilirubine UDP-glucuronosyltransférase sur la face luminale du réticulum endoplasmique hépatique de rat

113 S. Dragacci, J. Magdalou, D. Bagrel, M. Roques, S. Fournel-Gigleux and G. Siest
Glucuronidation in human hepatoma cell lines and liver microsomes

Glucuronoconjugaison dans les cellules d'hépatomes et les microsomes hépatiques chez l'homme

121 **C.A. McQueen and G.M. Williams**
Conjugation of chemical carcinogens in cultured hepatocytes
Conjugaison des carcinogènes chimiques dans les hépatocytes en culture

129 **M.H. Grant, H. Doostdar, M. Maley, W.T. Melvin, J. Engeset and M.D. Burke**
Glucuronidation in rat and human hepatocyte cultures and in human HEP G2 hepatoma cells
Glucuronoconjugaison dans les hépatocytes en culture de rat et d'homme, ainsi que dans les cellules d'hépatomes humains HEP G2

137 **M. Diez Ibanez, M. Chessebeuf-Padieu and P. Padieu**
Production of free and glucuronoconjugated ring hydroxylated metabolites of 2-acetylaminofluorene in rat liver epithelial cell lines upon cocarcinogen induction
Production de métabolites hydroxylés sur le noyau, libres et glucuronoconjugués, du 2-acétylaminofluorène dans les cellules épithéliales hépatiques de rat après induction par un co-carcinogène

141 **H. Matern, H.U. Marschall, H. Wietholtz and S. Matern**
Glucuronidation and glucosidation of bile acids in normal tissues and carcinoma of man
Glucuronoconjugaison et glucosidation des acides biliaires dans les tissus normaux et cancéreux chez l'homme

151 **A.Sj. Koster, M.H. de Vries, F.A.M. Redegeld, R.P.J. Oude Elferink and P.L.M. Jansen**
Formation and transport of glucuronide-conjugates in the isolated perfused rat liver, intestine and kidney
Formation et transport des glucuronoconjugués dans le foie de rat isolé perfusé, l'intestin et le rein

159 **C.D. Klaassen and D. Goon**
Saturation of glucuronidation in the in situ intestine
Saturation de la glucuronoconjugaison dans l'intestin in situ

169 **J.-F. Ghersi-Egea, Y. Tayarani, J.M. Lefauconnier and A. Minn**
Enzymatic protection of the brain : role of 1-naphthol UDP-glucuronosyltransferase from cerebral tissue and cerebral microvessels
Protection enzymatique dans le cerveau : rôle de l'UDP-glucuronosyltransférase (1-naphtol) dans les tissus et microvaisseaux cérébraux

177 **Z. Jayyosi, B. Antoine, J. Thomassin, J. Magdalou, A.M. Batt and G. Siest**
Difference in UDP-glucuronosyltransferases between rat and hamster
Différence dans les activités UDP-glucuronosyltransférases entre rat et hamster

ANALYTICAL AND BIOTECHNOLOGIC APPROACHES/APPROCHES ANALYTIQUES ET BIOTECHNOLOGIQUES

185 J. Caldwell, N. Grubb, S. Nicholls, K.A. Sinclair, A.J. Hutt, A. Weil, S. Fournel-Gigleux
Structural and stereochemical aspects of acylglucuronide formation and reactivity
Aspects structuraux et stéréochimiques de la formation et de la réactivité des acylglucuronides

193 H.H.G. Van Es, W.H.M. Peters, B.G. Goldhoorn, M. Paul-Abrahamse, R.P.J. Oude Elferink and P.L.M. Jansen
Immunochemical characterization of UDP-glucuronyl transferase by monoclonal antibody techniques
Caractérisation immunochimique de l'UDP-glucuronyl transférase par les techniques d'anticorps monoclonaux

201 A. Nicolas and P. Leroy
New chromatographic methods for *in vitro* glucuronidation studies
Nouvelles méthodes chromatographiques pour étudier la glucuronoconjugaison in vitro

211 R.B. Van Breemen
Fast atom bombardment mass spectrometry with B/E linked scanning of ether- and thiophenol-linked glucuronides
Spectrométrie de masse FAB avec balayage asservi B/E pour l'étude des glucuronides d'éther et de thiophénol

221 J. Magdalou, B. Faye, B. Antoine and G. Siest
Modulation of UDP-glucuronosyltransferase kinetic by the lipid composition of the microsomal membranes in rat liver
Modulation de la cinétique de l'UDP-glucuronosyltransférase par la composition lipidique des membranes microsomales hépatiques de rat

225 A. Ury, P. Ullmann, P. Bouvier-Nave and P. Benveniste
Reconstitution of UDP-glucose-sterol-beta-D-glucosyltransferase into lipid vesicles and regulation by phospholipids
Reconstitution de l'UDP-glucose-sterol-beta-D-glucosyltransférase dans des vésicules lipidiques et régulation par des phospholipides

229 L. Von Meyerinck, C. Augustin, M. Schulz, F. Donn, H.F. Benthe and A. Schmoldt
Monoclonal antibodies to rat liver 4-nitrophenol UDP-glucuronosyltransferase
Anticorps monoclonaux envers la 4-nitrophénol UDP-glucuronosyltransférase

233 A. Weil, J.P. Guichard and J. Caldwell
Interactions between fenofibryl glucuronide and human serum albumin or human plasma
Interactions entre le fénofibryl glucuronide et l'albumine sérique humaine

TOXICOLOGICAL, PHARMACOLOGICAL AND PHYSIOPATHOLOGICAL APPLICATIONS/*APPLICATIONS EN TOXICOLOGIE, PHARMACOLOGIE ET EN PHYSIOPATHOLOGIE*

239 **K.W. Boc, S. Krull, U. Jongepier and G. Schirmer**
Rat and human liver UDP-glucuronosyltransferases inducible by 3-methylcholanthrene-type inducers
UDP-glucuronosyltransférases induites par des inducteurs de type 3-méthylcholanthrène chez le rat et l'homme

249 **J.P. Cano, G. Fabre, P. Maurel, N. Bichet, Y. Berger and P. Vic**
Inter-individual variability and induction of cytochromes P-450 and UDP-glucuronosyltransferases in human liver microsomes and primary cultures of human hepatocytes
Variation inter-individuelle et induction des cytochromes P-450 et des UDP-glucuronosyltransférases dans les microsomes hépatiques humains et les cultures primaires d'hépatocytes humains

261 **L.Z. Benet and H. Spahn**
Acyl migration and covalent binding of drug glucuronides — potential toxicity mediators
Migration du groupement acyle et fixation covalente des glucuronides des médicaments — médiateurs possibles de toxicité

271 **G.J. Mulder, F.C.J. Wierckx, P.L.M. Jansen and A. Warrander**
Acyl-glucuronidation of ponalrestat in the rat in vivo and its role in the sex difference in urinary excretion of the drug
Formation d'acyl-glucuronide du ponalrestat chez le rat in vivo et son rôle dans la différence d'excrétion du médicament selon le sexe

279 **J. Fevery, V. Mesa, M. Muraca and W. Van Steenbergen**
Effects of drugs and of bilirubinostasis on glucuronidation of bilirubin
Effets des médicaments et de la cholestase sur la glucuronoconjugaison de la bilirubine

285 **G. Carrera, S. Forgues, J. Alary and H. Lapontarique**
Effects of an experimental hepatitis induced by D-galactosamine on the metabolism and toxicity of chlorpropham : *in vivo* and *in vitro* studies
Effets d'une hépatite expérimentale provoquée par la D-galactosamine sur le métabolisme et la toxicité du chlorpropham : étude in vivo *et* in vitro

289 **C. Celier, S. Marie, T. Cresteil and J.P. Leroux**
Hepatic drug-metabolizing enzymes and prenatal exposure to clofibrate
Enzymes hépatiques du métabolisme des médicaments et exposition prénatale au clofibrate

293 **A. Devaux and J.L. Rivière**
Study of UDPG-transferases in the carp, *Cyprinus carpio*
Etude des UDP-glucuronosyltransférases chez la carpe, Cyprinus carpio

297 **A. Durand, J.P. Thenot, G. Gillet, M. Beauvallet and P.L. Morselli**
Influence of repeated administration of fengabine, a new antidepressant on its own metabolism — *in vitro* study with rat hepatic microsomes

Influence d'une administration répétée de fengabine, un nouveau antidépresseur sur son propre métabolisme — étude in vitro avec des microsomes hépatiques de rat

301 **A. Foliot, A. Myara, D. Touchard and F. Trivin**
Effects of various drugs on microsomal UDP-glucuronosyltransferase activity in hamster liver
Effets de nombreux médicaments sur l'activité UDP-glucuronosyltransférase hépatique chez le hamster

305 **S. Fournel-Gigleux, J. Magdalou, C. Lafaurie, G. Siest, L. Grislain, M.H. Garnier, J.F. Dabé, W. Luijten, N. Bromet and M. Devissaguet**
Glucuronidation of perindopril by hepatic microsomes : inter-species comparison
Glucuronoconjugaison du périndopril par les microsomes hépatiques : comparaison inter-espèces

311 **H. Goudonnet, J. Mounié, J. Magdalou, A. Escousse and R.C. Truchot**
Comparative induction of rat liver bilirubin UDP-glucuronosyltransferase by ciprofibrate and other hypolipidaemic agents belonging to the fibrate series : influence of the thyroid status
Induction comparée de l'UDP-glucuronosyltransférase hépatique de rat par le ciprofibrate et d'autres agents hypolipémiants appartenant à la série des fibrates : influence de l'état thyroïdien

317 **M. Totis, A.M. Batt and G. Siest**
Induction of different forms of UDP-glucuronosyltransferases by 52028 RP, an isoquinoleine derivative
Induction de différentes formes d'UDP-glucuronosyltransférases par le RP 52028, un dérivé de l'isoquinoléine

321 **G.M. Pacifici, M. Franchi, L. Vannucci, F. Mosca**
Sulphation and glucuronidation of ethinyloestradiol in human issues
Sulfo-et glucuronoconjugaison de l'éthinyloestradiol dans les tissus humains

325 Author Index
Index des auteurs

Molecular basis of multiplicity and regulation of UDP-Glucuronosyltransferases

Bases moléculaires de la multiplicité et de la régulation des UDP-Glucuronosyltransferases

Cloning and characterization of 3-methylcholanthrene inducible rat liver UDP-Glucuronosyltransferase mRNA

T. Iyanagi

Division of Biochemistry, Institute of Basic Medical Sciences, University of Tsukuba, Ibaraki 305, Japan

ABSTRACT

We have purified 3-methylcholanthrene (MC) inducible UDP-glucuronosyltransferase (GT_{MC}) from rat liver microsomes, and determined the amino acid sequences of fragments of the enzyme including the amino terminus. On the basis of this information, we isolated and sequenced a cDNA clone. The deduced amino acid sequence of this cDNA contains a putative signal sequence and stop transfer signal containing a hydrophobic segment (Iyanagi et al. (1986) J. Biol. Chem., 261, 15607-15614).

Specific cDNA probes were used to analyse the induction of the enzyme in normal Wistar rat livers by treatment with MC. RNA blot analysis showed that MC increased the amount of hybridizable mRNA in the liver. The mRNA levels in the livers of heterozygous and homozygous Gunn rats were also increased by MC.

Southern blot analysis of genomic DNA in normal Wistar rats suggests that there is a unique coding for the MC-inducible GT isoenzyme. Similar restriction fragments of genomic DNA were observed in heterozygous and homozygous Gunn rat genomic DNA.

KEYWORDS

Hepatic UDP-glucuronosyltransferase, cDNA cloning and sequence structure, 3-methylcholanthrene induction, genomic DNA, hyperbilirubinemic Gunn rat, cytochrome P-450.

INTRODUCTION

Hepatic UDPGTs are a family of enzymes that catalyse the conjugation of endogenous substrates and xenobiotics with UDP-glucuronic acid (Siest et al., 1986). The enzymes, which exhibit different substrate specificities, have been purified in several laboratories. Some forms are increased in amount by treatment of animals with inducers such as 3-methylcholanthrene (MC) and 2,3,7,8,-tetrachloro-dibenzo-p-dioxin (TCDD). These inducers are also known to induce the synthesis of cytochromes P-450, DT-diaphorase, glutathione S-transferases and other drug metabolizing enzymes.

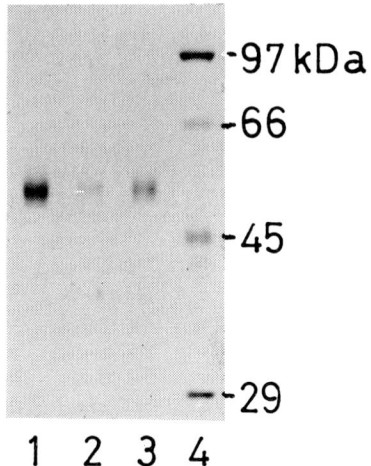

Fig 1. SDS/polyacrylamide gel electropheresis of GT_{MC}. Lanes: 1, 2μg; 2, 0.4μg; 3, 1μg of purified GT_{MC}. Lane 4, Mr, protein standards.

Structural Characteristic of GT_{MC}. For the structural analysis of GT_{MC}, tryptic peptides of the purified enzyme were separated by HPLC and sequenced, and one of them with minimal codon degeneracy was used as the cDNA probe. The rat liver cDNA library was constructed in pBR322 and screened for a GT_{MC} specific sequence using the mixture of 18-base oligonucleotides. The full-length clones eventually obtained were found by sequencing to be 1927 nucleotides long with untranslated region of 124 and 216 base pairs in the 5'- and 3'-terminal regions, respectively. The cDNA insert contained 1,587 base pairs that encode a complete primary sequence of a putative precursor form of GT_{MC} with a calculated molecular weight of 60,114.

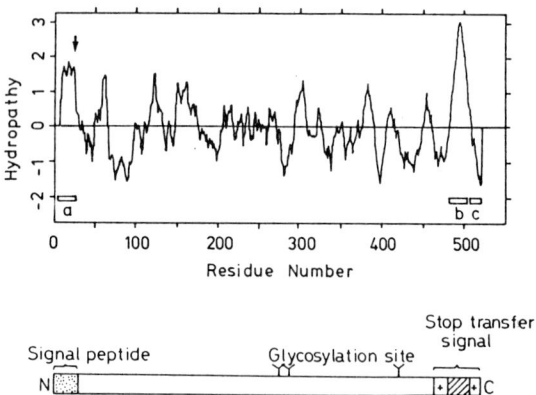

Fig 2. Hydropathy analysis of the deduced amino acid sequence of GT_{MC}. The highly hydrophobic (a and b) and positively charged amino acid (c) segments are designated. The NH2-terminal region of the mature enzyme is indicated by the arrow.

Cloning and characterization of 3-methylcholanthrene inducible rat liver UDP-Glucuronosyltransferase mRNA

T. Iyanagi

Division of Biochemistry, Institute of Basic Medical Sciences, University of Tsukuba, Ibaraki 305, Japan

ABSTRACT

We have purified 3-methylcholanthrene (MC) inducible UDP-glucuronosyltransferase (GT_{MC}) from rat liver microsomes, and determined the amino acid sequences of fragments of the enzyme including the amino terminus. On the basis of this information, we isolated and sequenced a cDNA clone. The deduced amino acid sequence of this cDNA contains a putative signal sequence and stop transfer signal containing a hydrophobic segment (Iyanagi et al. (1986) J. Biol. Chem., 261, 15607-15614).

Specific cDNA probes were used to analyse the induction of the enzyme in normal Wistar rat livers by treatment with MC. RNA blot analysis showed that MC increased the amount of hybridizable mRNA in the liver. The mRNA levels in the livers of heterozygous and homozygous Gunn rats were also increased by MC.

Southern blot analysis of genomic DNA in normal Wistar rats suggests that there is a unique coding for the MC-inducible GT isoenzyme. Similar restriction fragments of genomic DNA were observed in heterozygous and homozygous Gunn rat genomic DNA.

KEYWORDS

Hepatic UDP-glucuronosyltransferase, cDNA cloning and sequence structure, 3-methylcholanthrene induction, genomic DNA, hyperbilirubinemic Gunn rat, cytochrome P-450.

INTRODUCTION

Hepatic UDPGTs are a family of enzymes that catalyse the conjugation of endogenous substrates and xenobiotics with UDP-glucuronic acid (Siest et al., 1986). The enzymes, which exhibit different substrate specificities, have been purified in several laboratories. Some forms are increased in amount by treatment of animals with inducers such as 3-methylcholanthrene (MC) and 2,3,7,8,-tetrachloro-dibenzo-p-dioxin (TCDD). These inducers are also known to induce the synthesis of cytochromes P-450, DT-diaphorase, glutathione S-transferases and other drug metabolizing enzymes.

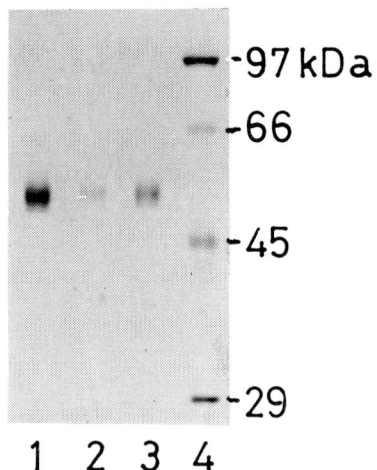

Fig 1. SDS/polyacrylamide gel electropheresis of GT_{MC}. Lanes: 1, 2μg; 2, 0.4μg; 3, 1μg of purified GT_{MC}. Lane 4, Mr, protein standards.

Structural Characteristic of GT_{MC}. For the structural analysis of GT_{MC}, tryptic peptides of the purified enzyme were separated by HPLC and sequenced, and one of them with minimal codon degeneracy was used as the cDNA probe. The rat liver cDNA library was constructed in pBR322 and screened for a GT_{MC} specific sequence using the mixture of 18-base oligonucleotides. The full-length clones eventually obtained were found by sequencing to be 1927 nucleotides long with untranslated region of 124 and 216 base pairs in the 5'- and 3'-terminal regions, respectively. The cDNA insert contained 1,587 base pairs that encode a complete primary sequence of a putative precursor form of GT_{MC} with a calculated molecular weight of 60,114.

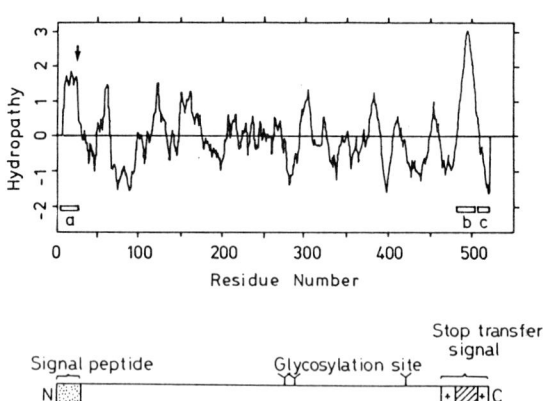

Fig 2. Hydropathy analysis of the deduced amino acid sequence of GT_{MC}. The highly hydrophobic (a and b) and positively charged amino acid (c) segments are designated. The NH2-terminal region of the mature enzyme is indicated by the arrow.

The UDPGT isoenzyme using 4-nitrophenol (NP) as substrate is inducible by MC (Bock et al., 1979). We have previously shown that the inductive effect of MC results in increases in the translational activity of GT_{MC} mRNA (Iyanagi et al., 1986). However, MC does not induce the UDPGT with impaired activity towards NP in the hyperbilirubinemic Gunn rat. The cytochrome P-450 isoenzyme in Gunn rats, on the other hand, is increased by treatment with MC (Vainio and Hietanen., 1974 and Coughtrie et al., 1987). These facts suggest that the MC-inducible UDPGT isoenzyme is absent in Gunn rats. The molecular basis for the different inducibilities of the GT_{MC} and cytochrome P-450 isoenzymes has not been elucidated.

In this manuscript we have summarized our previous work aimed at characterizing the structure of GT_{MC}. Furthermore, we have extended these studies to examine the differences in the inducibility of the GT_{MC} and cytochrome P-450 isoenzymes in normal Wister and Gunn rat tissues.

MATERIAL AND METHODS

Enzyme preparation. Hepatic microsomes were prepared from female Wister rats injected daily for 3 days with MC (4 mg/100g body weight). The enzyme was purified from MC-treated rat liver microsomes by the method of Falany and Tephly (1983) with some modifications (Iyanagi et al., 1986).

Animal treatment. Female Wistar (W) and female Sprague-Dawley (SD) rats were obtained from Doken Inc (Ibaraki, Japan). Adult female heterozygous and homozygous Gunn rats (8-12 weeks, 100-200 g) were from colonies maintained in the Sankyo Company Ltd (Laboratory animal science and toxicology laboratory, Shizuoka, Japan) (Nagai et al., 1987). For induction studies, MC (4 mg/100g body weight) was injected intraperitoneally for 2 days, and animals were sacrificed on the third day.

cDNA cloning. Cloning of cDNA coding for GT_{MC} was as described in a previous publication (Iyanagi et al., 1986).

RNA blot analysis. Total RNA was extracted from the livers of untreated or MC-treated female rats by the guanidine thiocyanate method. Total RNA was denatured for electrophoresis on a 1.2% agarose gel containing 0.66M formaldehyde, and then transferred to a nitrocellulose filter. The filter was hybridized with 32P labeled cDNA probes of GT_{MC}. The detection of cytochrome P-450c was performed using an oligonucleotide probe as described by Giachelli and Omiecinski (1987).

DNA blot analysis. High-molecular-weight genomic DNA was prepared according to the method of Maniatis et al. (1982). Southern blot analysis was carried out at 65°C for 18h as described by Maniatis et al. (1982) using nick-translated cDNA as probes.

RESULTS AND DISCUSSION

Purification and characterization of GT_{MC}. The MC-inducible UDPGT (GT_{MC}) was purified to homogeneity from liver microsomes of MC-treated female Wistar rats. The purified enzyme had a high activity for 4-nitrophenol (NP) as a substrate and an Mr of 55-KDa as determined by SDS-PAGE (Fig. 1). For the amino acid sequence analysis, the enzyme was further purified by HPLC. The sequence of the amino terminal 26 amino acids of the enzyme was determined by automated microsequence analysis. The histidine at the COOH-terminal was detected by hydrazinolysis.

The amino acid sequence deduced from the cDNA revealed a sequence of positively charged amino acids at the COOH-terminus that could serve as a stop-transfer signal (Fig. 2, domain b). On the other hand, the NH2-terminal sequence, amino acids 1-25 (Fig. 2, domain a) is hydrophobic, and is cleaved to form the mature enzyme.

The amino acid sequences of 5 isoenzymes including GT_{MC} have been deduced from cDNA clones (Fig. 3). A comparison of the 5 isoenzymes reveals the following structural characteristics, (1) all transferase clones encode 528-530 amino acids, (2) the putative signal sequence and stop transfer sequence are found in all isoenzymes, (3) homologous and variable amino acids are not evenly distributed along the sequence as and clustering of homologous amino acid are noted in the COOH-terminal region, (4) GT_{MC} is approximately 40% similar to that of the other isoenzymes. These results suggest that these 5 species of GT diverged from a common ancestor.

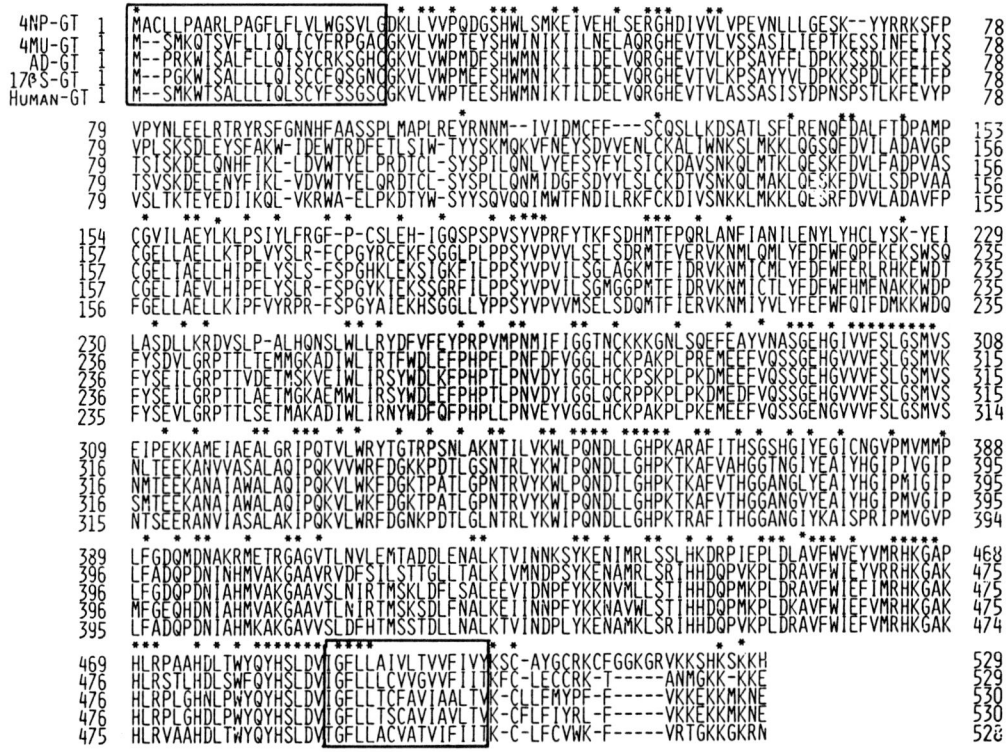

Fig 3. Sequence homology of UDPGT isoenzymes. The putative signal sequence and stop transfer signal region are enclosed in a box. Identical amino acids in the 5 isoenzymes are indicated by asterisk. 4NP-GT, 4-nitrophenol UDPGT (Iyanagi et al., 1986); 4MU-GT, 4-methylumbelliferone UDPGT (Mackenzie, 1986); AD-GT, androsterone UDPGT (Jackson and Burchell, 1986 and Mackenzie, 1986); 17β-hydroxysteroid UDPGT (Harding et al., 1987 and Mackenzie, 1987); Human-GT, Human UDPGT (Jackson et al., 1987).

Regulation of GT_{MC} mRNA. MC administration to rats resulted in an elevation in the translational activity of GT_{MC} mRNA (Iyanagi et al., 1986). This data is further supported by the results presented in Fig. 4. RNA blot analysis showed that MC increased the amount of hybridizable mRNA in livers of SD, normal Wistar, heterozygous (j/+) and homozygous (j/j) Gunn rats (Fig. 4, GT_{MC}). The levels of mRNA isolated from untreated rats were extremely low in all rat livers. Cytochrome P-450c, which is an MC-inducible isoenzyme, was also increased by MC treatment of the animals (Fig. 4, P-450c).

Vainio and Hietanen (1974) and Coughtrie et al. (1987) suggested that the isoenzyme of MC-inducible GT is absent in homozygous Gunn rats. The present data, however, indicate that MC-inducible mRNA is present in homozygous Gunn rats liver. Possible explanations for these observations are: mRNA is increased by the treatment of MC, but no emzyme or a "defective" GT_{MC} is synt   ized. To confirm this idea, the enzyme activity and the existence of enzyme protein must be clarified. Such a study is under investigetion in our laboratory.

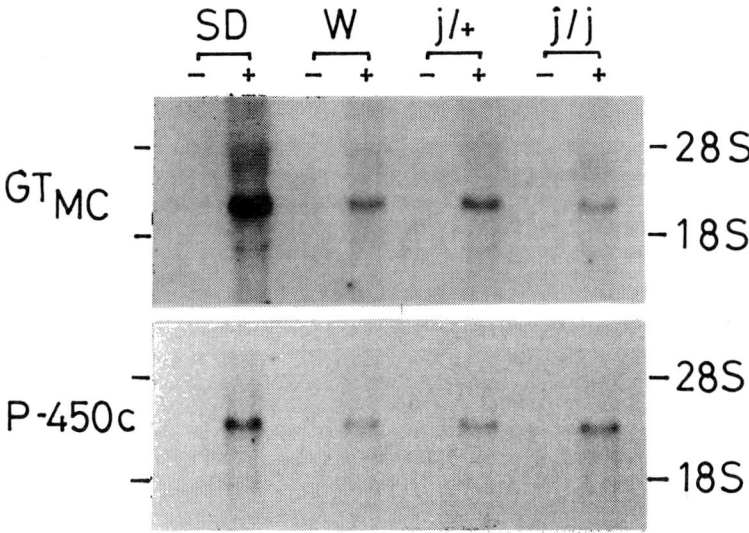

Fig 4. Blot analysis of RNA from rat liver. The GT_{MC} mRNA (10μg of total RNA) was detected using an EcoRI-Hind III fragment (nucleotide -110-371 of cDNA) labeled with 32P by nick translation. The cytochrome P-450c mRNA (10μg of total RNA) was detected using an oligonucleotide probe, as described under Materials and Methods. MC (- or +), untreated (-) or MC-treated (+); SD, Sprague-Dawley rat; W, normal Wister rat; j/+, heterozygous Gunn rat; j/j, homogzygous Gunn rat.

Southern blot analysis of rat liver genomic DNA. High-molecular-weight DNA isolated from normal Wistar, and heterozygous and homozygous rat liver was digested with several restriction endonucleases and Southern blotted from an agarose gel. The 5' EcoRI-Hind III fragment hybridized to one band from the EcoRI, BamHI and KpnI digests (Fig. 5,A) whereas the mixture of cDNA probes, which encompassed most of the cDNA hybridized to two or three band in normal Wistar and heterozygous and homozygous Gunn rat genomic DNA (Fig. 5,B). These results suggest that the MC-inducible GT is encoded by a single gene spanning approximately 15kb, and that a large deletion in the Gunn rat genome involving the area encoding GT_{MC} has not occured.

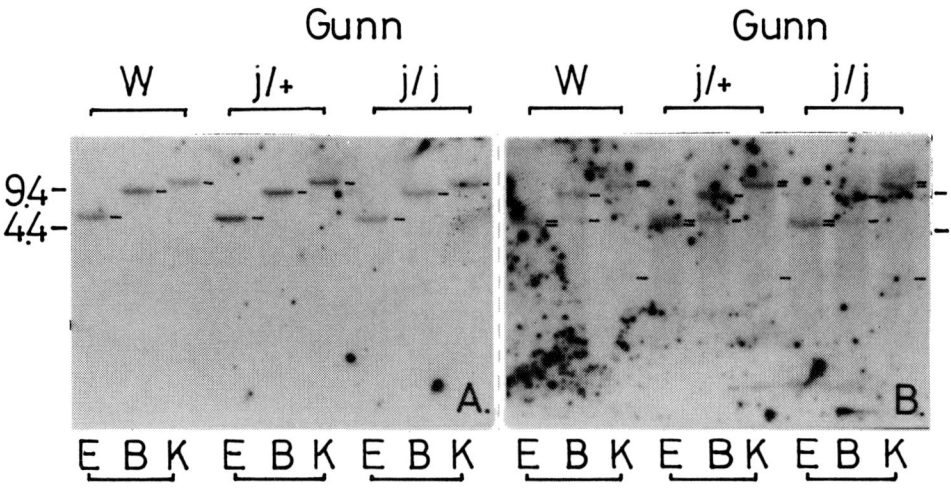

Fig 5. Southern blot analysis of rat liver genomic DNA. The 32P-labeled probes used were the EcoRI-Hind III fragment (nucleotide -110-371) and the Pvu II-Dra I fragment (nucleotide 371-1777) of the cDNA. In panel A the EcoRI-Hind III fragment was used whereas in panel B the mixture of EcoRI-Hind III and Pvu II-Dra I fragments were used as probes. E,EcoRI digest; B,BamHI digest; K,Kpn I digest.

Further studies. UDPGTs are membrane-bound enzymes that are localized in the endoplasmic reticulum (Roy Chowdhury et al., 1985). The enzyme activity of UDPGTs in isolated microsomes is markedly stimulated by treatment with detergents which affect the integrity of the membrane. These observations suggest that the enzyme is located on the luminal side of the ER. The amino acid sequence predicted from the cDNA support this proposed disposition of the enzyme in the ER membrane (Fig. 2 and 3).

UDPGTs are known to be involved in drug metabolism in concert with cytochrome P-450, that is, phase I and II reactions take place successively in the ER. The asymmetrical arrangement of these drug metabolizing enzymes in the membrane may ensure the vectorial excretion of drug metabolites from cytosol compartments to the lumen of the ER, as shown in Fig. 6. Furthermore, this model proposes the existence of the translocator (T) for transport across the membrane, of UDP-glucuronic acid (UDPGA), a substrate for UDPGT, that is synthesized in the cytosol compartments.

Cytochromes P-450, located in the ER, are also induced by treatment with MC, and the presence of both cis-acting regulatory genetic elements (Gonzalez et al., 1985; Sogawa et al., 1986) and a trans-acting receptor gene (Hankinson et al., 1985) have been comfirmed. The mechanism of induction of GT_{MC} by MC, however, has not been clarified. Therefore, it will be interesting to study the mechanism underlying the coinduction of these two kinds of drug metabolizing enzymes by MC.

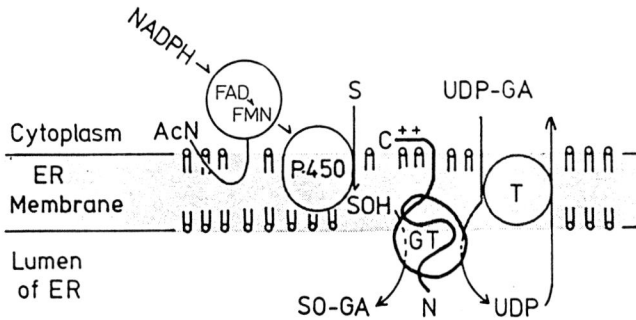

Fig 6. The vectorial transport model for drug biotransformation catalyzed by both the cytochrome P-450 system and UDPGT in the membrane of the ER. The model indicates that a drug substrate (S) is hydroxylated by the cytochrome P-450 system (Phase I reaction) (Iyanagi et al., 1981; Iyanagi et al., 1981) and the hydroxylated product (SOH) is glucuronized by UDP-GT (Phase II reaction), which is located in the luminal side of the ER membrane (Iyanagi et al., 1986). The postulated translocation protein (T) catalyzes a translocatio reaction of UDP-GA from the cytoplasmic compartment by a coupled exchange with UDP. The charged segment at the COOH-terminal of the GT is marked with a +. FAD-FMN, NADPH-cytochrome P-450 reductase; P-450, cytochrome P-450; GT, glucuronosyltransferase; T, translocation protein for UDP-GA; S, drug substrate; SOH, hydroxylated product; SO-GA, glucuronide conjugate of SOH; ER, endoplasmic reticulum.

Acknowledgments - I am deeply indebted to Dr. H. Tanase, (Laboratory animal science and toxicology laboratory, Shizuoka, Japan) for supplying of the Gunn rats and also Drs. P.I. Mackenzie, K. Sogawa, Y. Fujii-Kuriyama and K.F. Anan, for helpful discussions and sugestions.

REFERENCES

Bock, K.W., Lilienblum, W. and Pfeil, H.(1979): Purification of rat liver microsomal UDP-glucuronosyltransferase. Separation of two enzyme forms inducible by 3-methylcholanthrene or phenobarbital. Eur. J. Biochem. 98, 19-26.

Coughtrie, M.W.H., Burchell, B., Shepherd, I.M. and Bend, J.R.(1987): Defective induction of phenol glucuronidation by 3-methylcholanthrene in Gunn rats is due to the absence of a specific UDP-glucuronosyltransferase isoenzyme. Mol. Pharmacol. 31, 585-591.

Falany, C.N. and Tephly, T.R.(1983): Separation, purification and characterization of three isoenzymes of UDP-glucuronosyltransferase from rat liver microsomes. Arch. Biochem. Biophys. 227, 248-258.

Giachelli, C.M. and Omiecinski, C.J.(1987): Developmental regulation of cytochrome P-450 genes in the rat. Mol. Pharmacol. 31, 477-484.

Gonzalez, F.J. and Nebert, D.W.(1985): Autoregulation plus upstream positive and negative control regions associated with transcriptional activation of the mouse P-450 gene. Nucleic Acids Res. 13, 7269-7288.

Hankinson, O., Anderson, R.D., Birreu, B.W., Sander, F., Negishi, M. and Nebert, D.W.(1985): Mutations affecting the regulation of transcription of the cytochrome P-450 gene in the mouse hepa-1 cell line. J. Biol. Chem. 260, 1790-1795.

Harding, D., Wilson, S.M., Jackson, M.R., Burchell, B., Green, M.D. and Tephly, T.R.(1987): Nucleotide and deduced amino acid sequence of rat 17β-hydroxysteroid UDP-glucuronosyltransferase. Nucleic Acids Res. 15, 3936.

Iyanagi, T., Haniu, M., Sogawa, K., Fujii-Kuriyama, Y., Watanabe, S., Shively, J.E. and Anan, K.F.(1986): Cloning and characterization of cDNA encoding 3-methylcholanthrene-inducible rat mRNA for UDP-glucuronosyltransferase. J. Biol. Chem. 261, 15607-15614.

Iyanagi, T., Suzaki, T. and Kobayashi, S.(1981): Oxidation-reduction states of pyridine nucleotide and cytochrome P-450 during mixed-function oxidation in perfused rat liver. J. Biol. Chem. 256, 12933-12939.

Iyanagi, T., Makino, R. and Anan, K.F.(1981): Studies on the microsomal mixed-function oxidase system: Mechanism of action of hepatic NADPH-cytochrome P-450 reductase. Biochemistry 20, 1722-1730.

Jackson, M.R. and Burchell, B.(1986): The full length coding sequence of rat liver androsterone UDP-glucuronyltransferase cDNA and comparison with other members of this gene family. Nucleic Acids Res. 14, 779-795.

Jackson, M.R., Mccarthy, L.R., Harding, D., Wilson, S., Coughtrie, M.W.H. and Burchell, B.(1987): Cloning of a human liver microsomal UDP-glucurono-syltransferase cDNA. Biochem. J. 242, 581-588.

Mackenzie, P.I.(1986): Rat liver UDP-glucuronosyltransferase; Sequence and expression of a cDNA encoding a phenobarbital-inducible form. J. Biol Chem. 261, 6119-6125.

Mackenzie, P.I.(1986): Rat liver UDP-glucuronosyltransferase; cDNA sequence and expression of a form glucuronidating 3-hydroy-androgens. J. Biol. Chem. 261, 14112-14117.

Mackenzie, P.I.(1987): Rat liver UDP-glucuronosyltransferase; Identification of cDNAs encoding two enzymes which glucuronidate testosterone, dihydrotestosterone, and ß-estradiol. J. Biol. Chem. 262, 9744-9749.

Maniatis, T., Fritsch, E.F. and Sambrook (1982): Molecular cloning: A laboratory Manual (Cold Spring Harbor, New York).

Nagai, F., Takahashi, M., Homma, H., Tanase, H. and Matsui, M.(1987): A comparison of uridine diphosphate-glucuronosyltransferase and other drug metabolizing enzyme activities between two mutant strains of wistar rats with a genetic deficiency in bilirubin or androsterone glucuronidation. J. Pharmacobio. Dyn. 10, 421-426.

Roy Chowdhury, J., Novikoff, P.M., Roy Chowdhury, N. and Novikoff, A.B.(1985): Distribution of UDP-glucuronosyltransferase in rat tissue. Proc. Natl. Acad. Sci. USA 82, 2990-2994.

Siest, G., Antoine, B., Fournel, S., Magdalou, J. and Thomassin, J.(1987): The glucuronosyltransferases: What progress can pharmachlogists expect from molecular biology and cellular enzymology? Biochem. Pharmacol. 36, 983-989.

Sogawa, K., Fujisawa-Sehara, A., Yamane, M. and Fujii-Kuriyama, Y.(1986): Regulatory DNA elements localized remotely upstream from the drug-metabolizing cytochrome P-450 gene. Proc. Natl. Acad. Sci. U.S. 83, 8044-8048.

Vainio, H. and Hietanen, E.(1974): Induction deficiency of the microsomal UDP-glucuronosyltransferase by 3-methylcholanthrene in Gunn rats. Biochim. Biophys. Acta. 362, 92-99.

Résumé

Nous avons purifié la forme d'UDP-glucuronosyltransférase (GT_{MC}) induite par le 3-méthylcholanthrène (MC) à partir de microsomes hépatiques de rat, et déterminé les séquences primaires des fragments NH_2 terminaux. Sur la foi de ces informations, nous avons isolé et séquencé un cDNA clone. Les acides aminés trouvés par déduction de la séquence de ce cDNA contiendraient une séquence signal et un signal d'arrêt de transfert possèdant un segment hydrophobique (Iyanagi et al. (1986) J. Biol. Chem., 261, 15607-15614).

Des sondes spécifiques à cDNA ont été utilisées pour analyser l'induction de l'enzyme dans le foie de rat Wistar après traitement par le MC. L'étude des blots d'ARN montre que le 3M augmente la quantité d'ARN messager hybridisable dans le foie. Ce taux d'ARN est aussi augmenté par le MC dans le foie de rats Gunn hétérozygotes et homozygotes. Une analyse par Southern blot de DNA génomique de rats Wistar contrôles suggère qu'il existe une région unique codant pour l'isoenzyme GT inductible par le MC. Des fragments de restrictions similaires des DNA génomiques ont été observés chez le DNA de rats Gunn homozygotes et hétérozygotes.

Cloning of human UDP-Glucuronosyltransferase cDNAs

D. Harding, M.R. Jackson, R. Wooster, S. Fournel-Gigleux and B. Burchell

Department of Biochemistry. University of Dundee, Dundee DD1 4HN, Scotland, UK

ABSTRACT
Seven different classes of human liver UDP-glucuronosyltransferase (UDPGT) cDNAs (HLUGs) were isolated from λgt11 cDNA libraries. The cDNA clones were separated into two sub-families on the basis of deduced amino acid sequence homology. Sub-family 1 contained 5 clones similar to rat androsterone and testosterone UDPGT and mouse m-1 GT. Sub-family 2 consisted of 2 cDNAs closely related to rat liver 4-nitrophenol-UDPGT (4-NP-GT). Inspection of the sequence of the sub-family 2 cDNAs, HLUGP1 and HLUGP2, indicates that a genetic recombination event may have occurred to enhance UDPGT substrate specificity. The UDPGT isoenzymes encoded by the full length cDNAs HLUG25 and HLUGP1 had characteristic N-terminal signal sequences. *In vitro* transcription/translation studies using the clone HLUG25 indicated that this signal sequence was cleaved, and that the UDPGT was glycosylated.The substrate specificities encoded by HLUG25 and HLUGP1 were determined after transient expression in COS 7 cells.

Key Words: Human UDP-glucuronosyltransferases/cDNAs/processing/expression.

INTRODUCTION
UDP-glucuronosyltransferase (UDPGT EC 2.4.1.17) is a family of integral membrane enzymes that catalyse the glucuronidation of many potentially toxic xenobiotics and endogenous compounds (Dutton, 1980). Overwhelming evidence indicates that glucuronidation in the rat is catalysed by a family of isoenzymes (see Siest *et al*, 1987; Burchell *et al*, 1987, for reviews). Very little direct data describing human UDPGTs exist. Immunoblotting of human liver microsomes identified at least 6 UDPGT isoenzymes (Jackson *et al*, 1987). Studies on the tissue specificity (Roy Chowdhury *et al*, 1985; M.W.H.Coughtrie, manuscript submitted), development (Leakey *et al*, 1987; Onishi *et al*, 1979), kinetics (Bock *et al*, 1978; Mahu *et al*, 1981; Parquet *et al*, 1985; Dragacci *et al*, 1987; Miners *et al*, 1988) and genetic deficiencies (Crigler and Najjar, 1952; Arias *et al*, 1969) of human UDPGT indicated that distinct isoforms may exist that specifically glucuronidate bilirubin, bile acids, morphine and 5-hydroxytryptamine. Recent protein purification has suggested that two distinct isoenzymes which glucuronidate a range of phenolic compounds are found in human liver (Irshaid and Tephly, 1987).

Cloned molecular probes are needed to define unique UDPGT isoenzymes and for studying the regulation, expression and inherited defects of human UDPGTs. In the present paper we report the molecular cloning of 7 different human UDPGT cDNA species. Comparisons of amino acid sequences deduced from these human UDPGT cDNAs have been made and are discussed with reference to rat UDPGT. Preliminary evidence for a genetic recombination event contributing to the range of human UDPGT substrate specificity is discussed. The processing during biosynthesis of the cloned UDPGT cDNAs has been examined and the substrate specificity encoded by two cloned human UDPGT cDNAs has been determined.

MATERIALS AND METHODS

Screening of Human Liver cDNA Libraries and Analysis of Human cDNA.

Human liver cDNA libraries constructed in the vector λgt11 were kindly provided by S. Woo (Baylor College of Medicine, Houston, Texas) and by Maloy Laboratories. HLUG25 cDNA, the 5' EcoRI fragment of HLUG 25 (Jackson *et al*) and RKUG39, a rat kidney 4-NP GT cDNA, (Iyanagi *et al*, 1987; Harding *et al*, unpublished data) were labelled by random oligonucleotide priming (Feinberg and Vogelstein, 1984.) and used as hybridisation probes for plaque screening. Low stringency conditions were employed (Maniatis *et al*, 1982).The cDNA inserts were isolated and subcloned into M13 mp18 and mp19 for sequence analysis as described previously (Jackson *et al*, 1987). DNA sequence analysis was performed using the UWGCG sequence analysis package (Devereux *et al*, 1986).

In Vitro Transcription/Translation of HLUG25.

HLUG25 cDNA was subcloned from λHLUG25 DNA (Jackson *et al*, 1987) into Gemini 1™ in both + and - orientations. Transcription was as described by Clemens (1984). p25+ and p25- were linearised with EcoRV prior to transcription and capped using G 5' ppp 5'. 0.05 µg of capped mRNA was added to a messenger-dependent reticulate lysate system with 15 µCi of ^{35}S methionine in the presence or absence of dog pancreas microsomes (Walter *et al*, 1981; Clemen *et al*, 1984). Immunoprecipitation was carried out by a method adapted from Fagan *et al* (1983) using an anti-rat liver UDPGT antibody (Burchell *et al*, 1984). Translation products were separated using 7.5% SDS PAGE and visualised after treatment with 2,5-diphenyloxazole (PPO) followed by autoradiography.

Transient Expression of Human UDPGT cDNAs in COS7 Cells.

HLUG25 and HLUGP1 were subcloned into the transient expression vector pKCRH2 and semi confluent COS7 cells were transfected with the recombinant plasmids. Growth of transfected cells in the presence and absence of tunicamycin, coupled with immunoprecipitation and SDS PAGE of newly synthesised radiolabelled proteins, was used to determine the glycosylation state of the expressed UDPGT isoenzymes. To determine the substrate specificties of the isoenzymes encoded by HLUG25 and HLUGP1, transfected cell homogenates were challenged with a wide range of agylcones in the presence of radiolabelled UDPGA. Reaction components were separated by thin layer chromatography as described by Bansal and Gessner (1980).

RESULTS AND DISCUSSION

Characterisation of Human Liver UDPGT cDNAS.

One human UDPGT cDNA (HLUG25) was isolated previously (Jackson *et al*, 1987). Four more closely-related UDPGT cDNAs have been isolated by screening human liver cDNA libraries at low stringency. Two additional, less homologous, human UDPGT cDNAs, HLUGP1 and HLUGP2, have been isolated using a rat kidney 4-NP GT cDNA probe. Three cDNA clones encode a full-length UDPGT coding region; HLUG25, HLUG4 and HLUGP1 (see Fig.1).

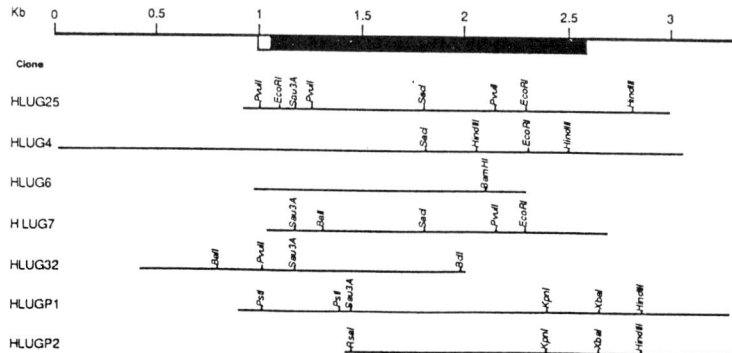

Fig. 1. Partial restriction maps of the human UDPGT cDNA classes isolated.

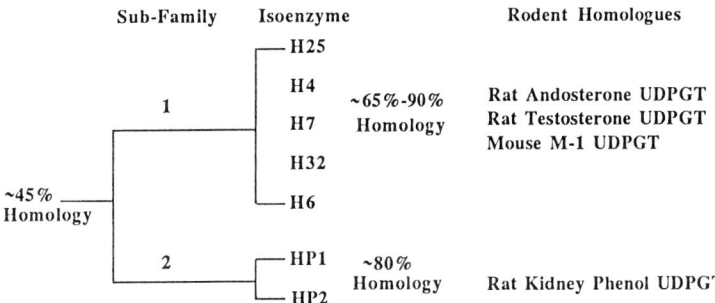

Fig.2. <u>Relationship of the human UDPGT cDNAs (derived from the deduced amino acid sequence identities).</u> *The isoenzyme encoded by the human UDPGT cDNA is prefixed with H and the number of the isoenzyme refers to the cDNA which encodes that isoenzyme. Thus HLUG25 encode the isoenzyme H25.*

The amino acid sequences encoded by the 7 cDNAs (HLUGS) have been deduced and analysed. The degree of identity between the 7 deduced amino acid sequences indicated that we have isolated human liver UDPGT cDNAs encoding isoenzymes from two sub-families (see Fig.2)

Sub-family 1, composed of the cDNAs HLUG25, HLUG4, HLUG7, HLUG32 and HLUG6, showed more than 70% homology to rat androsterone UDPGT (Jackson and Burchell, 1986; Mackenzie, 1986) rat testosterone UDPGT (Harding *et al*, 1987; Mackenzie, 1987) and Mouse m-1 GT (Kimura end Owens, 1987). Similarity between members of sub-family 1 is spread throughout the coding region although homology is greater in the C-terminal half than in the N-terminal half. Analysis of the nucleotide sequnces of this sub-family showed a similar pattern (see Fig 3a). Less significant nucleotide identity was observed within the non-coding regions of these cDNAs.

A very different pattern of amino acid and nucleotide sequence conservation was seen on analysis of the clones HLUGP1 and HLUGP2. HLUGP1 is 77% similar to rat liver 4-NP GT. Identity between HLUGP1 and HLUGP2 was ~80%. The 5'-145 amino acids of HLUGP2 were 48% similar to the comparable area in HLUGP1. The 3'-246 amino acids of both isoforms were identical as was the coding nucleotide sequence. Significantly the 3'-untranslated region of these two human cDNAs was also identical (see Fig 3b). This situation is analogous to that found for rat liver cytochrome P-450 b/e in which a gene conversion event was postulated to have occurred in order to enhance substrate specificity (Atchison and Adesnik, 1985). Further investigation is required to determine the mechanism by which these 2 UDPGTs have evolved, but it appears that the 5' region of HLUGP2 may represent part of another related UDPGT gene of unknown function. A recombination event may have occurred between the unknown UDPGT gene and the HP1 gene resulting in an increase in the range of substrates conjugated by UDPGTs.

Comparison of the amino acid sequences between 2 isoenzymes from different sub-families (HLUG25-HLUGP1) revealed an overall similarity of 44%. Closer inspection revealed that >65% identity between HLUG25 and HLUGP1 was found in the C-terminal half of the sequences; very poor homology <23% was found within the N-terminal half of the proteins.

Inspection of the amino acid sequence of the UDPGT isoenzymes encoded by the clones HLUG25 and HLUGP1 revealed that the amino-terminal area of the open reading frames encoded peptides similar to the cleaved signal sequences of the rat UDPGT proteins. This indicated that human UDPGTs may also be modified in this way. Human UDPGTs may also be glycosylated as both HLUG25 and HLUGP1 contain potential N-glycosylation sites (Hanover and Lennarz, 1981).

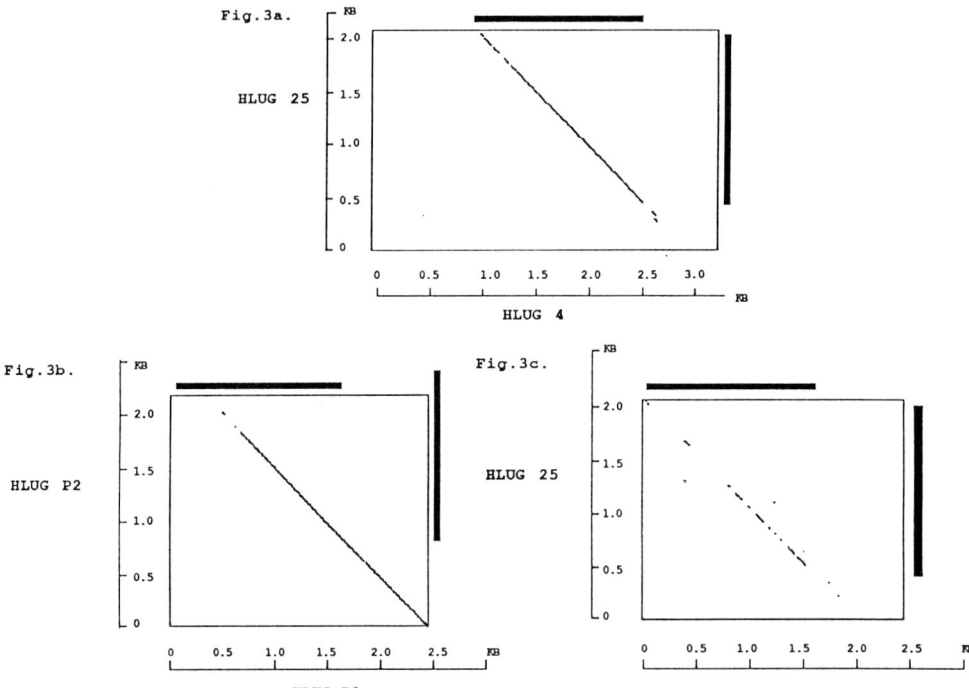

Fig. 3., Comparison of Nucleotide Sequence Identity of Human UDPGT cDNAs.
Fig. 3a shows the distrubution of sequence identity between 2 cDNAs of human UDPGT sub-family 1. Fig. 3b is the comparison between HLUGP1 and HLUGP2. Fig. 3c indicates the area of homology between human UDPGT sub-families 1 and 2. The coding region is indicated by ▬▬▬ .

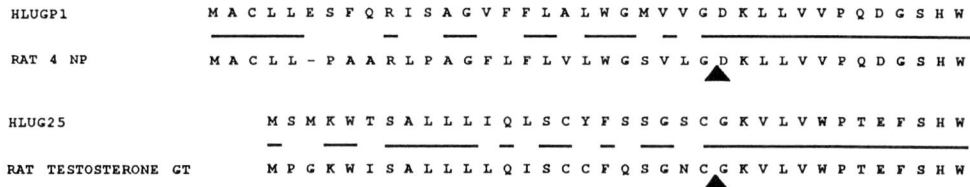

Fig. 4. Comparison of the Amino Teminal Sequences encoded by the cDNAs HLUGP1, Rat kidney phenol UDPGT, HLUG25 and Rat Testosterone UDPGT, ▲ indicates the amino terminus of the mature rat UDPGT protein (Iyanagi et al, 1986, Harding et al, 1987). Sequence identity between rat and human UDPGTs is shown by ▬▬▬ .

Processing of a Human UDPGT Glucuronosyltransferase.
HLUG25 was used as a model for studying the processing of human UDPGTs by coupling the cDNA to an *in vitro* transcription/translation system. Only *in vitro* translation of HLUG25 mRNA in the correct orientation produced radiolabelled proteins immunoprecipitable with anti-UDPGT antisera (see Fig. 5). The main immunoprecipitated translation product was a 53 kDa protein - the putative full-length product of HLUG25. Other minor products precipitated with this antibody are products of initiation of translation within the mRNA (R Wooster, unpublished data). Dog pancreas microsomes are known to possess signal peptidase and glycosyl transferase which modify the initial translation product (Walter *et al*, 1981; Clemens, 1984). The addition of dog pancreas microsomes to the translated p25+ mRNA resulted in the appearance of two

additional products of 50 and 53 kDa and translation was more efficient in the presence of dog pancreas microsomes. The two additional proteins appear to be post-translationally modified products of HLUG25. The 50 kDa protein may be the full length translation product after cleavage of the signal sequence and the 53 kDa protein may be the cleaved and glycosylated product. One putative N-glycosylation site was observed within the deduced amino acid sequence (-Asn-Thr-Ser-) at residues 315-317.

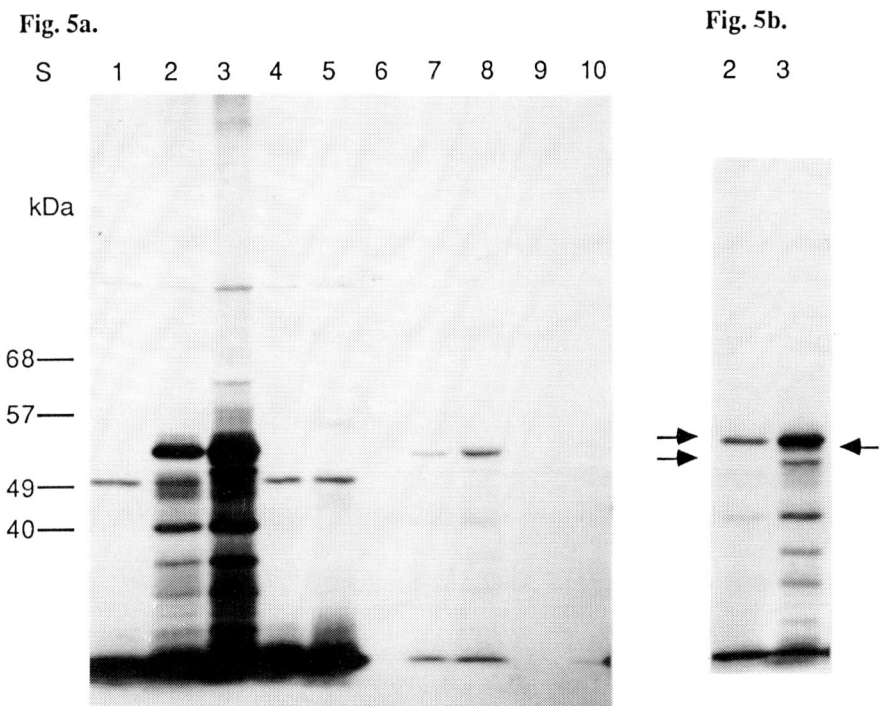

Fig. 5. *In vitro transcription/translation analysis of the UDPGT isoenzyme encoded by HLUG25.* Fig.5a; translation products were separated by SDS PAGE and visualised by autoradiography. Lane 1 is the translation products of p25- mRNA. Lanes 2 and 3 are the products of p25+ mRNA; dog pancreas microsomes were added to lane 3. Tracks 4 and 5 are as lanes 2 and 3 except no RNA was added. Lanes 6-10 show the immunoprecipitated products of lanes 1-5 respectively. Exposure was for three days at -80 C. The translation products of, <50kDa were due to internal initiation of translation. Fig.5b. is as for lanes 2 and 3 of Fig.5a. except that exposure was overnight. The arrows represent molecular weights of 54kDa, 50kDa, (left) and 53kDa (right), these are the unmodified, partially modified and fully modified UDPGT respectively. Molecular weight standards are indicated on the left.

Expression of HLUG25 and HLUGP1.
HLUG25 was expressed as a 53kDa glycoprotein. No activity towards androsterone or testosterone was found after transfection with HLUG25 despite high homolgy to rat androsterone UDPGT (Jackson and Burchell, 1986; Mackenzie, 1986) and rat testosterone UDPGT (Harding et al 1987, Mackenzie 1987). However HLUG25 did encode an isoenzyme capable of glucuronidating hyodeoxycholic acid but not lithocholic acid (Fournel-Gigleux et al, unpublished data). HLUGP1 encoded a human liver UDPGT isoenzyme, expressed as a 55kDa glycoprotein, with catalytic activity restricted to the glucuronidation of small planar phenolic compounds such as 1-naphthol and 4-NP (Harding et al, manuscript submitted).

Acknowledgements.
Financial support for this work was obtained from the Medical Research Ccouncil and the Wellcome Trust. BB is a Wellcome Trust Senior Lecturer.

Footnote.
1. The following abbreviations were used; UDPGT- UDP-glucuronosyltransferase, human UDP-glucuronosyltransferase cDNA- HLUG, 4NP- 4-nitrophenol, SDS-PAGE- Sodium dodecyl sulphate polyacrylamide gel electrophoresis.

References.
Arias, I.M., Gartner, L.M., Cohen, M., Esser, J.B. and Levi, A.J. (1969) Chronic non-haemolytic unconjugated hyperbilirubinaemia with glucuronosyltransferase deficiency Am.J.Med. **47**, 395-409.

Atchison, M. and Adesnik, M. (1986) Gene conversion in a cytochrome p450 gene family. Proc.Natl.Acad.Sci., **85**, 2300-2304

Bansal, S.K. and Gessner, T. (1980) A unified method for assay of uridine-diphosphoglucuronyltransferase activities towards various aglycones using uridine diphospho {U-C^{14}] glucuronic acid. Anal.Biochem. **109**, 321-329.

Bock, K.W., Brunner, G., Hoensch, H., Huber, E. and Josting, D. (1978) Determination of microsomal UDP-glucuronosyltransferase in needle-biopsy specimens of human liver. Eur.J.Clin.Pharmacol. **14**, 367-376.

Burchell, B., Kennedy, S.M.E., Jackson, M.R., McCarthy, L.R. and Barr, G.C. (1984) The Biosynthesis and induction of microsomal UDP-glucuronyltransferase in avian liver. Biochem.Soc.Trans. **12**, 50-53.

Burchell, B., Coughtrie, M.W.H., Jackson, M.R., Shepherd, S.R.P., Harding, D. and Hume, R. (1987) Genetic deficiency of bilirubin glucuronidation in rats and humans. Molec.Aspects Med. **6**, 429-455.

Clemens, M.J. (1984) Translation of eukaryotic messenger RNA in cell-free extracts. In Transcription and Translation: a Practical Approach, ed. B.D. Hames and S.J. Higgins, pp. 231-270. Oxford, Washington, IRL Press.

Crigler, J.F. and Najjar, V.A. (1952) Congenital familial non-haemolytic jaundice with kernicterus. Paediatrics, **10**, 169-180.

Devereaux, J., Haeberli, P. and Smithies, O. (1984) A comprehensive set of sequence analysis programs for the VAX. Nucleic Acids Res., **12**, 387-395.
Dragacci, S., Hamer-Hansen, C., Fournel-Gigleux, S., Lafaurie, C., Magdalou, J. and Siest, G. (1987). Comparative study of clofibric acid and bilirubin in human liver microsomes. Biochemical Pharmacology, **136**, 3923-3927.

Dutton, G.J. (1980) Glucuronidation of Drugs and Other Compounds, CRC Press, Boca Raton, Florida, USA.

Fagan, J., Pasteuka, J., Guengerich, F., Gelboin, H. (1983) Multiple cytochrome p450s are translated from multiple messenger ribonucleic acids. Biochemistry, **22**, 1927-1934.

Feinberg, A.P. and Vogelstein, B. (1984). A technique for radiolabelling DNA restriction endonuclease fragments to high specific activity. Anal.Biochem., **137**, 266-267.

Harding, D., Wilson, S.M., Jackson, M.R., Burchell, B., Green, M.D. and Tephly, T.R. (1987) Nucleotide and deduced amino acid sequence of 17ß-hydroxy-steroid UDP-glucuronosyltransferase. Nucleic Acid Res. **15,** 3936

Hanover, J.A. and Lennarz, W.J. (1981) Transmembrane assembly of membrane and secretory glycoproteins. Arch.Biochem.Biophys. **211,** 1-19.

Irshaid, Y.M. and Tephly, T.R. (1987) Isolation and purification of two human liver UDP-glucuronosyltransferases. Molecular Pharmacology, **31,** 27-34.

Iyanagi, T., Haniu, M., Sugawa, K., Fujii-Kuriyama, Y., Watanabe, S, Shively, J.E. and Anan, K.F. (1986) Cloning and characterisation of cDNA encoding 3-methylcholanthrene inducible rat mRNA for UDP-glucuronosyltransferase. J.Biol.Chem. **261,** 15607-15614.

Jackson, M.R. and Burchell, B. (1986) The full length coding sequence of rat liver androsterone UDP-glcuronosyltransferase cDNA and comparison with other members of this gene family. NucleicAcid Res., **14,** 779-795.

Jackson, M.R., McCarthy, L.R., Harding, D., Wilson, S., Coughtrie, M.W.H. and Burchell, B. (1987) Cloning of a human liver microsomal UDP-glucuronosyltransferase cDNA. Biochem.J., **242,** 581-588.

Kimura, T. and Owens, I.S. (1987) Mouse UDP-glucuronosyltransferase: cDNA and complete amino acid sequence and regulation. Eur.J.Biochem., **168,** 515-521.

Leakey, J.E.A., Hume, R. and Burchell, B. (1987). Development and multiple activities of UDP-glucuronosyltransferase in human liver. Biochem.J. **245,** 859-861.

Mackenzie, P. (1986). Rat liver UDP-glucuronosyltransferase: cDNA sequence and expression of a form glucuronidating 3-hydroxy androgens J.Biol.Chem., **261,** 14112-14117.

Mackenzie, P. (1987). Rat liver UDP-glucuronosyltransferase: Identification of cDNAs encoding two enzymes which glucuronidate testosterone, dihydrosterone and ß-estradiol..J. Biol. Chem. **262,** 9744-9749.

Mahu, J., Preaux, A., Mavier, P. and Berthelot, P. (1981) Characterization of microsomal bilirubin and p-nitrophenol uridine diphospho glucuronosyltransferase activities in human liver: a comparison with rat liver. Enzyme **26,** 93-102.

Maniatis, T., E. Fritsch and J. Sambrook (1982). Molecular cloning: A laboratory manual. Cold Spring Harbor Laboratory, New York, USA.

Miners, J.O., Lillywhite, K.J., Matthews, A.P., Jones, E. and Birkett, D.J., (1988) Kinetic and inhibitor studies of 4-methylumbelliferone and 1-naphthol glucuronidation in human liver microsomes. Biochemical Pharmacology, **37,** 665-671.

Onishi, S., Kawade, N., Itoh, S., Isobe, K. and Suguyama, S. (1979) Postnatal development of uridine-diphosphate glucuronyltransferase activity towards bilirubin and 2-aminophenol in human liver. Biochem.J., **184,** 705-707.

Parquet, M., Pessah, A., Mavier, P. and Berthelot, P. (1985) Glucuronidation of bile acids in human liver intestine and kidney. FEBS Lett., **189,** 183-187.

Roy-Chowdhury, J. and Arias, I.M. (1986) in Bile Pigments and Jaundice: Molecular, Metabolic and Medical Aspects, ed. Ostrow, J.D., New York, USA, Marcel Dekker, 318-324.

Siest, G., Antoine, B., Fournel, S., Magdalou, J. and Thomassin, J. (1987). The glucuronosyltransferases: what progress can pharmacologists expect from molecular biology and cellular enzymology? Biochemical Pharmacology., 36, 983-987.

Walter, P., Ibrahimi, I. and Blobel, G. (1981) Translocation of proteins across the endoplasmic reticulum. 1. Signal Recognition Protein (SRP) binds to in vitro assembled polysomes synthesizing secretory protein. J.Cell Biol, 91, 545-551

Résumé

Nous avons isolé l'ADN$_c$ codant pour différentes formes d'UDPGT humaines. Chaque ADN$_c$ correspond à une forme distincte d'ARNm d'UDPGT humaine - ceci demontrant définitivement la multiplicité des UDPGT chez l'homme. Les clones ADN$_c$ peuvent être separés en deux sous-familles possédant environ 45% de similarité entre elles; le degré de similarité à l'interieur de chaque sous-famille est superior à 65%. Les membres de la sous-famille no. 1 sont trés similaires à l'UDPGT androsterone de rat, l'UDPGT testosterone de rat et autres membres de ce groupe, et similaires également a l'UDPGT m-1 de souris. La sous-famille no. 2 posséde deux sortes do cDNA et code pour les formes d'UDPGT ayant une forte homologie de séquence avec l'UDPGT 4-nitrophenol de rat. La distribution des séquences homologues le long de la séquence nucléotidique de ces 2 ADN$_c$ suggére qu'une recombination génétique soit responsable de l'augmentation de spécificité de substrat des UDPGT.

La séquence primaire N-terminale des isoenzymes correspondantes aux "full length" ADN$_c$ possède des séquences caracteristiques de "signal séquences", et ces isoformes sont dotées de sites possibles de N-glycosylation. Nous avons etudié la maturation d'une isoforme et montré que celle-ci est effectivement glycosylée et al "séquence-signal" clivée.

La transfection de deux clones d'ADN$_c$ d'UDPGT humaines "full-length" (HLUG 25 et HLUG P$_1$) dans des coflutes COS-7 permet l'expression de deux glycoproteins de 53 et 55 kDa respectivement. HLUG 25 code pour une forme d'UDPGT catalysant la glucuronidation de l'acid hydeoxycholique mais non lithocholic alors que HLUG P$_1$ code pour une isoenzyme a specificité de substrat restreinte aux phenols plans de petite taille.

Expression of UDP-Glucuronosyltransferase cDNA

Peter I. Mackenzie

Department of Clinical Pharmacology, Flinders Medical Centre, Bedford Park S.A. 5042 Australia

ABSTRACT

Attempts at producing catalytically-active UDP glucuronosyltransferase from cDNA expression in bacteria were unsuccessful. The coding regions of four UDP glucuronosyltransferase cDNAs (UDPGTr-2,3,4 and 5) were therefore placed under transcriptional control of the SV40 viral promotor and transfected into mammalian cells (green monkey kidney COS) in culture. Nascent enzyme produced from each transfected cDNA was characterized with respect to its size on SDSPAGE gels and the occurrence of posttranslational processing events. UDPGTr-2 and UDPGTr-4 had molecular weights of 53K daltons and contained endoglycosidase H-sensitive carbohydrate moieties whereas UDPGTr-3 and UDPGTr-5 had molecular weights of 50K daltons and were not glycosylated. Using a battery of chemicals, the aglycone preference of each nascent enzyme was determined. UDPGTr-2 glucuronidated 4-hydroxybiphenyl, 4-methylumbelliferone and chloramphenicol. This enzyme was also active in the deconjugation of 4-methylumbelliferone glucuronide. Testosterone was a substrate of all four forms whereas androsterone and bile acids were mainly glucuronidated by UDPGTr-4. Chimeras of UDPGTr-2 and 4 cDNAs were made and transfected into COS cells. Although chimeric UDPGTs with subunit molecular weights of 53K daltons were synthesized, these proteins were inactive in the glucuronidation of substrates typical of the parent forms. These studies demonstrate the potential of recombinant DNA technology for characterizing UDPGT forms and investigating the domains and amino acid residues involved in catalysis.

KEYWORDS

UDP glucuronosyltransferase cDNAs, expression in culture, chimeric proteins.

INTRODUCTION

Determining the substrate specificities of individual forms of UDP glucuronosyltransferase (UDPGT) and developing reagents specific for each form are projects basic to an understanding of the heterogeneity and regulation of this complex family of conjugating enzymes. Characterization of UDPGT forms in terms of their primary and secondary structures and substrate preferences has classically involved the isolation of pure proteins. The synthesis of cataly tically active proteins from cDNAs is an alternative approach to characterizing UDPGTs that avoids the problems of purifying sufficient quantities of a membrane-bound enzyme which is stable and unaffected by contaminating detergents.

The cDNAs to several forms of UDPGT have been synthesized and cloned (Iyanagi et al., 1986; Jackson & Burchell, 1986; Mackenzie, 1986a,b, 1987; Harding et al., 1987). These include clones encoding 3-methylcholanthrene-inducible (4NPGT; Iyanagi et al., 1986) and phenobarbital-inducible (UDPGTr-2; Mackenzie, 1986a) forms and forms which are relatively unaffected by these prototypic inducers (UDPGTr-3,4,5; Mackenzie, 1986b, 1987, unpublished data). This paper will describe experiments utilizing bacterial and mammalian expression vectors containing the coding regions of UDPGTr-2,3,4 and 5 in investigations of the substrate preferences and catayltic domains of UDPGTs.

EXPRESSION OF UDPGT cDNA IN BACTERIA

Expression of mammalian genes in bacteria is less costly and generally yields higher amounts of protein than expression in eukaryotic cells. For these reasons the bacterial expression vector pKK223-3 (Amann et al., 1983) containing the coding region of UDPGTr-2 was constructed (Fig. 1A) and used to transform E.coli JM105. In this bacteria, transcription of UDPGTr-2 RNA which is under the control of the TAC promoter is repressed unless isopropyl β-D-thiogalactoside (IPTG) is present. Individual bacterial colonies harbouring the plasmid construct were grown in the presence of this compound and protein analyzed on SDSPAGE gels. A protein with a relative molecular mass (Mr) of 35K daltons was synthesized from IPTG treated-cells containing UDPGTr-2 coding sequence in the correct orientation with respect to transcription signals (Fig. 1B). This protein which constituted about 5% of the total cellular protein, was inactive in the glucuronidation of 1-naphthol, 4 methylumbelliferone and chloramphenicol and appeared to be a truncated form of UDPGT. Whether this 35K dalton protein was a consequence of proteolysis of UDPGTr-2 (Mr 53K) or utilization of an internal methionine residue as an initiation codon is unknown. Attempts at producing a functional full-length protein by deletion of 5' and 3' noncoding regions from the UDPGTr-2 cDNA insert of the expression plasmid and assaying in the presence of protease inhibitors were unsuccessful.

As certain eukaryotic posttranslational processing events (e.g. glycosylation, protein phosphorylation), which may be important for glucuronidating activity, do not occur in bacteria, experiments were initiated to express UDPGT cDNA in mammalian cells.

EXPRESSION OF UDPGT cDNA IN MAMMALIAN CELLS

UDPGT cDNA, when inserted in an SV40 expression vector and placed in green monkey kidney COS cells, resulted in the synthesis of UDPGT polypeptides (Fig. 2). In this system, the vector is replicated 100-1000 fold due to the presence of the large T antigen in the COS cell chromosomes and transcription of UDPGT cDNA is driven by the viral SV40 promoter. The nascent UDPGT protein constituted about 0.05% of total cellular protein, as determined by radiolabelling experiments. Although all forms of UDPGT cloned to date have Mrs of 60.5K when calculated from their deduced amino acid sequences, analysis by

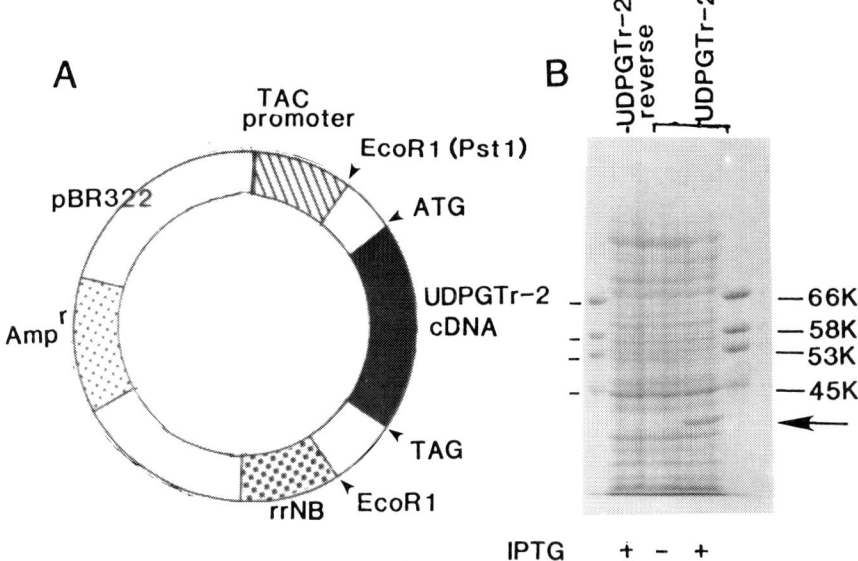

Fig. 1. Expression of UDPGTr-2 cDNA in E. coli. (A) Transcription of insert DNA in the expression vector pKK223-3 (Pharmacia) is driven by the IPTG-inducible TAC promotor (▨) and is terminated by the rrNB ribosomal RNA transcription terminator (▦). The PstI site of the PstI/EcoR1 fragment of pUDPGTr-2F (Mackenzie, 1986a) which contains the coding region (■), was converted to an EcoR1 site by the addition of EcoR1 linkers and ligated to EcoR1-digested pKK223-3 using established methods (Maniatis et al., 1982). Plasmids containing UDPGTr-2 cDNA in the correct orientation (as illustrated above) and reverse orientation were isolated and used to transform E. coli JM105. (B) Colonies harbouring the plasmids were grown in the presence (+) or absence (-) of IPTG and the protein analyzed by SDSPAGE and visualized by staining with coomassie blue. The molecular weight markers, albumin (66K), catalase (58K), glutamate dehydrogenase (53K) and ovalbumin (45K) are indicated. The 35K dalton protein formed in IPTG-treated bacteria transformed with UDPGTr-2 in the sense orientation is denoted with an arrow.

SDSPAGE revealed that UDPGTr-2 and UDPGTr-4 had Mrs of 53K daltons whereas the experimental values for UDPGTr-3 and UDPGTr-5 were 50K daltons (Fig. 2B). Both UDPGTr-2 and UDPGTr-4 contained asparagine-linked complex carbohydrate moieties as their treatment with endoglycosidase H resulted in the production of proteins with Mrs of about 50K daltons (Fig. 2B). UDPGTr-3 and UDPGTr-5 (not shown) proteins were unaffected by this treatment. These results are in agreement with the presence of potential N-linked glycosylation sites (Asn-x-ser/thr) in the UDPGTr-2 and -4 deduced amino acid sequences and their absence in those of UDPGTr-3 and -5.

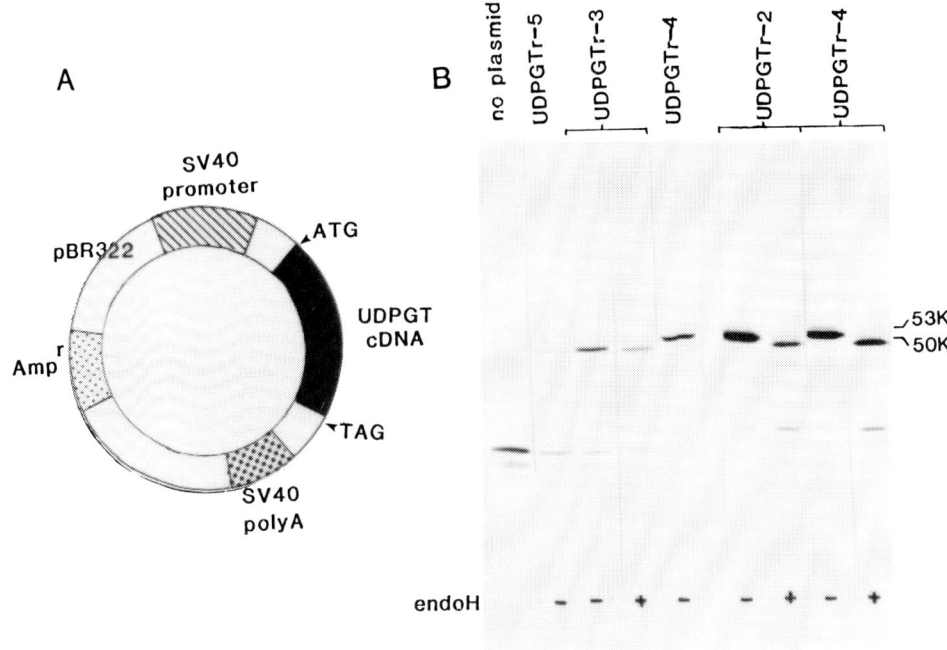

Fig. 2. Expression of UDPGT cDNA in Green Monkey kidney (COS) cells. The mammalian expression vectors pcD containing UDPGT cDNAs (A) were constructed as previously described (Mackenzie, 1986a). Nascent UDPGT was radiolabelled with ^{35}S-L-methionine, 72h after transfection into COS cells and analyzed by immunoadsorption and SDSPAGE (Mackenzie, 1986a). Labelled protein was visualized by autoradiography (B). In some cases, immunocomplexes were treated with endoglycosidase H (endo H+) at 37°C for 10h to remove N-linked complex carbohydrate before electrophoretic analysis.

Conjugation and Deconjugation Reactions of cDNA-Encoded UDPGT

A battery of 20 representative endogenous and exogenous substrates has been used to characterize the aglycone preferences of the four cDNA-encoded UDPGTs (Mackenzie 1986a, 1987). The results of one experiment is shown in Fig. 3. Testosterone was glucuronidated by all four forms. Of the four forms, however, UDPGTr-2 was the most active when activity was related to the amount of protein synthesized from the transfected expression vector. Etiocholanolone, androsterone and the bile acids, on the other hand, were preferentially glucuronidated by UDPGTr-4. Dihydrotestosterone and β-estradiol were also substrates of these enzymes whereas activity towards estrone could not be detected.

UDPGTr-2 glucuronidated the exogenous substrates 4-hydroxybiphenyl, 2-hydroxybiphenyl, chloramphenicol and 4-methylumbelliferone. It was also active in the conversion of 4-methylumbelliferone glucuronide to aglycone and glucuronic acid. This result confirms those reported for microsomal preparations (Peters et al., 1986, Roy Chowdhury et al., 1986) and furthermore, demonstrates that deconjugation of a glucuronide is preferentially catalyzed by that enzyme form involved in its formation rather than another UDPGT form.

Phenolphthalein is preferentially glucuronidated by UDPGTr-4. Other exogenous substrates such as 1-naphthol, 4-nitrophenol and thiophenol were not glucuronidated to any significant extent by the cDNA-encoded UDPGTs synthesized in this transfection system.

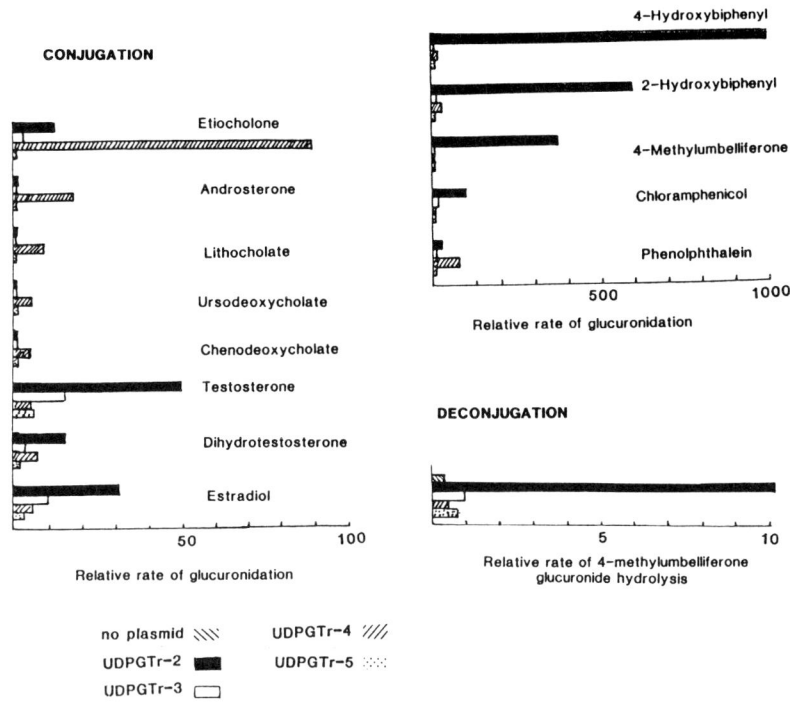

Fig. 3. Activities of cDNA-encoded UDPGT. UDPGTr-2,3,4 and 5 cDNAs were transfected into COS cells and nascent UDPGT assayed with ^{14}C-UDP glucuronic acid and the substrates listed (Mackenzie 1986a, 1987). Deconjugation of 4-methylumbelliferone was also determined (Peters et al., 1986). Relative rates are calculated as the amounts of radioactive glucuronide or 4-methylumbelliferone fluorescence formed per amount of nascent enzyme present (determined by labelling with ^{35}S-L-methionine) in the assay mixture.

Synthesis of Chimeric Proteins Using UDPGT cDNAs

The ability to produce an active enzyme from a cDNA expressed in cell culture has raised the possibility of manipulating the cDNA in order to synthesize chimeric proteins which contain portions of different UDPGT forms in the same polypeptide chain. In this manner the regions of the enzyme involved in substrate binding and catalysis may be identified. To this end, a restriction site common to UDPGTr-2 and UDPGTr-4 (SacI) was utilized to ligate the 5'-half of UDPGTr-2 cDNA to the 3'-half of UDPGTr-4 cDNA and the 3'-half of UDPGTr-2 to the 5'-half of UDPGTr-4 cDNA (Fig. 4A). The two chimeric cDNAs which both contain an uninterrupted open-reading frame together with the parent cDNAs, were expressed in cell culture and nascent protein labelled with ^{35}S-L-methionine. As shown in Fig. 4B parent and chimeric proteins with Mrs of 53K daltons were synthesized from the transfected cDNAs. In contrast to the parent proteins, however the chimeric proteins, were inactive in the glucuronidation of the substrates of UDPGTr-2, (4-hydroxybiphenyl, testosterone) and UDPGTr-4 (androsterone) (Fig. 4B), possibly as a result of the disruption of domains or tertiary structures critical to catalysis. The construction of other chimeric UDPGT cDNAs which preserve these proposed critical regions and their expression in cell culture is in progress.

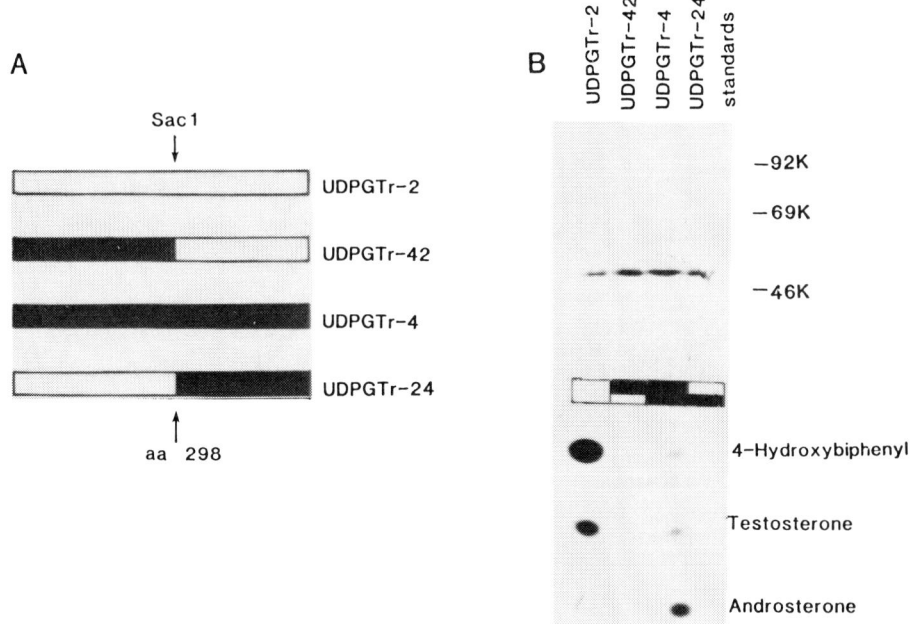

Fig. 4. Expression of chimeric UDPGT cDNA in COS cells. (A) The pcD-based vectors, pUDPGTr-2F and pUDPGTr-4 (Mackenzie, 1986a,b) were digested with the restriction enzyme SalI and SacI. The SalI/SacI fragments that included the SV40 promoter and region coding for the first 298 residues of UDPGT were interchanged and religated to the vector fragment, to produce the chimeric plasmids pUDPGTr-42, which encodes the first 298 residues of UDPGTr-4 joined to the terminal 231 residues of UDPGTr-2 and pUDPGTr-24 encoding the first 298 residues of UDPGTr-2 and last 232 residues of UDPGTr-4. (B) The parent and chimeric plasmids were transfected in COS cells and levels of nascent UDPGT (B-top panel) and activities towards 4-hydroxybiphenyl, testosterone and androsterone were measured radiochemically as described previously (Mackenzie 1986a, 1987). Autoradiographs of the regions of TLC plates containing radio-labelled glucuronides are depicted in B (lower panel).

CONCLUSION

The synthesis of a single form of UDPGT from cDNA expressed in mammalian cell culture is a suitable means of determining the substrate specificities and subunit molecular weights of individual forms of this complex family of enzymes. This technique obviates the need to purify each form and avoids problems of enzyme purity and stability and deleterious effects of detergents on catalytic activities. Furthermore, amino acid residues and polypeptide domains critical to catalytic activity and substrate preference can be assessed by manipulation of the cDNA to produce chimeric proteins or proteins altered at specific sites. Although the synthesis of an active protein in the bacterial system described in this work was unsuccessful, it does have the potential for making small peptides to various regions of the UDPGT polypeptides chain that can be used as antigens for the production of form-specific antisera.

ACKNOWLEDGEMENTS

The author is grateful for the support of Dr. Dan Nebert, Dr. Frank Gonzalez, Professor Don Birkett and colleagues and the financial assistance of the National Institutes of Health, U.S.A. and the National Health and Medical Research Council of Australia. The author is a NH & MRC Research Fellow.

REFERENCES

Amann, E., Brosius, J. and Ptashne, M. (1983): Vectors bearing a hybrid trp-lac promoter useful for regulated expression of cloned genes in Escherichia coli. Gene. 25, 167-178.

Harding, D., Wilson, S.M., Jackson, M.R., Burchell, B., Green, M.D. and Tephly, T.R. (1987): Nucleotide and deduced amino-acid sequence of rat liver 17-hydroxysteroid UDP-glucuronosyltransferase. Nucl. Acids Res. 15, 3936.

Iyanagi, T., Haniu, M., Sogawa, K., Fujii-Kuriyama, Y., Watanabe, S., Shively, J.E. and Anan, K.F. (1986): Cloning and characterization of cDNA encoding 3-methylcolanthrene inducible rat mRNA from UDP-glucuronosyltransferase. J. Biol. Chem. 261, 15607-15614.

Jackson, M.R. and Burchell, B. (1986): The full length coding sequence of rat liver androsterone UDP-glucuronyltransferase cDNA and comparison with other members of the gene family. Nucl. Acids Res. 14, 779-795.

Mackenzie, P.I. (1986a): Rat liver UDP-glucuronosyltransferase. Sequence and expression of a cDNA encoding a phenobarbital-inducible form. J. Biol. Chem. 261, 6119-6125.

Mackenzie, P.I. (1986b): Rat liver UDP-glucuronosyltransferase. cDNA sequence and expression of a form glucuronidating 3-hydroxyandrogens. J. Biol. Chem. 261, 14112-14117.

Mackenzie, P.I. (1987): Rat liver UDP-glucuronosyltransferase. Identification of cDNAs encoding two enzymes which glucuronidate testosterone, dihydrotestosterone and β-estradiol. J. Biol. Chem. 262, 9744-9749.

Maniatis, T., Fritsch, E.F. and Sambrook, J. (1982): <u>Molecular Cloning, a Laboratory Manual</u>, CSH press.

Peters, W.H.M., Jansen, P.L.M., Cuypers, H.T.M., de Abreu, R.A. and Nauta, H. (1986): Deconjugation of glucuronides catalyzed by UDP glucuronyltransferases. <u>Biochim. Biophys. Acta</u> <u>873</u>, 252-259.

Roy Chowdhury, N., Arias, I.M., Lederstein, M. and Roy Chowdhury, J. (1986): Substrates and products of purified rat liver bilirubin UDP-glucuronosyltransferases. <u>Hepatology</u> <u>6</u>, 123-128.

Résumé

Nous n'avons pas réussi à exprimer une UDP-glucuronyltransférase catalytiquement active à partir d'un cDNA dans les bactéries. Les régions codant pour quatre cDNAs (UDPGTr-2,3,4 et 5) ont été alors placées sous contrôle transcriptionnel d'un promoteur viral SV40 et transfectées dans des cellules de mammifères en culture (COS de rein de singe vert). L'enzyme produite pour chaque cDNA transfecté est caractérisée en taille par électrophorèse en gel de polyacrylamide avec SDS, et selon les évènements postranslationnels observés. Les UDPGTr-2 et UDPGTr-4 ont un poids moléculaire de 53K daltons et contiennent une partie sucre sensible à l'endoglycosidase H, tandis que les UDPGTr-3 et UDPGTr-5 ont un poids moléculaire de 50K daltons et ne sont pas glycosylées. La préférence des enzymes vis-à-vis d'un très grand nombre de substrats a été déterminée. L'UDPGTr-2 conjugue le 4-hydroxybiphényle, la 4-méthylombelliférone et le chloramphénicol. Cette enzyme peut déconjuguer le glucuronide du 4-methylombelliférone. La testostérone est un substrat des quatre formes, tandis que l'androstérone et les acides biliaires sont surtout conjugués par l'UDPGTr-4. Des chimères d'UDPGTr-2 et des 4 cDNas sont fabriquées et transfectées dans des cellules COS. Bien que les UDPGTs chimères synthétisées aient un poids moléculaire de 53K daltons, elles sont incapables de conjuguer les substrats représentatifs de protéines parentales. Ces études démontrent l'utilité potentielle de la technologie des recombinants génétiques pour caractériser les différentes formes d'UDPGT et définir les régions et acides aminés impliqués dans la catalyse.

Expression of UDP-Glucuronosyltransferase isoforms during development and carcinogen-induced preneoplastic transformation of liver in rats

Jayanta Roy Chowdhury*, Pulak Lahiri*, Peter I. Mackenzie*, Frederick F. Becker** and Namita Roy Chowdhury*

*Liver Research Center, Albert Einstein College of Medicine, Bronx, New York 10461, USA, **The Flinders University of South Australia School of Medicine, Bedford Park, South Australia 5042 and ***The University of Texas System Cancer Center, Houston, Texas, USA

ABSTRACT

To study the regulation of individual isoforms of UDP-glucuronosyltransferases (UDPGT) we developed two specific antisera that recognize a 3-methylcholanthrene-inducible (3-MC-I) UDPGT isoform, and UDPGT isoforms that are active toward steroid substrates, respectively. By comparing the mRNA sequences of various UDPGT isoforms, we synthesized two oligonucleotide probes, that are specific for the 3-MC-I form and androsterone-UDPGT, respectively. We used these probes to determine the abundance of the enzyme proteins and their corresponding mRNAs in the liver and kidney by blotting techniques, immunocytochemistry and in situ hybridization. The 3-MC-I form (Mr 57000) and the corresponding mRNA were abundant in the renal tubular epithelium; only a minor amount was present in the hepatocyes of untreated rats. This isoform and the corresponding mRNA in the liver were induced 15-fold, 24 hr after 3-MC administration. The steroid-UDPGTs and corresponding mRNAs were abundant in hepatocytes, but not in the kidney, and were not induced by 3-MC. The 3-MC-I mRNA appeared in the liver during the third week of gestation; peak levels were reached on the 17 day of gestation. The abundance was reduced to the low adult levels 7 days after birth. Only traces of steroid-UDPGT mRNAs were present in the liver in the third week of gestation; adult levels of abundance were reached in 7 days after birth. Livers with 2-acetylaminofluorane-induced preneoplastic nodules contained 10-fold more mRNA for the 3-MC-I isoform compared to control, whereas mRNA's for the androsterone-UDPGT isoforms were reduced by approximately 30%. In situ hybridization using biotinylated probes showed a marked increase in the 3-MC-I mRNA in the nodules, compared to the adjacent liver tissue. A parallel increase in the enzyme protein was observed by immunocytochemistry. Androsterone-UDPGT mRNA and the steroid-UDPGT enzyme protein was not increased in the nodules. These results demonstrate differential expression of independent UDPGT isoforms and suggest that the 3-MC-I form is oncofetal.

KEY WORDS

UDP-glucuronosyltransferase, 3-methylcholanthrene, androsterone, development, in situ hybridization, preneoplastic liver nodules

INTRODUCTION

UDP-glucuronosyltransferase (UDPGT) consists of a number of isoforms that have distinct but partially overlapping substrate specificity (Roy Chowdhury, et al, 1986). Comparison of the peptides produced by tryptic digestion of the proteins suggested that the isoforms have unique regions, as well as regions of homology (Roy Chowdhury, et al, 1986). The lack of availability of antibodies that are specific for individual isoforms has limited the study of regulation of the individual transferases in the past. In this study, we report the development of two antisera, which recognize a 3-methyl-cholanthrene-inducible (3-MC-I) UDPGT isoform and the constitutive steroid-UDPGT isoforms, respectively. These antisera were used to study the regulation of the transferase isoforms in rat liver during ontogenic development and carcinogen-induced preneoplastic transformation.

During the last few years, cDNAs for several UDPGT isoforms have been cloned and sequenced (Jackson and Burchell, 1986; Mackenzie, 1986a,1986b,1987; Iyanagi, 1986). Comparison of the nucleotide sequences of these cDNAs confirm that UDPGT isoforms differ in primary structure, but have extensive regions of homology. By computer matching of the sequences we identified the regions that are unique to specific UDPGT cDNAs, as well as regions that are common to all isoforms, and developed oligonucleotide probes to quantitate mRNAs for these two isoforms in rat liver during development and preneoplastic transformation. Relative abundances of the isoform-specific mRNAs were compared with contents of the corresponding immunoreactive enzyme proteins.

MATERIALS AND METHODS

Materials:
Inbred Wistar-RHA rats maintained on standard laboratory chow in a 12 hr light/dark cycle at the Central Animal Institute of the Albert Einstein College of Medicine, were used for this study. Female New Zealand White rabbits (2 kg), purchased from Dutchland Farm, New York, were used for immunization. Staphylococcal protein A, 2-acetylaminofluorane and 3-MC were obtained from Sigma (St. Louis, MO).

Development of Antisera:
Rats (250 g, male) were treated with 3-MC, 40 mg/kg intraperitoneally, for one day and the 3-MC inducible isoform (Mr 57000) was purified from the liver as described by Iyanagi et al (1986). An antiserum was developed in rabbits as previously described (Roy Chowdhury, et al, 1983). UDPGT isoforms with activities toward testosterone, androsterone and bilirubin were purified as previously described (Roy Chowdhury, et al, 1986), immobilized on cyanogen bromide-activated Sepharose 4B (Pharmacia, Nutley, NJ) and packed into a column. The antiserum against the 3-MC-I isoform was passed through this column to absorb out the components of the polyclonal antibodies that cross-react with the constitutive forms of UDPGT. When tested by immunotransblot methods, this absorbed antiserum recognized the 3-MC-I UDPGT isoform, but not the isoforms that are active toward testosterone, androsterone and bilirubin. Another antiserum was raised against purified androsterone-UDPGT, and absorbed against the 3-MC-I UDPGT immobilized on cyanogen bromide-activated Sepharose 4B. This absorbed antiserum recognized the constitutive forms of UDPGT, but not the 3-MC-I isoform.

Synthesis of Isoform-specific Oligonucleotide Probes:
Two 40-mer oligonucleotides with aminolinkers for biotinylation at the 5' end, complimentary to unique regions of the cDNA for the 3-MC-I isoform and the androsterone-UDPGT isoform, respectively, were synthesized in an automated DNA

synthesizer. Two 30-mer nucleotides, without aminolinkers, complimentary to the unique regions of the above two UDPGT isoforms were also synthesized. The 40-mer oligonucleotides with aminolinkers were used for biotinylation using NHS-biotin. The 30-mer oligonucleotides were radiolabeled by enzyme-catalyzed phosphorylation of the 5' end using γ-^{32}P-ATP.

"Northern Blot" Hybridization
RNA was resolved by agarose gel electrophoresis and blotted to cellulose nitrate sheets; hybridization was performed using ^{32}P-labeled 30-mer oligonucleotides specific for the 3-MC-I or androsterone-UDPGT isoform. Relative RNA abundance was determined by densitometry of autoradiograms.

Immunocytochemical Studies
Antisera against the 3-MC-I form and androsterone-UDPGT were used for localization of the respective transferase isoforms in normal liver tissue and in livers containing preneoplastic nodules as previously described (Roy Chowdhury, et al, 1985).

In situ Hybridization:
Localization of isoform-specific UDPGT mRNAs in normal liver and in livers with preneoplastic nodules was performed using the biotinylated 40-mer oligonucleotide probes, specific for the 3-MC-I form and androsterone-UDPGT, respectively (Singer, et al, 1986).

Enzyme Induction
For mRNA analysis, rats (250 g male) were injected with 40 mg/kg of 3-MC in corn oil, intraperitoneally. Livers and kidneys were removed 24 hours after the injection and RNA was extracted. For determination of enzyme activity and immunological quantification of UDPGT, livers were removed 3 days after the injection of 3-MC.

Developmental Studies
Wistar-RHA rats were time-mated. Fetuses were removed by hysterotomy at 15th, 17th and 20th day of gestation and livers were collected. Livers were also harvested from pups on the day of birth and 7, 14 and 60 days after birth. RNA from the livers were extracted for quantification by Northern blot hybridization.

Development of Preneoplastic Liver Nodules
Preneoplastic liver nodules were induced in rats by administration of three 3-week cycles of 2-acetylaminofluorane, at weekly intervals, as previously described (Teebor and Becker, 1971). Livers from the rats bearing the preneoplastic nodules and those from control rats were removed. A portion was excised for RNA extraction. The remainder was cut into small pieces, and fixed in 4% paraformaldehyde. Vibratome sections were used for immunocytochemical studies or in situ hybridization.

Enzyme Assay and Immunotransblot Studies
UDPGT activity toward 4-nitrophenol, testosterone, androsterone and bilirubin were determined (Roy Chowdhury, et al, 1986) and immunotransblot was performed (Roy Chowdhury, et al, 1987) on microsomal fractions of liver and kidney homogenates as previously described. For the immunotransblot experiments, antisera against the 3-MC-I form or the androsterone-UDPGT form was used.

RESULTS

Organ Localization
Northern blot hybridization assay using the isoform-specific 30-mer oligo-

nucleotide probes indicated that the mRNA for androsterone-UDPGT was abundant in the liver and was hardly detectable in the kidney. In contrast, mRNA for the 3-MC-I form was abundant in the kidney and present in only minor amounts in the liver.

Immunotransblot studies using the antiserum against the 3-MC-I form also indicated that the 3-MC-I form was present mainly in the kidney, and only minor amounts were present in the liver. When the antiserum against the steroid-UDPGT isoforms was used, the corresponding proteins were not detectable in the kidney, but was found to be abundant in the liver.

In situ hybridization of untreated liver and kidney with the isoform-specific biotinylated 40-mer probes indicated that the mRNA for the 3-MC-I form is predominantly present in the renal tubular epithelium. Messenger RNA for the androsterone-UDPGT was present in the liver, exclusively in the hepatocytes.

These findings were consistent with the very low level of androsterone-UDPGT activity in the kidney. However, liver has a high level of UDPGT activity toward 4-nitrophenol, suggesting that the bulk of 4-nitrophenol-UDPGT activity in the untreated liver is not due to the 3-MC-I form.

Induction with 3-MC
Administration of 3-MC resulted in a 15-fold induction of the mRNA for the 3-MC-I form in the liver; in the kidney the induction was 2-3-fold. Immunotransblot studies using the antiserum specific for the 3-MC-I form showed a 10-fold induction of the immunoreactive protein in the liver. However, the enzyme activity toward 4-nitrophenol was increased by only 200%. This suggests that all forms of 4-nitrophenol-UDPGT are not induced by 3-MC administration. The androsterone-UDPGT and its corresponding mRNA did not increase after 3-MC administration.

Development
Messenger RNA for the 3-MC-I form appeared in the liver during the third week of gestation. A peak level of relative abundance of this isoform, that was approximately 10-fold higher than the adult level, was reached on the 17th day of gestation. After birth, the mRNA level rapidly decreased to the low adult levels in 7 days. In contrast, mRNA for the androsterone-UDPGT was barely detectable in the liver during the third week of gestation, and progressively increased to adult levels two weeks after birth.

Preneoplastic Nodules
Northern blot hybridization of RNA extracted from livers with preneoplastic nodules with the 30-mer probe for the 3-MC-I form showed a 10-fold increase in the corresponding mRNA over control liver. A similar increase was observed by immunotransblot studies using the antiserum specific for the 3-MC-I form. UDPGT activity toward 4-nitrophenol was increased 2.5-fold. Northern blot hybridization with the oligonucleotide probe for the androsterone-UDPGT isoform showed no increase in the abundance of the corresponding mRNA in the liver with preneoplastic nodules. Similarly, UDPGT activity toward testosterone and androsterone, and the immunoreactive steroid-UDPGT isoforms were not increased in the livers with preneoplastic nodules.

In situ hybridization with the biotinylated 40-mer oligonucleotide probe for the 3-MC-I form (Fig. 1) showed a marked increase in the corresponding mRNA in the nodules, compared to the surrounding liver tissue. However, the apparently normal regions in the nodule-bearing livers showed higher mRNA levels compared to livers from untreated rats. An increase in the corresponding UDPGT isoform in the nodules was demonstrated by immunocytochemistry using the antiserum specific for this isoform. In contrast, no increase in androsterone-UDPGT mRNA was observed by in situ hybridization (Fig. 2). Similarly, immunocytochemistry using the antiserum against the steroid-UDPGT isoforms did not show any increase of these forms in the nodules.

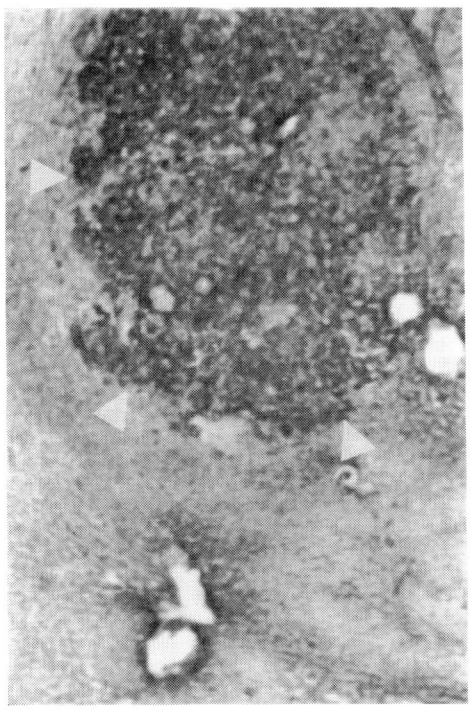

Fig. 1. In situ hybridization of preneoplastic nodules (white arrow heads) with the biotinylated probe for the 3-MC-I form.

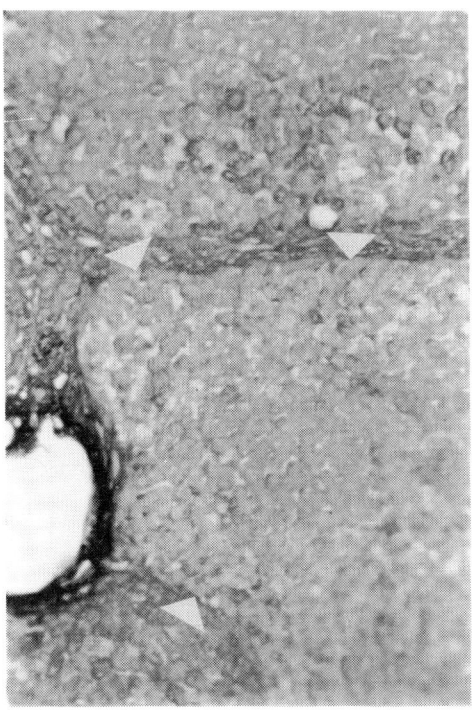

Fig. 2. In situ hybridization of preneoplastic nodules (white arrow heads) with the biotinylated probe for the androsterone-UDPGT.

DISCUSSION

Because of the partial structural homology among the various UDPGT isoforms, antiserum raised against one purified isoform almost invariably cross-reacts with other isoforms. Despite the use of hybridoma technique for raising monoclonal antibodies, it has not been possible to obtain isoform-specific antibodies. In this study, specificity of the antisera was increased by absorption against the other isoforms immobilized on Sepharose 4B. The absorbed antiserum against androsterone-UDPGT cross-reacts with testosterone-UDPGT, but not with the 3-MC-I form (Mr 57000) or the transferase isoform that is predominantly active toward 4-nitrophenol (Mr 51000). The absorbed antiserum against the 3-MC-I form recognized the carcinogen-inducible form; in addition the constitutive 4-nitrophenol UDPGT (Mr 51000) was weakly recognized. This antiserum did not recognize the other constitutive transferases. Availability of these two polyclonal antibodies allowed us to independently quantify the 3-MC-I form and the androsterone/testosterone UDPGTs, respectively. Transblot studies using these antisera clearly demonstrate that the 3-MC-I form differs in organ distribution, ontogenic development and expression in preneoplastic nodules from the constitutive steroid-UDPGT isoforms. The level of protein expression in each organ and all experimental conditions used in this study correlated well with the relative abundance of the corresponding mRNAs, as determined by Northern blot hybridization using isoform-specific probes. This suggests that the UDPGT isoforms are regulated by modulation of transcription rates or stabilization of respective mRNAs. Determination of nuclear transcription rate under the various experimental conditions will be required to differentiate between the two possibilities.

The use of immunocytochemistry and in situ hybridization has enabled us to determine relative concentrations of the transferases and their corresponding mRNAs at tissue and cellular levels. Although the nodules had much higher levels of the 3-MC-I isoform and its corresponding mRNA compared to the adjacent tissue, the apparently normal areas in the nodule-bearing livers expressed this isoform at a much higher level than does liver from untreated rats. This indicates that the effect of 2-AAF on induction of this isoform persists long after the withdrawal of the carcinogen.

Although hepatic UDPGT activity toward 4-nitrophenol was increased in all situations in which the 3-MC-I form was increased, the extent of enhancement of the transferase activity was always much lower than the increase in the inducible enzyme protein and its specific mRNA. This suggests that the 3-MC-I form is not responsible for the bulk of the constitutive 4-nitrophenol-UDPGT activity in the rat liver. The surge of the 3-MC-I form in late fetal life and its hyperexpression in the preneoplastic nodules qualify it as an oncofetal protein.

Our findings confirm the observation of Iyanagi, et al (1986) that the probe for the hepatic 3-MC-I form recognizes an abundant constitutive mRNA in the kidney. However, at this time it is not known whether the hepatic 3-MC-I UDPGT is identical with the UDPGT isoform that is abundant in the renal tubules of untreated rats.

ACKNOWLEDGEMENT

This work was supported in part by the National Institutes of Health grants DK 34357 to JRC, DK 39137 to NRC, DK 35652 and a grant from the Gail Zuckerman Foundation.

REFERENCES

Teebor, G.W. and Becker, F.F. (1971): Regression and persistence of hyperplastic hepatic nodules induced by N-2-fluorenylacetamide and their relationship to hepatocarcinogenesis. Cancer Res. 31:1-3.

Iyanagi, T., Haniu M., Sogawa, K., Fujii-Kuriayama, Y. and Watanabe, S., Shively, J.E. and Anan, K.F. (1986): Cloning and characterization of cDNA encoding 3-methylcholanthrene-inducible rat mRNA for UDP-glucuroosyltransferase. J. Biol. Chem., 15607-15614.

Jackson, M.R. and Burchell, B. (1986): The full length coding sequence of rat liver androsterone UDP-glucuronosyltransferase cDNA and comparison with other members of this gene family. Nucleic Acid Res., 14:779-795.

Mackenzie, P.I. (1986a): Rat liver UDP-glucuronosyltransferase: Sequence and expression of a cDNA encoding a phenobarbital inducible form. J. Biol. Chem., 261:6119-6125.

Mackenzie, P.I. (1986b): Rat liver UDP-glucuronosyltransferase: cDNA sequence and expression of a form glucuronidating 3-hydroxyandrogens. J. Biol. Chem., 261:14112-14117.

Mackenzie, P.I. (1987): Rat liver UDP-glucuronosyltransferase: Identification of cDNAs encoding two enzymes which glucuronidate testosterone, dihydrotestosterone and beta-estradiol. J. Biol. Chem., 262:9744-9749.

Roy Chowdhury, J., Novikoff, P.M., Roy Chowdhury N. and Novikoff, A.B. (1985): Distribution of uridine diphosphateglucuronate glucuronosyltransferase in rat tissues. Proc. Natl. Acad. Sci., USA, 82:2990-2994.

Roy Chowdhury, J., Roy Chowdhury N., Falany, C.W., Tephley, T.W. and Arias, I.M. (1986): Isolation and characterization of multiple forms of rat liver UDP-glucuronate glucuronosyltransferase. Biochem. J., 233:827-837.

Roy Chowdhury, J., Roy Chowdhury N., Moscioni, A.D., Tukey, R., Tephly, T.R. and Arias, I.M. (1983): Differential regulation by triiodothyronine of substrate-specific uridinediphosphoglucuronate glucuronyltransferases in rat liver. Biochim. Biophys. Acta, 761:58-65.

Roy Chowdhury, N., Gross, F., Moscioni, A.D., Kram M., Arias, I.M. and Roy Chowdhury, J. (1987): Isolation and purification of multiple normal and funcionally defective forms of UDP-glucuronosyltransferase from livers of inbred Gunn rats. J. Clin. Invest., 79:327-334.

Singer, R.H., Lawrence, J.B. and Villnave, C. (1986): Optimization of in situ hybridization using isotopic and non-isotopic detection methods. Biotechniques, 4:230-250.

Résumé

Pour étudier la régulation des isoformes de l'UDPGT, nous avons préparé deux antisérums : l'un contre la forme inductible par le 3-méthylcholanthrène (3.MC.I) et l'autre contre celle conjuguant les substrats stéroïdiens. En comparant les séquences des mRNA des isoformes de l'UDPGT, nous avons synthétisé deux sondes oligonucléotidiques spécifiques respectivement des formes 3-MC-I et UDPGT-androstérone.

Nous avons utilisé ces sondes pour déterminer l'abondance de ces protéines et leurs mRNAs correspondants dans le foie et le rein par blotting, immunocytochimie et hybridation in situ. La forme 3-MC-I (57 000) et le mRNA correspondant sont abondants dans l'épithélium tubulaire rénal, seule une quantité mineure est présente dans les hépatocytes des rats non traités. Cette isoforme et le mRNA correspondant sont induits de 15 fois en 24 heures après l'administration du 3-MC. Les UDPGT-stéroïdes et les mRNA correspondants sont abondants dans les hépatocytes, et non pas dans le rein, et ne sont pas inductibles par le 3-MC. Le mRNA 3-MC-I apparaît dans le foie pendant le 3ème semaine de gestation, et le niveau maximum est atteint au 17ème jour de gestation. Cette abondance est réduite jusqu'au faible niveau de l'adulte pendant 7 jours après la naissance. Le mRNA de l'UDPGT stéroïdes est présent seulement à l'état de trace à la 3ème semaine de gestation ; la concentration de l'adulte est atteinte 7 jours après la naissance. Comparés aux foies contrôles, les foies présentant des nodules préneoplastiques induits au 2-acetylaminofluorène contiennent 10 fois plus de mRNA de l'isoforme 3 MC-I, alors que le mRNA des isoformes UDPGT-androstérone est réduit approximativement de 30 %. L'hybridation in situ utilisant des sondes biotinylées a montré une augmentation prononcée du mRNA 3-MC-I dans les nodules, comparé au tissu hépatique adjacent. Une augmentation parallèle de l'enzyme correspondante est observée par immunocytochimie. Le mRNA de l'UDPGT-androstérone et l'enzyme correspondante ne sont pas augmentés dans les nodules. Ces résultats démontrent une expression différentielle des isoformes de l'UDPGT et suggèrent que la forme 3-MC-I est oncofoetale.

Characterization of UDP-Glucuronosyltranferases from animal and human liver

Thomas Tephly, Marcy Townsend, Birgit Coffman, Jaime Puig and Mitchell Green

Department of Pharmacology, University of Iowa, City, Iowa 52242, USA

ABSTRACT

UDP-Glucuronosyltransferases (UDPGTs) have been isolated to apparent homogeneity from rabbit, rat and human hepatic microsomes. A UDPGT which reacts with 4-hydroxybiphenyl has been isolated from liver microsomes of phenobarbital-treated rats and its substrate specificity has been determined. This enzyme displayed a monomeric molecular weight of about 52,500 k-Da on SDS-PAGE. This protein as well as rabbit liver p-nitrophenol and estrone UDPGTs; rat liver, p-nitrophenol, 3α-hydroxysteroid, 17β-hydroxysteroid and morphine UDPGTs; and human liver pI 7.4 and pI 6.2 UDPGTs were reacted with an endoglycosidase in order to determine the presence of carbohydrate. Human liver pI 7.4 and pI 6.2 UDPGTs and rat liver 17β-hydroxysteroid UDPGT did not react with endoglycosidase H. All other UDPGTs tested did react with endoglycosidase H. N-Terminal amino acid sequences are presented for rabbit liver estrone UDPGT and for rat liver p-nitrophenol, 17β-hydroxysteroid, 3α-hydroxysteroid and morphine UDPGTs.

KEYWORDS

UDP-glucuronosyltransferases, glycoproteins, N-terminal amino acid sequence, 4-hydroxybiphenyl (UDP-glucuronosyltransferase).

INTRODUCTION

Evidence exists for the presence of at least 20 different UDP-glucuronosyltransferases (UDPGTs) in rabbit, rat, mouse, pig and human hepatic microsomes. Of these, about 11 have been purified to apparent homogeneity in our laboratory. It is apparent from the substrate specificities of purified UDPGTs that each species has a different pattern of constituent UDPGTs. To date, it has not been possible to directly compare UDPGTs between different species because UDPGTs with similar substrate specificities or inducibility have not been purified from any two species. Rat liver UDPGTs have been studied extensively because of the relatively large number of isoenzymes available. In this paper a comparison of these proteins for certain of their physical properties with several UDPGTs isolated from rabbit and human liver will be made. In addition, we will report on the purification and partial characterization of a phenobarbital-inducible UDPGT which glucuronidates 4-hydroxybiphenyl.

RESULTS AND DISCUSSION

We have purified a 4-hydroxybiphenyl (4-HBP) UDPGT to apparent homogeneity from liver microsomes of rats treated with sodium phenobarbital (80 mg/kg for 4 days). Procedures employed were similar to those described by Puig and Tephly (1986) with an additional affinity chromatographic step using UDP-hexanolamine Sepharose 4-B. 4-HBP-UDPGT activity elutes from the chromatofocusing column with an apparent pI of 5.5. Using a pH 6.5 bis-tris buffer this enzyme was bound to the UDP-hexanolamine column and eluted with UDPGA. Figure 1 shows the results of an experiment where purified 4-HBP-UDPGT from two different preparations were analyzed by SDS-PAGE. The apparent subunit molecular weight is approximately 52,500 k-Da. In Table 1 a preliminary study of the substrate specificity is summarized.

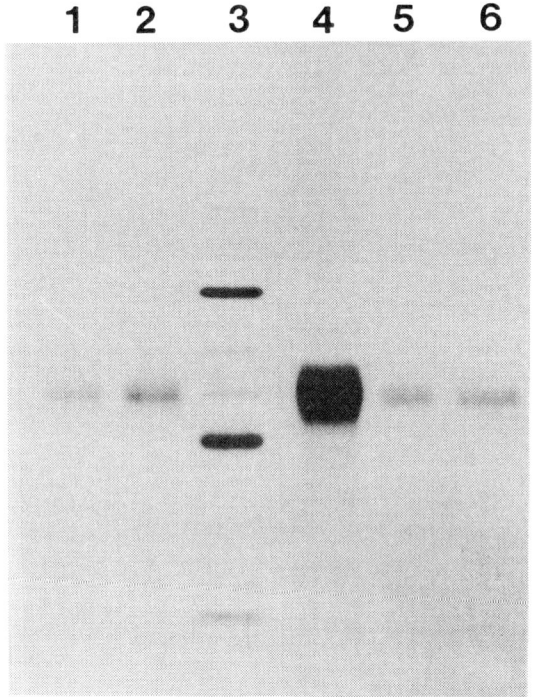

Figure 1. SDS-PAGE of 4-hydroxybiphenyl UDPGT. Lanes 1 and 2 represent 1.0 and 2.0 µg of 4-hydroxybiphenyl UDPGT protein from one preparation and lanes 4, 5 and 6 represent 50 µg, 1 µg and 2 µg of 4-hydroxybiphenyl UDPGT from a second preparation, respectively. Lane 3 shows molecular weight standards of 94,000, 67,000, 58,000, 53,000, 43,000 and 30,000 k-Da.

Table 1. Substrate Specificity of Purified
Rat Hepatic 4-Hydroxybiphenyl UDPGT

Substrate	Specific Activity[1]
4-Hydroxybiphenyl	853
4-Methylumbelliferone	693
Testosterone	0
Androsterone	0
Chloramphenicol	0
Acetaminophen	0

[1] nmoles/min/mg protein

It is interesting to note that this protein does not react with chloramphenicol or morphine (Puig and Tephly, 1986) although morphine and chloramphenicol UDPGTs are induced in rats by phenobarbital treatment (Bock et al., 1979). Although 3α-hydroxysteroid UDPGT has a similar monomeric molecular weight (52,000 k-Da), no activity was observed with androsterone. However, it can be seen that this enzyme has activity toward 4-methylumbelliferone. These data indicate that, in rat liver, 2 UDPGTs, p-nitrophenol UDPGT (Falany and Tephly, 1983) and 4-HBP-UDPGT, can react with 4-methylumbelliferone. The former is induced by 3-methylcholanthrene while the latter is induced by phenobarbital.

Glycosylation of membrane-bound proteins can have a significant effect on both the structure and function of these proteins. For example, the carbohydrate moiety of a glycoprotein may serve as a recognition site for substrate binding on receptors, it may stabilize the protein conformation during synthesis or may allow for orientation and anchoring of the protein within the membrane. Nine highly purified hepatic UDPGTs from 3 different species (rat, rabbit and human) were subjected to treatment with endo-β-N-acetylglucosaminidase H (Endo H) (from Streptomyces plicatus) and then SDS-PAGE was performed. A decrease in the subunit molecular weight was taken as evidence their reactivity with Endo H thus leading to removal of a carbohydrate moiety. Table 2 summarizes this information.

Table 2. Glycosylation of Purified Hepatic UDPGTs

	Presence of Carbohydrate
Rat UDPGTs	
p-Nitrophenol	+
17β-OH steroid	−
3α-OH steroid	+
Morphine	+
4-OH biphenyl	+
Rabbit UDPGTs	
p-Nitrophenol	+
Estrone	+
Human UDPGTs	
pI 7.4	−
pI 6.2	−

The decrease in subunit molecular weights ranged between 2000-4500 k-Da when reactivity with Endo H was observed. Rat liver 17β-hydroxysteroid UDPGT does not react with Endo H suggesting that the purified protein is not glycosylated. This finding is in agreement with the reported deduced amino acid sequence for this enzyme which indicated no potential glycoslation sites (Harding et al., 1987). It is interesting that the human hepatic UDPGTs studied do not react with Endo H suggesting that these proteins are not glycosylated.

Removal of the carbohydrate moieties from rabbit liver p-nitrophenol and estrone UDPGTs and rat liver 3α-hydroxysteroid UDPGT did not reduce the catalytic activities of these enzymes. This indicates that glycosylation of these UDPGTs is not necessary for expression of enzymatic activity of these proteins. Thus, it is possible (but not obligatory) for glycosylation to play a role in the membrane orientation of these proteins. However, more studies are required in order to determine the role of glycosylation in UDPGT biology and chemistry.

The availability of highly purified UDPGTs has allowed us to determine the N-terminal amino acid sequence of these proteins. Table 3 summarizes information for 5 purified UDPGTs.

Table 3. N-Terminal Amino Acid Sequences of Purified Hepatic UDPGTs

AA#	Rat				Rabbit
	17β-HS	3α-HS	PNP	Morphine	Estrone
1	Gly	Gly	Asp	Asp	Gly
2	Lys	Lys	Lys	?	Lys
3	Val	Val	Leu	Leu or Val	Val
4	Leu	Leu	Leu	Leu	Leu
5	Val	Val	Val	Val	Val
6	Trp	Trp	Val	Phe or Ile	Trp
7	Pro	Pro	Pro	Pro	Pro
8	Met	Met	Gln	Ile	Met
9	Glu	Asp	Asp	Glu or Leu	Glu
10	Phe	Phe	Gly	Phe or Tyr	?
11	Ser	Ser	Ser	Ser	Ser
12	His	His	His	His	His
13	Trp	Trp	Trp	?	Trp
14	Met	Met	Leu	Ile or Leu	Met
15	Asn	Asn	?	Asn	Asn

Marked similarities in the N-terminal amino acid sequences can be observed for the 5 UDPGTs. However, with the rat liver UDPGTs it can be seen that amino acids 8-10 are unique and can distinguish between the individual UDPGTs. The sequence for p-nitrophenol UDPGT agrees with that reported by Iyanagi et al. (1987). The N-terminal sequence for 17β-hydroxysteroid UDPGTs agree with the deduced sequences reported by Harding et al. (1987), Jackson and Burchell (1986), and Mackenzie (1986), assuming that there is a 23 amino acid leader sequence which is removed during insertion into the membrane. The data presented here for morphine UDPGT should be regarded as preliminary but indicate that morphine UDPGT also has a different sequence in the 8-10 position than that determined for p-nitrophenol UDPGT. Both p-nitrophenol and morphine UDPGTs have very similar monomeric molecular weights (56,000 k-Da) on SDS-PAGE (Falany and Tephly, 1983; Puig and Tephly, 1986). Rabbit liver estrone UDPGT has an N-terminal sequence (through the first 15 amino acids) that appears to be identical to rat liver 17β-hydroxysteroid UDPGT. Since the substrate specificity of these proteins is quite different, it would appear that more work is needed to determine the sequence at or about the active sites of these proteins. With these data as well as with deduced amino acid sequences from cDNAs of othe UDPGTs, it is clear why it is difficult to generate specific polyclonal antibodies towards these proteins.

REFERENCES

Bock, K.W., Josting, W., Lilienblum, W. and Pfeil, H. (1979): Purification of rat liver microsomal UDP-glucuronyltransferase. Separation of two enzyme forms inducible by 3-methylcholanthrene or phenobarbital. Eur. J. Biochem. 98, 19-26.

Falany, C.N. and Tephly, T.R. (1983): Separation, purification and characterization of three isoenzymes of UDP-glucuronosyltransferase from rat liver microsomes. Arch. Biochem. Biophys. 227, 248-258.

Harding, D., Wilson, S.M., Jackson, M.R., Burchell, B., Green, M.D. and Tephly, T.R. (1987): Nucleotide and deduced amino acid sequence of rat liver 17β-hydroxysteroid UDP-glucuronosyltransferase. Nucleic Acids Res. 15, 3936.

Iyanagi, T., Haniu, M., Sogawa, K., Fujii-Kuriyama, Y., Watanabe, S., Shively, J.F. and Anan, K.F. (1986): Cloning and characterization of cDNA encoding 3-methylcholanthrene inducible rat mRNA for UDP-glucuronosyltransferase. J. Biol. Chem. 261, 15607-15614.

Jackson, M.R. and Burchell, B. (1986): The full length coding sequence of rat liver androsterone UDP-glucuronosyltransferase cDNA and comparison with other members of this gene family. Nucleic Acids Res. 14, 779-795.

Mackenzie, P.I. (1986): Rat liver UDP-glucuronosyltransferase. cDNA sequence and expression of a form glucuronidating 3-hydroxyandrogens. J. Biol. Chem. 261, 14112-14117.

Puig, J.F. and Tephly T.R. (1986): Isolation and purification of rat liver morphine UDP-glucuronosyltransferase. Mol. Pharmacol. 30, 558-565.

Résumé

Des UDP-glucuronosyltransferases (UDPGT)s ont été isolées jusqu'à l'homogénéité apparente à partir de microsomes hépatiques de lapin, rat et d'homme.

Une UDPGT capable de conjuguer le 4-hydroxybiphényle a été isolée de microsomes hépatiques de rats traités par le phénobarbital, et sa spécificité enzymatique a été déterminée. Cette enzyme présente un poids moléculaire monomérique de 52500 k-Da après électrophorèse en gel de polyacrylamide (SDS). Cette protéine ainsi que les UDPGT hépatiques de lapin (p-nitrophénol, estrone), de rats (p-nitrophénol, 3 α-hydroxy-stéroïde, 17 β-hydroxystéroïde, morphine), d'homme (pI 7,4 et 6,2) sont soumises à l'action d'une endoglycosidase pour déterminer la présence de glucides. Les UDPGT hépatiques humaines (pI 7,4 et 6,2) et de rats (17 B-hydroxystéroïdes) ne réagissent pas avec l'endoglycosidase H. Toutes les autres UDPGT testées réagissent avec l'endoglycoside H.

Nous présentons les séquences des acides aminés N-terminaux, correspondant pour l'UDPGT hépatique de lapin (estrone) et de rat (p-nitrophénol, 17 β-hydroxystéroïde, 3 α-hydroxystéroïde et morphine).

Carboxylic Acids as inhibitors and substrates of UDP-Glucuronosyltransferases

S. Fournel-Gigleux* ***, J. Magdalou*, G. Siest*, M.C. Carré**, S.R.P. Shepherd***, M.R. Jackson***, D. Harding*** and B. Burchell***

* Centre du Médicament, UA CNRS n° 597, 30 rue Lionnois, 54000 Nancy, France
** Laboratoire de Chimie Organique, Université de Nancy I, 54500 Vandœuvre lès Nancy, France
*** Department of Biochemistry, University of Dundee, DD1 4HN Dundee, Scotland, UK

SUMMARY

Substrate specificity of individual isoforms of UDP-glucuronosyltransferase (UDPGT,EC 2.4.1.17) has been assessed using different sources of enzyme, namely purified bilirubin UDPGT, catalytically active rat kidney phenol UDPGT expressed in mammalian cell cultures from its corresponding cDNA and specifically induced or deficient rat liver microsomal isoenzymes.

The study focused on the formation of acylglucuronides with regard to their metabolic reactivity and potential toxicity in human. The glucuronidation of four aryloxy- and arylacetic acids with therapeutic relevance was strongly induced by phenobarbital treatment, but was not deficient in the Gunn rat. This suggests that these aglycones may be glucuronidated by the (-)-morphine conjugating enzyme or a closely regulated form. Kinetic evidence confirmed this hypothesis. In agreement, these compounds were not substrates for a rat kidney phenol UDPGT isoform expressed in COS -7 cells, which exhibited a restricted specificity towards small (length < 6.3Å) and planar (bulkiness < 4.5Å) phenols. In addition the investigation of the glucuronidation of twenty alkylphenols and naphthols enabled us to give a crude description of the molecular conformation of the aglycones accepted in the active site of this cloned UDPGT.

Finally we designed an original series of potential inhibitors of the bilirubin UDPGT isoenzyme, with triphenylalkanoic structure. Among them 7,7,7-triphenylheptanoic acid exerted the strongest inhibition both on microsomal and purified bilirubin UDPGT. Interestingly this compound was actively glucuronidated by the purified preparation. This indicates that the selectivity of this isoenzyme may not be restricted to the endogenous substrate bilirubin. We propose that this series of triphenylalkanoic acids could be useful tools to investigate the molecular basis of glucuronides formation for bilirubin and other carboxylic acids.

Key words. UDP-glucuronosyltransferase / Carboxylic acids / Substrate-specificity / Acylglucuronides / Expression / Inhibition / Bilirubin

INTRODUCTION

Arylalkanoic acids represent a broad class of pharmacological agents including hypolipidemic, anti-inflammatory and diuretic drugs, possibly responsible for adverse reactions via the formation of acylglucuronides (Stogniew and Fenselau,1982;Smith *et al* ,1986). Bilirubin IXα , the final product of heme breakdown,is also metabolized to unstable acylglucuronides which may become irreversibly bound to albumin in pathological conditions(Weiss et al , 1983; McDonagh et al , 1984). The recent finding that acylglucuronides represent reactive metabolites, potentially toxic by formation of protein adduct,emphasizes the need for a thorough investigation of the molecular basis of the glucuronidation of arylcarboxylic substrates, all the more since conjugation to glucuronic acid constitutes a primary metabolic pathway for most of these compounds (Caldwell,1982). Functional heterogeneity of UDPGT has been defined in early studies (Dutton,1980;Siest et al ,1987; Boutin, 1987), which describe at least two groups of activities differentially regulated and presenting separate but overlapping substrate specificity towards hydroxylated molecules. The known substrate specificity of bilirubin UDPGT is limited to the obvious endogenous substrate bilirubin and bilirubin monoglucuronides, although this UDPGT which catalyses the formation of ester glucuronides would seem to have the potential to accept mono- and dicarboxylic acids as substrates. The formation of acylglucuronides in which glucuronic acid is conjugated through an acetal linkage to the carboxylic group of the substrate, is relatively poorly understood,except for bilirubin.

In this work, a multi-faceted approach including the use of specifically induced or deficient microsomal activities, purified preparations and expressed protein in mammalian cell cultures from its corresponding cDNA is described to assess the substrate specificity of the different isoforms of UDPGT. In addition we show the development of novel arylalkanoic inhibitors and substrates for this enzymatic system .

MATERIALS AND METHODS

Male Wistar rats 180-200g were treated with either phenobarbital (80 mg/kg body weight/day ip during 4 days), 3-methylcholanthrene (80 mg/ kg body weight, one single ip injection 4 days before sacrifice), clofibrate (200 mg/kg body weight/day, by gastric intubation, once a day for five days). Congenic homozygous Gunn rats (RAfd- j/j) were provided by Dr R Leyten (Neverlee, Belgium)(Leyten et al , 1986). Microsomes were prepared and protein content measured as previously described;bilirubin, 1-naphthol, androsterone, testosterone, morphine UDPGT activities were evaluated using published procedures (see Fournel et al,1986 and Coughtrie et al, 1987 for references).

Acylglucuronides formed in vitro from $[^{14}C]$ UDPGA were quantitatively analysed by high performance liquid chromatography on a C18 reverse phase column as described by Hamar-Hansen et al (1986) and Fournel-Gigleux et al (1988). A thin layer chromatography method, similarly based on the use of radiolabelled UDPGA ,was also used. Conditions were similar to that reported by Bansal and Gessner (1980) except the concentration of cold UDPGA was reduced to 18 µM in order to increase the sensitivity of the method by increasing the rate of radioactivity incorporated in the glucuronide.

Purification of bilirubin UDPGT from clofibrate treated rat liver included the following steps : rat liver microsomes were solubilized in 1% Lubrol PX, a 20-60% ammonium precipitate was dissolved in 0.05% Lubrol PX and applied to a DEAE cellulose anion exchange column. The proteins eluted by a KCl gradient were then separated by chromatofocusing (MonoP column) (pH gradient, 9 to 6) on a FPLC system (Pharmacia), (for details see Burchell et al ,1987). The purity of the enzymes was assessed by SDS-polyacrylamide gel electrophoresis. The two purest fractions (homogenous on 7.5% SDS-polyacrylmide gels) were used for the following studies, after reconstitution of the catalytic activity with egg lecithin liposomes (2mg/mg portein).

A cDNA clone was isolated from a rat kidney cDNA library in the expression vector λ gt 11 with a polyclonal antibody (Harding et al., unpublised data). The full length insert was subcloned in M13mp18 and mp19M ,and the coding sequence was found to be identical to that reported by Iyanagi et al (1986). This RKUG39 cDNA was inserted in the correct and incorrect orientation with respect to the SV40 promoter of the transient expression vector pKCRH2 and then transfected to semi-confluent monkey kidney fibroblasts (COS-7 cells) by the $CaPO_4$ / glycerol shock procedure (Jackson et al , manuscript submitted). The proteins expressed were radiolabelled in vitro with $[^{35}S]$ methionine and the UDPGT specifically immnoprecipitated and analysed on 7.5% SDS- polyacrylamide gels and fluorography as previously described (Jackson et al, 1986). The substrate specificity of the UDPGT expressed was investigated in homogenates of the whole cells harvested 72 hours after transfection.

RESULTS AND DISCUSSION

Specific inducers of different UDPGT isoforms and the Gunn rat strain were used to define the substrate specificity of acylglucuronide formation. The glucuronidation of these arylacetic acids (1-, 2-naphthylacetic acids, RS-2-phenylpropionic acid) and one aryloxyacetic acid (clofibric acid) was compared to the glucuronidation of known type-substrates for identified isoforms. Results are shown in Fig 1.

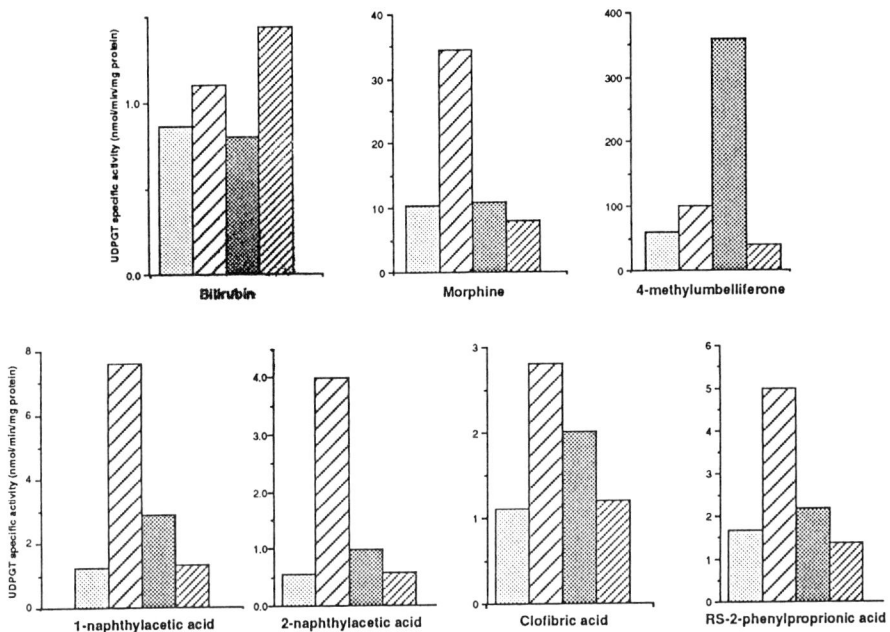

Figure 1. Effects of several inducers on the glucuronidation of carboxylic and hydroxylated substates in rat liver microsomes.
▓ control rat liver, ＼＼ phenobarbital treated rat liver, ▓ 3-methylcholanthrene treated rat liver, ＼＼＼＼ clofibrate treated rat liver. Details concerning the treatment of the animals are given under Materials and Methods section.

3-Methylcholanthrene and clofibrate had little effect on the glucuronidation of either of the four carboxylic acids tested. By contrast phenobarbital strongly induced carboxylic acid UDPGT activities, particularly towards 1- and 2-naphthylacetic acids, which were respectively 6 and 7 fold increased compared to control values in untreated rat liver microsomes. Moreover the conjugation of these carboxylic substrates was not changed in the Gunn rat with regard to the congenic Wistar strain (Fournel-Gigleux et al,1988). The latter result, together with the lack of induction by clofibrate strongly suggests that these compounds are not glucuronidated by bilirubin UDPGT. In contrast, these carboxylic substrates exhibit a similar behaviour as (-)-morphine. The finding that (-)-morphine UDPGT activity is competitively inhibited by 1-naphthylacetic acid (M.Coughtrie, personal communication), indicates that the arylcarboxylic acids are likely to be glucuronidated by the (-)-morphine conjugating enzyme forming 3-O-glucuronides, or a closely related form of enzyme. The neonatal ontogenic development observed for clofibric acid UDPGT activity in the rat is in full agreement with this asumption (Odum and Orton, 1983 and table1).

Table 1. Hepatic glucuronidation of arylcarboxylic substrates

Chemical Class	aryloxycarboxylic acids	arylacetic acids
Type-Substrate	clofibric acid	2-phenylpropionic acid 1-naphthylacetic acid 2-naphthylacetic acid
in vivo metabolic pathway[a]	conjugation to glucuronic acid	conjugation to glucuronic acid or to glycine
Inducibility[b]	2-3 x fold induction by phenobarbital	5-7 x fold induction by phenobarbital
Ontogenic development[b]	neonatal	unknown
Glucuronidation in the Gunn rat[b]	no deficiency	no deficiency
Inhibition kinetics[d]	unknown	competitive inhibition of (-)morphine glucuronidation by 1-naphthylacetic acid
Isoform of UDPGT[e]	no glucuronidation by a rat kidney phenol cDNA expressed in COS-7 cells	no glucuronidation by a rat kidney phenol cDNA expressed in COS-7 cells

[a] Emudianughe et al, 1983
[b] Fournel et al, 1988
[c] Odum and Orton, 1983
[d] Coughtrie et al (personal communication)
[e] Jackson et al (submitted manuscript)

Expression of the cDNAs corresponding to the individual isoforms of UDPGT in mammalian cell cultures supplies the appropriate source of enzyme to study the substrate specificity of the different UDPGTs. For this purpose we have used a rat kidney cDNA (Harding et al, unpublished work). The coding sequencewas identical to the clone reported by Iyanagi et al (1986), (4-nitrophenol UDPGT) based on comparison with limited amino-acid sequence from purified enzyme). Infection of COS - 7 cells with a recombinant plasmid including the coding sequence of RKUG39 resulted in the efficient expression of a 54 kDa glycopeptide specifically immunoprecipitated by polyclonal anti-UDPGT antibodies. The newly synthesized proteins displayed a glucuronosyltransferase activity towards 4-methylumbelliferone, 1-naphthol and 4-nitrophenol but not towards morphine, chloramphenicol or any steroid tested (androsterone, testosterone,oestrone). The enzymatic activity towards 4-hydroxybiphenyl was detectable but low (Fig.2). Moreover, we observed that the isoform encoded by this clone is not the UDPGT glucuronidating the four arylcarboxylic acids tested (results not shown). This confirmed the validity of the analysis based on indirect criteria to discriminate between different isoform. The identification of the cDNA(s) encoding the isoform(s) of UDPGT responsible for the metabolism of these aryl- and aryloxyacetic acids is currently under investigation.

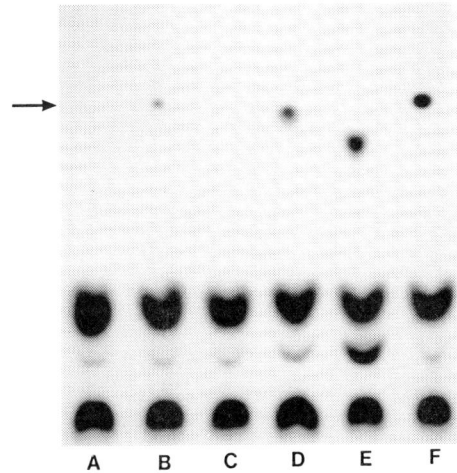

Figure 2. Autoradiogram of a chromatogram on tlc plate
A, B, C, D, E, F correspond to the analysis of incubation mixtures using respectively cloramphenicol, 4-hydroxybiphenyl, morphine, 4-nitrophenol, 4-methylumbelliferone and 1-naphthol as aglycones. The radioactive spots showed by an arrow represents the glucuronides formed ($R_f = 0.8$ except for morphine and 4-methylumbelliferone, $R_f = 0.7$ and 0.25 respectively). No radioactive spot was observed when UDP-glucuronic acid was omitted from the incubation mixture.

Moreover this approach is very informative for the characterization of the chemical criteria required for a substrate to fit in the active site of a UDPGT isoenzyme. The examination of the glucuronidation of more than twenty structurally related alkylphenols and naphthols by the expressed RKUG39 enabled us to describe at least three critical features determining their metabolism by this isoform. They are the following: the length of the molecule (< 6.3Å as defined by Boutin et al, 1985), the bulkiness (< 4.5Å as defined by Okulicz-Kozaryn et al, 1981) and the presence of an aromatic ring on which the hydroxyl is fixed (Jackson et al, 1988, manuscript submitted).

In addition we have designed a series of arylalkanoic acids related to triphenylacetic acid as structural probes for different isoforms of UDPGT. We previously showed that triphenylacetic acid is a competitive inhibitor of in vitro rat liver microsomal bilirubin UDPGT (Fournel et al, 1986). The structural requirements for its inhibitory potency have been examined using a wide range of arylalkanoic acids. We established that the inhibition depends at least on three factors (i) the presence of three phenyl rings, (ii) the length of the aliphatic chain between the phenyl rings and the carboxylic group and (iii) the presence of a carboxyl group. Among the molecules tested, 7,7,7-triphenylheptanoic acid was the most effective inhibitor. The spatial arrangement of this molecule is shown in Fig. 3.

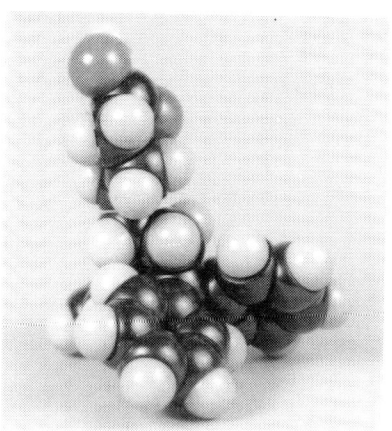

Figure 3. Spatial organization of 7,7,7-triphenylheptanoic acid

It exhibited stronger and more specific inhibitory potency towards bilirubin UDPGT activity than towards any other activity tested (1-naphthol, testosterone, androsterone). Moreover it strongly and competitively inhibited purified bilirubin UDPGT, with a Ki in the µM range.
Finally, the glucuronidation of eight triphenylalkanoic acids differing from each other by the length of their aliphatic chain was investigated with several enzyme sources. In rat liver microsomes, 3,3,3-triphenylbutanoic acid was the best substrate, while UDPGT towards 7,7,7-triphenyl-heptanoic acid was hardly detectable (data not shown). Most interestingly, only the latter molecule was glucuronidated by a purified form of bilirubin UDPGT. In addition the glucuronidation of this substrate was induced by clofibrate and deficient in the Gunn rat.
These results suggest that 7,7,7-triphenyl-heptanoic acid is likely to represent a new substrate for bilirubin UDPGT and that this molecule and its derivatives could be useful probes for the isoforms of UDPGT.

REFERENCES

Bansal, S.K. and Gessner, T. (1980): A unified method for assay of uridine-diphosphoglucuronyltransferase activities towards various aglycones using uridine-diphospho [U-^{14}C] glucuronic acid. Anal.Biochem. **109**, 321-329.

Boutin,J.A., Thomassin,J., Siest,G.and Cartier,A.(1985): Heterogeneity of hepatic microsomal UDP-glucuronosyltransferase activities. Conjugations of phenolic and monoterpenoid aglycones in control and induced rats and guinea-pigs. Biochem.Pharmacol.**34**,2235-2249

Boutin,J.A.(1987): Indirect evidences of UDP-glucuronosyltransferase heterogeneity: How can it help purification? Drug Metab.Rev.**18**,517-551

Burchell, B., Coughtrie M.W.H., Jackson, M.R., Shepherd S.R.P., Harding D. and Hume, R. (1987): Genetic deficiency of bilirubin glucuronidation in rats and humans. Molec.Aspects Med. **6**, 429-455

Caldwell,J.(1982),in "Metabolic Basis of Detoxification" (W.B.Jakoby, J.R. Bend and J.Caldwell, eds.), Academic Press, New York.

Coughtrie,M.W.H., Burchell, B., Sheperd, I.M. and Bend, J.R.(1987): Defective induction of phenol glucuronidation by 3-methylcholanthrene in Gunn rats is due to the absence of a specific UDP-glucuronosyltransferase isoenzyme. Mol.Pharmacol., **31**, 585-591

Dutton, G.J. (1980): Glucuronidation of Drugs and Other Compounds, CRC Press, Boca Raton, Florida, U.S.A.

Emudianughe, T.S., Caldwell, J., Sinclair, K.A. and Smith, R.L. (1983): Species differences in the metabolic conjugation of clofibric acid and clofibrate in laboratory animals and man. Drug Metab.Dispos. **11**,97-102

Fournel,S., Gregoire,B., Magdalou,J., Carre, M.C., Lafaurie, C., Siest, G. and Caubere, P. (1986): Inhibition of bilirubin UDP-glucuronosyltransferase activity by triphenylacetic acid and related compounds.Biochim.Biophys.Acta.**883**,190-196

Fournel-Gigleux, S., Hamar-Hansen, C., Motassim, N., Antoine, B., Mothe, O., Decolin, D., Caldwell, J. and Siest,G.(1988): Substrate-specificity and enantioselectivity of arylcarboxylic acid glucuronidation. Drug Metab.Dispos.(in press)

Hamar-Hansen, C., Fournel, S., Magdalou, J., Boutin, J.A. and Siest, G. (1986): Liquid chromatographic assay for the measurement of glucuronidation of arylcarboxylic acids using uridine diphospho -[U ^{14}C]-glucuronic acid. J.Chromatogr.,**383**, 51-60

Jackson, M.R., Kennedy, S.M.E., Lown, G. and Burchell, B. (1986): Induction of UDP-glucuronosyltransferase mRNA in embryonic chick livers by phenobarbital. Biochem.Pharmacol., **35**, 1191-1198

Iyanagi, T., Haniv, M., Sugawa, K., Kujii-Kuriyama, Y., Watanabe, S., Shively, J.E. and Anan, K.F. (1986): Cloning and characterization of cDNA encoding 3-methylcholanthrene inducible rat mRNA for UDP-glucuronosyltransferase. J.Biol.Chem.,**261**, 15607-15614

Leyten, R., Vroemen, J.P.A.M., Blanckaert, N.and Heirweigh, K.P.M.(1986): The congenic normal R/APfd and jaundiced R/APfd-j/j rat strains:a new animal model of hereditary non-haemolytic hyperbilirubinaemia due to defective bilirubin conjugation. Lab.Animals, **20**, 335-342

Mishina, M., Kurosaki, T., Tobimatsu, T., Morimoto, Y., Noda, M., Yamamoto, T.Terao, M., Lindstrom, J., Takahashi, T., Kuno, M.and Numa, S.(1984): Expression of functional acetylcholine receptor from cloned cDNAs. Nature, **307**, 604-608

McDonagh, A.F., Palma, L.A., Lauff, J.J.and Wu, T.W. (1984): Origin of mammalian biliprotein and rearrangement of bilirubin glucuronides in vivo in the rat. J.Clin.Invest. **74**,763-770

Okulicz-Kozaryn, Shaefer, M.,Batt, A.M., Siest,G.and Loppinet, V. (1981): Stereochemical heterogeneity of hepatic UDP-glucuronosyltransferase activity in rat liver microsomes. Biochem.Pharmacol. **30**, 1457-1461

Odum, J. and Orton, T.C. (1983): Hepatic microsomal glucuronidation of clofibric acid in the adult and neonate albino rat. Biochem.Pharmacol. **23**, 3565-3569

Siest, G., Antoine, B., Fournel, S., Magdalou, J. and Thomassin, J. (1987): The glucuronosyltransferases: what progress can pharmacologists expect from molecular biology and cellular enzymology ? Biochem. Pharmacol. **36**, 983-987

Smith, P.C., McDonagh, A.F.and Benet, L.Z. (1986): Irreversible binding of Zomepirac to plasma protein in vitro and in vivo.J.Clin.Invest.**77**, 934-939

Stogniew, M.and Fenselau, C.C. (1982): Electrophilic reaction of acyl-glucuronides.Drug Metab.Dispos. **10**, 609-613

Weiss, J.S., Gautmam, A., Lauff, J.J., Sunderg, M.W., Jatlow, P., Boyer, J.L.and Seligson, D. (1983): The clinical importance of a protein-bound fraction of serum bilirubin in patients with hyperbilirubinemia. N.Engl.J.Med. **309**, 147-150.

Acknowledgements
We are grateful to Chantal Lafaurie for excellent technical assistance. S.F-G thanks the European Science Foundation and the European Medical Research Council, la Fondation pour la Recherche Médicale and the Wellcome Trust for financial support. BB is a Wellcome Trust Senior Lecturer.

RESUME

Nous avons étudié la specificité de substrat des isoformes de l'UDPGT au moyen de différentes sources d'enzymes : de l'UDPGT bilirubine purifiée, de l'UDPGT phenol de rein de rat exprimée dans des cellules en culture à partir du clone ADNc correspondant et des isoformes microsomales spécifiquement induites ou génétiquement déficientes.

Notre travail porte plus particulièrement sur la formation des acylglucuronides, qui du fait de leur réactivité métabolique, seraient responsables de phénomènes toxiques lors de l'administration de composés carboxyliques en thérapeutique humaine. On observe que la conjugaison de quatre acides aryloxy- et arylacetiques, choisis en raison de leur interêt thérapeutique, est fortement induite par le phenobarbital et n'est pas déficiente chez le rat Gunn. Ce profil d'activité suggère que ces aglycones sont conjuguées par la même UDPGT que la morphine ou une forme proche. Les études cinétiques confirment cette hypothèse.

Egalement en accord, nous observons que ces composés ne sont pas substrats d'une isoforme d'UDPGT de rein de de rat, qui possède une spécificité restreinte vis à vis des phenols de longueur < 6.3Å et d'épaisseur < 4.5Å. De plus, au moyen d'une série de vingt alkylphenols et naphthols, nous donnons une description schématique de la conformation moléculaire des substrats pris en charge par le site actif de cette isoforme.

Enfin nous avons développé une série originale d'inhibiteurs potentiels de la forme d'UDPGT conjugant la bilirubine, qui possèdent une structure arylalcanoique. Parmi ces molécules, l'acide 7,7,7-triphenylheptanoique possède le meilleur pouvoir inhibiteur à la fois sur l'UDPGT bilirubine microsomale et purifiée. Ces résultats suggèrent que cette série d'acides triphenylhalcanoiques constituedes outils moléculaires intéressants dans l'etude de la formation des glucuronides de bilirubine et d'autres acides carboxyliques.

Mechanistic and stereochemical investigations of UDP-Glucuronosyltransferases

Richard N. Armstrong, Jon C. Andre and Jos G. M. Bessems

Department of Chemistry and Biochemistry. University of Maryland, College Park, MD 20742, USA

ABSTRACT

The design of several types of alternative substrates and inhibitors of UDP-glucuronosyltransferase are described. The six kinetically stable conformational isomers of 3,4,5,6-tetramethyl-9,10-dihydroxy-9,10-dihydrophenanthrene have been used to help define the conformational selectivity of the enzyme. A marked preference of the purified enzyme for the pseudo-diequatorial diastereomers of the trans-diols is observed. The corresponding cis-diols react exclusively at the pseudo-equatorial hydroxyl group. The purified enzyme also exhibits enantioselective kinetics toward the chiral conformers of 1,1'-bi-2-naphthol. A combined enzymatic and chemical approach to the synthesis of analogues of UDP-glucose and UDP-glucuronate is described. The phosphono analogue of UDP-glucose (UDPCH$_2$G) is found to be a competitive inhibitor of UDP-glucuronosyltransferase.

KEY WORDS

Stereochemistry of UDP-glucuronosyltransferase, dihydrodiols, phenols, polycyclic aromatic hydrocarbons, UDP-glucuronate analogues.

INTRODUCTION

Biochemical investigations of the UDP-glucuronosyltransferases have been primarily focused on the identification and characterization of the numerous isoenzymic species by both classical and molecular biological techniques. The tremendous advances made in the high-resolution purification of isoenzymes, the structural characterization of the polypeptides by cDNA clones and the prospect for overproduction of the proteins suggest that detailed investigations of the physical-organic chemistry of reaction mechanism are now feasible. In this regard we have set about to develop a number of alternative substrate molecules to probe the mechanistic and stereochemical features of catalysis by the UDP-glucuronosyltransferases. These efforts have been focused on determining the molecular details of xenobiotic substrate recognition, with particular emphasis on metabolites of polycyclic aromatic hydrocarbons, and, more recently, on the development of alternative substrates for the physiological cofactor, UDP-glucuronate.

In this paper we review progress and outline some preliminary results in the design of alternative substrates for UDP-glucuronosyltransferase. First, the use of kinetically stable conformational isomers of dihydrodiols of polycyclic aromatic hydrocarbons to define the conformational specificity of the enzyme toward this class of substrates is described. Second, the ability of the enzyme to catalyze the glucuronidation of sterically hindered phenolic substrates is explored. Finally, some preliminary results in the design and synthesis of substrate analogues of UDP-glucuronate are presented.

MATERIALS AND METHODS

Substrates, reagents and enzymes
Dihydrodiols of 3,4,5,6-tetramethylphenanthrene were prepared as previously described (Armstrong et al., 1985a). 3,4,5,6-Tetramethyl-9-hydroxyphenanthrene was prepared by acid-catalyzed dehydration of cis-3,4,5,6-tetramethyl-9,10-dihydro-9,10-dihydroxyphenanthrene (Armstrong et al., 1987). Enantiomers of 1,1'-bi-2-naphthol were from Aldrich Chemical Co. UDP-glucuronate, inorganic pyrophosphatase, UTP:glucose-1-phosphate pyrophosphorylase, UDP-glucose dehydrogenase, NAD, buffer salts and detergents were from Sigma or Aldrich Chemical Co. Solubilized rat-liver microsomes and purified UDP-glucuronosyltransferase were prepared as described by Lewis & Armstrong (1983).

Enzyme assays
Solubilized microsomes and purified UDP-glucuronosyltransferase were assayed spectrophotometrically with 4-nitrophenol at pH 7.5 essentially as described by Lewis & Armstrong (1983). Kinetics of the glucuronidation of dihydrodiols and other phenols were followed by HPLC procedures as before (Lewis & Armstrong, 1983; Armstrong et al., 1985a). Inhibition of the solubilized microsomal glucuronidation of 4-nitrophenol was carried-out as described above at constant, 6 mM, $MgCl_2$. Kinetics of the UTP:glucose-1-phosphate pyrophosphorylase reactions were monitored by HPLC. UTP concentration was held constant (4 mM).

Synthesis of substrate analogues
Enzymatic synthesis of $UDPCH_2G$ was carried out on a 0.3 mmol scale in 28 mL of 0.1 M MOPS buffer (pH 7.5) containing 400 units each UTP:glucose-1-phosphate pyrophosphorylase and inorganic pyrophosphatase, 18 mM $MgCl_2$, 0.45 mmol UTP at room temperature for 6 hr. Product was purified by ion exchange chromatography. Difluoromethane diphosphonate was prepared as described by Davisson et al. (1986). This molecule was coupled to suitably protected glucose using dicyclohexylcarbodiimide (Myers et al., 1965). After deprotection the glucose-1-pyrophosphonate was coupled to 5'-O-tosyl-uridine by the general method of Davisson et al. (1987).

RESULTS AND DISCUSSION

Conformational specificity toward dihydrodiols
UDP-glucuronosyltransferase has been shown to exhibit a high degree of kinetic discrimination toward stereoisomeric dihydrodiol substrates (Lewis & Armstrong 1983) as illustrated for the trans and cis stereoisomers of 9,10-dihydroxy-9,10-dihydrophenanthrene (1-3) in Fig. 1 (R=H) and Table 1. The two enantiomeric trans-diols, 1 and 2 exist, as do most dihydrodiols, as two rapidly interconverting conformational diastereomers, one with pseudo-diaxial and the other with pseudo-diequatorial hydroxyl groups. The thermodynamic distribution of conformers may depend on substituents or on the solvent environment (Cobb et al., 1983). It should be readily apparent that any attempt to define the substrate selectivity of UDP-glucuronosyltransferase toward dihydrodiol substrates must examine the conformational requirements of the enzyme. To do this, the four kinetically

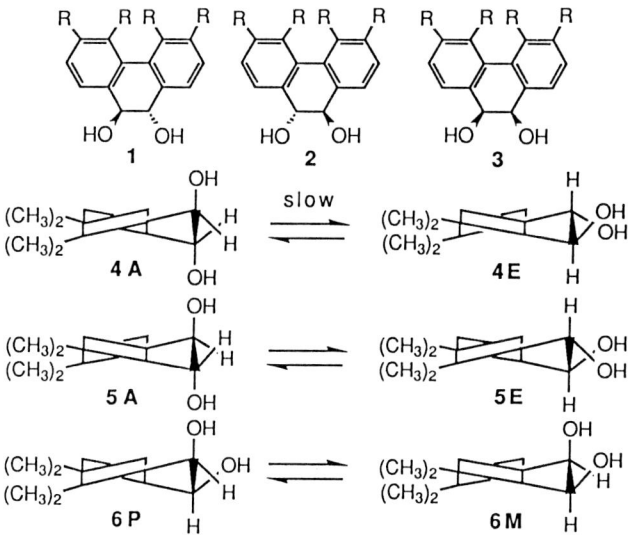

Figure 1. Structures of conformational isomers of phenanthrene 9,10-dihydrodiols

stable conformational diastereomers of trans-3,4,5,6-tetramethyl-9,10-dihydroxy-9,10-dihydrophenanthrene (R=CH$_3$) (4A-5E, Fig. 1) and the two conformational enantiomers of the cis-diol (6M and 6P) were synthesized (Armstrong et al., 1985a). Steric hindrance between the methyl groups at the 4- and 5-positions, buttressed by those in the 3- and 6-positions provides a barrier of close to 30 kcal/mol to pseudorotation or mutarotation of the pairs of conformational isomers. The remarkable conformational stability of these isomers is best illustrated by the fact that the t1/2 for racemization of 6 is about two years at room temperature (Armstrong & Lewis, 1985b).

The kinetic results for the trans-diols, 4 and 5, clearly indicate that the two pseudo-diequatorial isomers are much better substrates for the 4-nitrophenol

Table 1. Kinetic constants for the mono-glucuronidation of phenanthrene and tetramethylphenanthrene 9,10-dihydrodiols.[a]

Substrate	Absolute Configuration	Relative Configuration	k_c (s^{-1})	k_c/K_{mapp} $(M^{-1}s^{-1})$
1	S,S	trans	1.4	1,100
2	R,R	trans	0.070	4,400
3	R,S	cis	0.037	18,000
4E	S,S,M	trans-dieq	0.41	980
5E	R,R,P	trans-dieq	0.20	910
4A	S,S,P	trans-diax	<0.0005	-
5A	R,R,M	trans-diax	0.0069	-
6M	R,S,M	cis	0.0058	-
6P	R,S,P	cis	0.020	-

[a]Data from Lewis & Armstrong (1983) and Armstrong et al. (1985a).

conjugating enzyme than are the corresponding pseudo-diaxial diastereomers. In fact 4A appears not to be a substrate at all. It is also interesting to note that whereas the enzyme shows a high degree of kinetic discrimination between the enantiomers 1 and 2, it exhibits only a modest ability to distinguish 4E and 5E. This observation tends to suggest that the much lower turnover number (k_c) observed with 2 as compared to 1 may be due to tight non-productive binding of the wrong (eg. diaxial) conformer of 2. It is reasonable to conclude from the 30- to 800-fold preference for 4E and 5E that the diequatorial diastereomers of conformationally labile dihydrodiols are those that participate in productive enzyme-substrate complexes.

Each conformational enantiomer of the cis-diols 3 and 6 has two chemically and stereochemically distinct carbinol groups. Thus there are four possible stereoisomeric products that can be derived from 6, two from each kinetically stable enantiomer. It is clear from product analysis of the monoglucuronides derived from the enzyme catalyzed reaction of 6M and 6P that only one product is obtained from each. It would also appear that it is the equatorial hydroxyl group in each instance that is glucuronidated.

Whether the conformer selectivity and stereoselectivity of UDP-glucuronosyltransferase toward the kinetically stable molecules 4-6 can be generalized to other structurally diverse dihydrodiols is questionable. Nonetheless the preference of the enzyme with the phenanthrene 9,10-dihydrodiols is reasonably clear.

Sterically hindered chiral phenols
The limits to which UDP-glucuronosyltransferase can discriminate between chiral substrate surfaces is not clear. In an attempt to test these limits we have developed a synthesis of the kinetically stable chiral 3,4,5,6-tetramethyl-9-hydroxyphenanthrenes 7 as illustrated for the P enantiomer in Fig. 2. Acid catalyzed dehydration of the cis-diol 6P at -15°C leads to the corresponding chiral phenol 7P. The phenols 7P and 7M have two interesting and important properties. First, the conformational enantiomers exhibit reasonable kinetic stability with a half life for racemization of about one hour at room temperature (Armstrong et al., 1987). A second property of 7 is the position of the

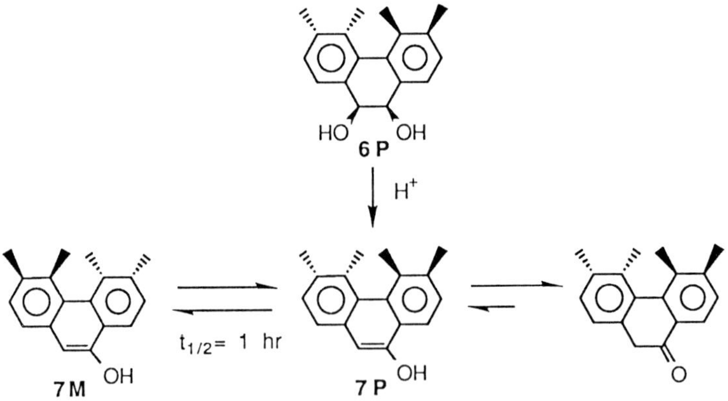

	R	enol	rel rate	ketone
7	CH₃	33	1	67
8	H	> 99	2	< 1

Figure 2. Conformer and tautomer equilibria for 9-hydroxyphenanthrene, 8 and 3,4,5,6-tetramethyl-9-hydroxyphenanthrene, 7.

enol-keto equilibrium. The tautomer equilibrium of 7 favors the ketone (Fig. 2) by about 2 to 1 (33% enol/67% ketone by NMR in CH$_3$CN) in marked contrast to the more usual case of 9-hydroxyphenanthrene, 8, which is $\geq$ 99% enol under the same conditions.

Solubilized microsomes catalyze the glucuronidation of 8 and racemic 7. Preliminary results suggest the relative rate of glucuronidation of 8 is twice that of racemic 7. It is perhaps no coincidence that the better substrate has a more favorable tautomeric equilibrium for reaction though other geometric effects may contribute to the altered reactivity as well (Lilienblum et al., 1987). Kinetic studies are in progress to examine this question as well as to determine if the enzyme is able to distinguish the two enantiomers of 7.

The purified p-nitrophenol-conjugating enzyme exhibits quite different kinetic properties toward the two enantiomers of 1,1'-bi-2-naphthol, 9. Reaction of 9M follows saturation kinetics with k_c = 0.19 s^{-1} and k_c/K_{mapp} = 150 M^{-1}s^{-1}. In contrast, the enzyme catalyzed reaction with 9P shows simple first-order kinetics up to the solubility limit of the substrate. The slope of the reciprocal plot of the kinetic data gives a value of k_c/K_{mapp} for 9P of 5.7 M^{-1}s^{-1}, 26-fold lower than the M-enantiomer. The preference for the M-enantiomer is considerably greater than that observed for the helical isomers of the <u>cis</u>- and <u>trans</u>-diols, perhaps due to the more exaggerated chiral substrate surface.

Analogues of UDP-glucuronate

There has been a noticeable lack of effective inhibitors and alternative substrates for kinetic and mechanistic studies of the UDP-glucuronosyltransferases. To fill this gap we have recently embarked on a program to prepare potentially useful analogues of UDP-glucuronate. Four of the target molecules are shown below. The phosphono analogues 10-13 represent a series of molecules in which the leaving group potential of UDP is varied from inert, as in 10, to something that theoretically could approach that of the natural substrate. Compound 10 would be expected to be an inhibitor of the enzyme, whereas 11-13 may be either substrates or inhibitors. Substitution of the methylene, fluoromethylene or difluoromethylene group in 11-13 should result in the systematic variation of the pKa of the leaving group, UMPXP. The relative pKa's with different X should

	X	Y
10	CH$_2$	O
11	O	CH$_2$
12	O	CHF
13	O	CF$_2$

follow the order $O \approx CF_2 > CHF > CH_2$. Thus, UMPCF$_2$P-glucuronate should, at least on electronic grounds, be as good a substrate as the natural one.

The initial synthetic targets in this series are compounds 10 and 13. Inasmuch as the phosphono analogue of glucose-1-phosphate (G-1-CH$_2$P) had been previously synthesized (Nicotra et al., 1982) it was thought that an enzymatic synthesis might be possible by the serial action of UTP:glucose-1-phosphate pyrophosphorylase and UDP-glucose dehydrogenase on this substance. The first step in the enzymatic synthesis works quite well, as is illustrated in the comparison of the initial velocity kinetics of the natural substrate, glucose-1-phosphate (G-1-P) (K_m = 22 μM, V_{max} = 92 μmol/min/mg) and G-1-CH$_2$-P (K_m = 330 μM, V_{max} = 56 μmol/min/mg) in Fig. 3. Yields of up to 80% can be achieved in preparative scale reactions which include inorganic pyrophosphatase to pull the equilibrium toward the product UDPCH$_2$G. However, oxidation of UDPCH$_2$G to the target compound 10 by UDP-glucose dehydrogenase is very inefficient, giving less than 2% conversion based on NADH formation. A chemical synthesis of 10 is in progress.

A preliminary, initial velocity kinetic investigation indicates that UDPCH$_2$G is itself a competitive inhibitor of UDP-glucuronosyltransferase vs UDP-glucuronate in the formation of 4-nitrophenol-β-glucuronide catalyzed by solubilized rat-liver microsomes as shown in Fig. 3. A replot of the slopes in Fig. 3 suggests UDPCH$_2$G is a parabolic rather than linear competitive inhibitor in this situation. The inhibition by UDPCH$_2$G is not particularly surprising given that a number of uridine-containing compounds do (eg. UDP and UMP). Whether 10 will, as expected, exhibit tighter binding than UDPCH$_2$G remains to be determined.

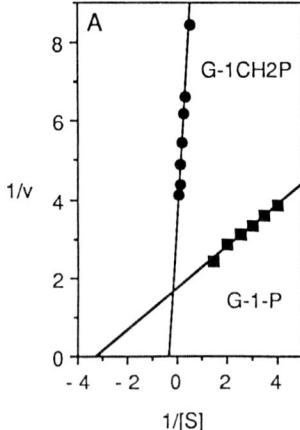 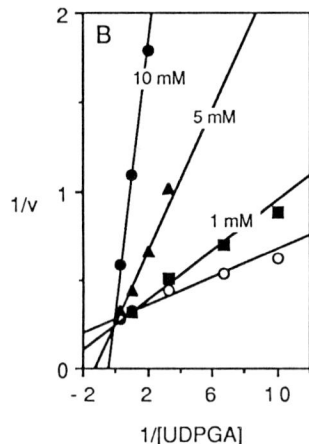

Figure 3. Initial velocity kinetics of formation of UDP-glucose and UDPCH$_2$-glucose (UDPCH$_2$G) catalyzed by UTP:glucose 1-phosphate pyrophosphorylase (panel A) and the inhibition of solubilized microsomal glucuronidation of 4-nitrophenol by UDPCH$_2$G (panel B). Units of reciprocal concentration are (A) 0.1 mM^{-1} and (B) mM^{-1}.

The synthesis of 13 has commenced along two routes as illustrated in Fig. 4. In anticipation that UMPCF$_2$PG might not be a good substrate for UDP-glucosedehydrogenase an alternate chemical oxidation prior to coupling of the uridine is being investigated. The 6-O-tritylated carbohydrate is used to selectively unmask the 6-position for oxidation. A somewhat different strategy based on the recent synthesis of UMPCH$_2$P-galactose using acyl protecting groups is another alternative

(Vaghefi et al., 1987). In the likely event that 11-13 are inhibitors of or substrates for UDP-glucuronosyltransferase these molecules should prove to be useful tools for the study of the chemical and kinetic mechanism of enzyme.

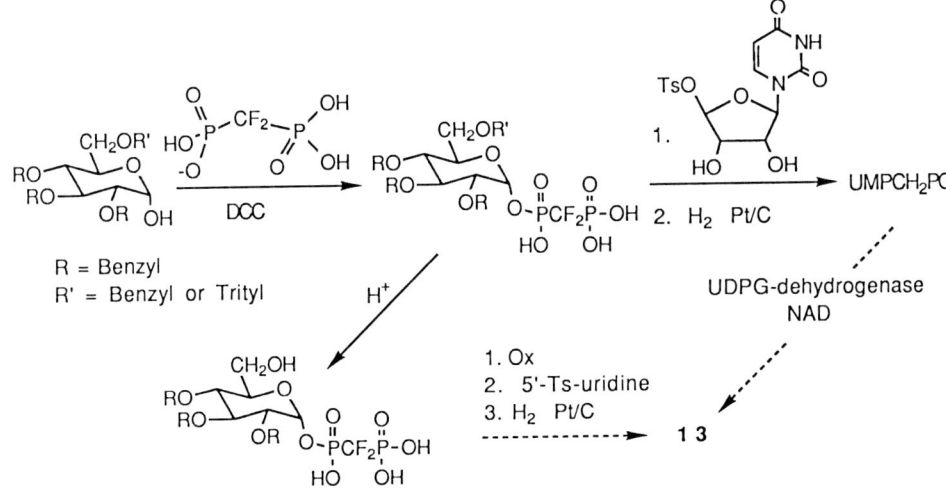

Figure 4. Proposed synthetic strategy for 13. Solid arrows indicate transformations already performed and dashed arrows reactions to be completed.

CONCLUSIONS

The design and use of alternative substrates and inhibitors of UDP-glucuronosyltransferase should become an increasingly valuable approach for mechanistic studies as our ability to purify or produce reasonable quantities of these enzymes improves. A number of laboratories have already demonstrated the value of delineating structure-activity relationships with aglycone substrates. The same may be possible for the glycosyl-donating substrate as well.

ACKNOWLEDGMENT

This research was supported in part by National Science Foundation Grant DMB 8716307 and by American Cancer Society Grant IN-147F to the Maryland Cancer Program.

REFERENCES

Armstrong, R. N., Lewis, D. A., Ammon, H. L. and Prasad, S. M. (1985a) Kinetically stable conformers of 3,4,5,6-tetramethyl-9,10-dihydroxy-9,10-dihydrophenanthrene as probes of the conformer specificity of UDPglucuronosyltransferase. J. Am. Chem. Soc. 107, 1057-1058.

Armstrong, R. N. and Lewis, D. A. (1985b) Pseudorotation barriers in cis-4,5-dimethyl- and cis-3,4,5,6-tetramethyl-9,10-dihydroxy-9,10-dihydrophenanthrene: Measurement of the buttressing effect. J. Org. Chem. 50, 907-908.

Armstrong, R. N., Ammon, H. L. and Darnow, J. D. (1987) Molecular geometry and conformational stability of 4,5-dimethyl- and 3,4,5,6-tetramethylphenanthrene: A look at the structural basis of the buttressing effect. J. Am. Chem. Soc. 109, 2077-2082.

Cobb, D. I., Lewis, D. A. and Armstrong, R. N. (1983) Solvent dependence of the conformation and chiroptical properties of trans-9,10-dihydroxy-9,10-dihydrophenanthrene and its monoglucuronides. J. Org. Chem. 48, 4139-4141.

Davisson, V. J., Woodside, A. B., Neal, T. R., Stremler, K. E., Muehlbacher, M. and Poulter, C. D. (1986) Phosphorylation of isoprenoid alcohols. J. Org. Chem. 51, 4768-4779.

Davisson, V. J., Davis, D. R., Dixit, V. M. and Poulter, C. D. (1987) Synthesis of nucleotide 5'-diphosphates from 5'-O-tosyl nucleosides. J. Org. Chem. 52, 1794-1801.

Lewis, D. A. and Armstrong, R. N. (1983) Stereoselectivity and regioselectivity of uridine-5'-diphosphoglucuronosyltransferase toward vicinal dihydrodiols of polycyclic aromatic hydrocarbons. Biochemistry 22, 6297-6303.

Lilienblum, W., Platt, K. L., Schirmer, G., Oesch, F. and Bock, K. W. (1987) Regioselectivity of rat liver microsomal UDP-glucuronosyltransferase activities toward phenols of benzo(a)pyrene and dibenz(a,h)anthracene. Mol. Pharmacol. 32, 173-177.

Myers, T. C., Nakamura, K. and Danielzadeh, A. B. (1965) Phosphonic acid analogs of nucleoside phosphates. III. The synthesis of adenosine-5'-methylenediphosphonate, a phosphonic acid analog of adenosine-5'-diphosphate. J. Org. Chem. 30, 1517-1520.

Nicotra, F., Ronchetti, F. and Russo, G. (1982) Stereospecific synthesis of the phosphono analogues of α- and β-D-glucose 1-phosphate. J. Org. Chem. 47, 4459-4462.

Vaghefi, M. M., Bernacki, R. J., Hennen, W. J. and Robins, R. K. (1987) Synthesis of certain nucleoside methylenediphosphonate sugars as potential inhibitors of glycosyltransferases. J. Med. Chem. 30, 1391-1399.

Résumé

La conception de plusieurs types de substrats et inhibiteurs potentiels de l'UDP-glucuronosyltransférase est décrite. Six isomères du phénanthrène (3,4,5,6-tétraméthyl-9,10-dihydroxy-9,10-dihydrophénanthrène) sont utilisés pour discriminer d'après leur cinétique de conjugaison, la sélectivité de la glucuronoconjugaison selon la conformation du substrat. Nous avons observé une préférence évidente de l'enzyme purifiée pour les diastéréoisomères trans-diols en position pseudo-diéquatoriale. Le composé cis-diol est glucuronoconjugué uniquement sur le groupement hydroxyle pseudo-équatorial. L'enzyme purifiée montre une cinétique énantiosélective envers les conformères chiraux du 1,1'-bi'2-naphtol. Une approche à la fois enzymatique et chimique a été utilisée pour synthétiser des analogues de l'UDP-glucose et de l'UDP-glucuronide. L'analogue phosphono de l'UDP-glucose ($UDPCH_2G$) est un inhibiteur compétitif de l'UDP-glucuronosyltransférase.

Genetic deficiency of UDP-Glucuronosyltransferase in the rat

Michio Matsui, Fusako Nagai and Hiroshi Homma

Kyoritsu College of Pharmacy, Shibakoen, Minato-ku, Tokyo 105, Japan

ABSTRACT

LA Wistar rats with genetic deficiency of androsterone UDP-glucuronosyltransferase (GT) have been established and inbred. Gunn rats which have defective bilirubin GT and low 4-nitrophenol GT activities were crossed with LA Wistar rats. The F1 hybrids showed normal GT activities toward bilirubin, androsterone and 4-nitrophenol. The F2 offsprings exhibited four different combinations of bilirubin and androsterone GT activities. These combinations were defects in both GT activities, a single defect in bilirubin GT activity, a single defect in androsterone GT activity, and normal two GT activities. They were segregated in approximate ratio of 1:3:3:9, which indicates that bilirubin GT and androsterone GT genes are located on different chromosomes. In F2 progeny, defective bilirubin GT and low 4-nitrophenol GT activities were not segregated, providing evidence that these two mutant genes are located on the same chromosome. Genes responsible for albino and hooded coat colors are not linked with bilirubin GT and androsterone GT genes.

KEYWORDS

UDP-glucuronosyltransferase, rat liver, deficiency, androsterone, bilirubin, chromosome, linkage

INTRODUCTION

Genetic deficiency of UDP-glucuronosyltransferase (GT) is known in some mutant rat strains. Gunn (1938) reported a mutant strain of Wistar rats which shows hereditary hyperbilirubinemia. It was reported subsequently that Gunn rats lack the ability to glucuronidate bilirubin (Lathe & Walker, 1957), due to the absence of bilirubin GT (Scragg et al., 1985). Gunn rats are a good animal model for the study of human Crigler-Najjar syndrome and have been extensively studied (Dutton, 1980).

Matsui & Hakozaki (1977) reported that Wistar rats showed marked individual variation in biliary excretion of exogenously administered androsterone. Some rats excreted large amounts of steroid glucuronides into the bile, whereas the other rats excreted predominantly steroid sulfates into the bile. Subsequent studies revealed the discontinuous variation in hepatic GT activity toward androsterone, the high GT activity (HA) to the low GT activity (LA) ratio being approximately 16:1 (Matsui & Hakozaki, 1979). Such a striking difference was not found in GT activities toward testosterone, bilirubin, 4-nitrophenol and phenolphthalein (Matsui et al., 1979). This variation was also found in Donryu and Wistar-King strains, but not in Sprague-Dawley and Long Evans strains (Matsui et al., 1979). Breeding experiments showed that genetic expression of LA phenotype is inherited as an autosomal recessive trait (Matsui & Watanabe, 1982a). Developmental study revealed that androsterone GT activity surged rapidly after 30 days of age in HA Wistar rats, while the activity remained low in LA Wistar rats (Matsui & Watanabe, 1982b). Purification of androsterone GT from HA and LA Wistar rats has provided evidence that androsterone GT protein is absent in LA Wistar rats (Matsui & Nagai, 1985, 1986). Green et al. (1985) found LA Wistar rats in their colony and obtained similar chromatographic profiles as we did. Corser et al. (1987) presented evidence that androsterone GT mRNA is absent in LA Wistar rats and that the genetic deficiency should be due to the deletion in androsterone GT gene. The occurrence of LA Wistar rats in Japan, the United States and England should imply that deficiency of androsterone GT must have taken place long ago in the genome of ancestral Wistar rats.

Six or more GT isoforms with partially overlapping substrate specificities exist in the rat liver (Siest et al., 1987). However, there is very little knowledge of the chromosomal organization of the GT gene family. To elucidate the linkage relationships for GT genes, we first compared GT activities between Gunn and LA Wistar rats and then raised recombinant rat strains by one outcross of Gunn rats with LA Wistar rats, followed by brother-sister inbreeding.

MATERIALS AND METHODS

Gunn rats were initially supplied to Sankyo Co., Shizuoka, Japan by Albert Einstein College of Medicine, New York, U. S. A. in 1964. Gunn rats were identified as icteric offsprings by matings of male homozygotes (genotype, jj) and female heterozygotes (j+) (Nagai et al., 1987). Wistar rats were classified into homozygous HA (genotype, HaHa) and LA (haha) Wistar rats in terms of hepatic androsterone GT activity (Matsui & Watanabe, 1982a).

Male Gunn rats (HaHa/jj) were crossed with female LA Wistar rats (haha/++). Hepatic GT activities of F1 hybrids were assayed by partial hepatectomy at 60 days of age or by decapitation at 150 days of age. F2 or F3 generation was obtained by matings of F1 or F2 offsprings at 4 weeks after the hepatectomy, respectively. Hepatic GT activities of F2 or F3 generation were determined by partial hepatectomy at 60 to 80 days of age.

Microsomal fractions were prepared by homogenization of livers with 0.25 M sucrose in 0.1 M Tris/HCl buffer, pH 7.4, followed by differential centrifugation (2000g for 10 min, 16000g for 45 min and 105000g for 60 min).

GT activities toward androsterone and 4-nitrophenol were assayed by a slight modification of the method described previously (Matsui et al., 1984). The standard incubation medium contained 0.17 mM [^{3}H]androsterone (13 nCi) or 0.36 mM 4-nitrophenol, 2 mM UDP-glucuronic acid, 10 mM $MgCl_2$ and 0.1 M Tris/HCl buffer, pH 7.4 in a total volume of 0.5 ml. To activate GT activities, 0.005-0.2% Triton X-100 and 1-30 mM concentrations of N-nitrosodiethylamine or N-nitrodiethylamine were added to the incubation media as described previously (Nagai et al., 1987). GT activity toward bilirubin was assayed according to the method described by Heirwegh et al. (1972).

RESULTS AND DISCUSSION

Comparison of hepatic GT activities between Gunn and LA Wistar rats

Gunn rat colonies appear to be genetically different from each other except for the jaundice locus, because of their crossbreeding with various rat strains. In fact, two Gunn rat populations appear to exist, one with low and one with high 4-nitrophenol GT activity (Dutton, 1980). Gunn rats used in this study were initially obtained from Albert Einstein College of Medicine, New York and had black pigment on heads and a black stripe on their backs similar to Long-Evans strain (Nagai et al., 1987). The occurrence of hooded Gunn rats was reported previously (Yeary & Grothaus, 1971; Leyten et al., 1986). Table 1 shows hepatic GT activities toward bilirubin, androsterone and 4-nitrophenol in Gunn and LA Wistar rats.

Table 1. Comparison of hepatic GT activities between Gunn and LA Wistar rats

Substrate	Activator	Gunn rat	LA Wistar rat
Bilirubin	Native	ND	0.15 ± 0.05
	Digitonin	ND	0.59 ± 0.13
Androsterone	Native	1.04 ± 0.06	0.08 ± 0.03
	Triton	4.91 ± 0.48	0.11 ± 0.04
4-Nitrophenol	Native	0.38 ± 0.07	1.26 ± 0.59
	Triton	1.72 ± 0.75	7.74 ± 3.05
	NEN	1.84 ± 0.09	1.97 ± 0.38
	Triton+NEN	14.68 ± 2.20	15.18 ± 4.18

Hepatic GT activities of female Gunn and LA Wistar rats are expressed as nmol/min per mg of protein. Each value is the mean $\pm$ S.D. for 4-5 animals. Triton: 0.02% Triton X-100. NEN: 10 mM N-nitrosodiethylamine. ND: not detectable. Reproduced from Nagai et al. (1987) with permission.

Gunn rats lacked bilirubin GT activity and showed normal androsterone GT activity, whereas LA Wistar rats had low androsterone GT activity and showed high bilirubin GT activity. In Gunn rats, native and Triton X-100-activated 4-nitrophenol GT activities were 20 to 30% of those of LA Wistar rats. However, their low 4-nitrophenol GT activities were restored to the high levels of LA Wistar rats by addition of N-nitrosodiethylamine. These results demonstrate that our Gunn rats have GT activities typical of Gunn rat populations (Dutton, 1980).

In a previous paper (Matsui et al., 1984), we reported that N-nitrodiethylamine activated GT activities toward 4-nitrophenol and 2-aminophenol in a way similar to N-nitrosodiethylamine. Figure 1 shows the effects of 0.005-0.2% Triton X-100 and 1-30 mM concentrations of N-nitrosodiethylamine and N-nitrodiethylamine on 4-nitrophenol GT activity in Gunn and LA Wistar rats. Addition of Triton X-100 alone stimulated the GT activity and the highest activity was attained at 0.02% concentration in both mutants (Fig. 1a, 1b), though the Gunn rat GT activity was much lower than that of LA Wistar rats. By the combined addition of Triton X-

100 and 10 mM concentration of N-nitrosodiethylamine (Fig. 1a) or N-nitrodiethylamine (Fig. 1b), the low Gunn rat GT activity was increased similarly to the high levels of LA Wistar rats. The addition of N-nitrosodiethylamine (Fig. 1c) or N-nitrodiethylamine (Fig. 1d) alone increased the low Gunn rat GT activity to the high levels of LA Wistar rats and the combined addition of 0.02% Triton X-100 and N-nitrosodiethylamine (Fig. 1c) or N-nitrodiethylamine (Fig. 1d) further stimulated the GT activity equally to high levels in both mutants. The maximal rate of the GT activity was attained at 10-30 mM concentrations of N-nitrosodiethylamine or N-nitrodiethylamine in the presence of 0.02% Triton X-100. N-Nitrodiethylamine appears to stimulate 4-nitrophenol GT activity more efficiently than does N-nitrosodiethylamine in the presence of 0.02% Triton X-100, epscially in Gunn rats. Based on these data, 4-nitrophenol GT activity was assayed in the presence of 0.02% Triton X-100 and by the combined addition of 0.02% Triton X-100 and 10 mM N-nitrodiethylamine in the subsequent studies.

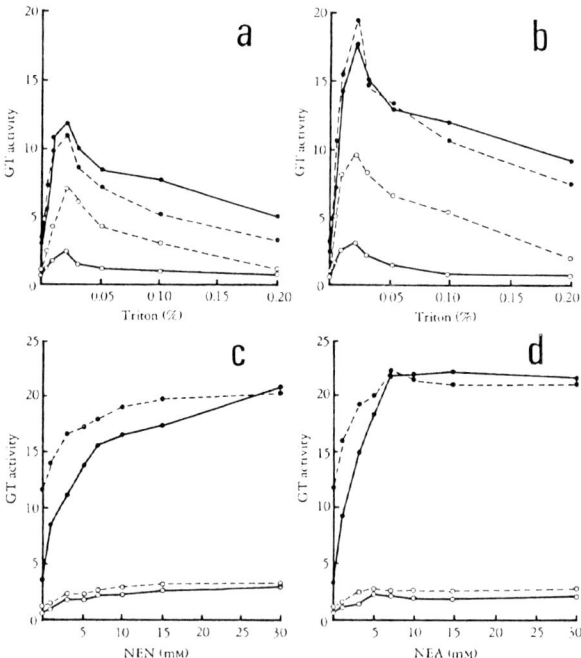

Fig. 1. Effects of Triton X-100, N-nitrosodiethylamine and N-nitrodiethylamine on hepatic 4-nitrophenol GT activity

GT activities from Gunn (—) and LA Wistar (- -) rats were determined at various concentrations of Triton X-100 in the absence (O) or the presence (●) of 10 mM N-nitrosodiethylamine (a) and 10 mM N-nitrodiethylamine (b), or at various concentrations of N-nitrosodiethylamine (c) and N-nitrodiethylamine (d) in the absence (O) or the presence (●) of 0.02% Triton X-100. GT activity is expressed as nmol/min per mg of protein. Triton: Triton X-100. NEN: N-nitrosodiethylamine. NEA: N-nitrodiethylamine. Reproduced from Nagai et al. (1987) with permission.

F1 hybrids derived from crosses between Gunn and LA Wistar rats

To elucidate the linkage relationships for bilirubin, androsterone and putative 4-nitrophenol GT genes, male Gunn rats were crossed with female LA Wistar rats. Table 2 shows the analysis of twenty-four F1 hybrids in GT activities toward bilirubin, androsterone and 4-nitrophenol. GT activities obtained by partial hepatectomy at 60 days of age and by decapitation at 150 days of age were not significantly different from each other, confirming that the partial hepatectomy at 60 days of age offers a good means for classification of GT activities. All the F1 hybrids showed normal GT activities toward bilirubin, androsterone and 4-nitrophenol. These results provide evidence that Gunn rats inherit homozygous dominant genotype (HaHa) for androsterone GT, whereas LA Wistar rats inherit homozygous dominant genotype (++) for bilirubin GT.

Table 2. Hepatic GT activities in F1 hybrids (Haha/j+) derived from crosses between male Gunn rats (HaHa/jj) and female LA Wistar rats (haha/++)

Substrate	Activator	60 days		150 days
		Male	Female	Female
Bilirubin	Native	0.21 ± 0.08	0.20 ± 0.10	0.32 ± 0.12
	Digitonin	0.48 ± 0.17	0.49 ± 0.27	0.86 ± 0.06
Androsterone	Native	0.44 ± 0.11	0.36 ± 0.10	---
	Triton	1.56 ± 0.47	1.41 ± 0.37	2.50 ± 0.89
4-Nitrophenol	Native	2.18 ± 0.56	1.29 ± 0.72	1.17 ± 0.18
	Triton	7.76 ± 0.95	5.60 ± 1.50	7.44 ± 2.59
	NEA	4.38 ± 0.59	3.15 ± 0.91	2.56 ± 0.19
	Triton+NEA	17.33 ± 2.42	14.63 ± 2.47	15.68 ± 1.57

GT activity is expressed as nmol/min per mg of protein. Each value is the mean ± S.D. for F1 hybrids at 60 days of age (hepatectomy, 6 males and 18 females) and at 150 days of age (decapitation, 3 females). Triton: 0.02% Triton X-100. NEA: 10 mM N-nitrodiethylamine.

F2 generation derived from crosses between Gunn and LA Wistar rats

GT activities toward bilirubin, androsterone and 4-nitrophenol in one hundred and thirty-five F2 offsprings are shown in Table 3. There were four different combinations of bilirubin and androsterone GT activities. These combinations were defects in both GT activities, a single defect in bilirubin GT activity, a single defect in androsterone GT activity and two normal GT activities. They were segregated in the ratio of 9:27:24:75, which is not significantly different from the expected ratio of 1:3:3:9 (χ^2=0.229, 0.98>P>0.95). This ratio is consistent with Mendel's second law, principle of independent assortment and provides evidence that bilirubin and androsterone GT genes are located on different chromosomes.

Defective bilirubin GT and low 4-nitrophenol GT activities were not segregated in F2 generation. These mutant genes are consequently located on the same chromosome. It is known that 4-nitrophenol is glucuronidated by several GT isoforms (Roy Chowdhury et al., 1986). Scragg et al. (1985) reported that bilirubin GT and possibly phenol GT (substrate: 2-aminophenol & 1-naphthol) were absent in Gunn rats. Furthermore, Coughtrie et al. (1987) described that the defective phenol GT was due to the absence of 3-methylcholanthrene-inducible phenol GT. Further study is required to elucidate the molecular basis of the deficiency in GT isoenzymes.

Gunn rats used in this study have black pigment on heads and a black stripe on their backs. F1 hybrids showed the similar coat color to that of Gunn rats. In F2 generation, the hooded rats showed the black pigment on heads with several variation in the black stripe. The hooded and albino rats were segregated in the ratio of 104:31, which is not significantly different from the expected ratio of 3:1 (χ^2=0.299, 0.7>P>0.5). This ratio is compatible with Mendel's first law, principle of segregation and confirms that albino coat color trait is inherited in an autosomal recessive fashion (Castle, 1947). In F2 progeny, albino rats were found as follows: four in the rats with defects in both GT activities, five in the rats with a defect in bilirubin GT activity, six in the rats with a defect in androsterone GT activity, and sixteen in the rats with two high GT activities. These data provide evidence that genes responsible for albino and hooded coat colors are not linked with bilirubin GT (Castle & King, 1940) and androsterone GT genes.

Table 3. Genetic expression of hepatic GT activities in F2 generation derived from crosses between Gunn (HaHa/jj) and LA Wistar (haha/++) rats

Animal	No	Bilirubin (Digitonin)	Androsterone (Triton)	4-Nitrophenol		Genotype
				(Triton)	(Triton+NEA)	
Male	7	ND	0.12 ± 0.05	1.82 ± 0.68	11.81 ± 1.37	
Female	2	ND	0.02, 0.13	1.72, 1.40	12.69, 13.77	
Total	9	ND	0.11 ± 0.05	1.76 ± 0.61	12.12 ± 1.37	haha/jj
Male	14	ND	1.65 ± 0.60	1.99 ± 0.57	11.88 ± 2.14	
Female	13	ND	1.71 ± 0.78	1.78 ± 0.49	12.48 ± 1.13	HaHa,Haha/
Total	27	ND	1.68 ± 0.69	1.89 ± 0.54	12.17 ± 1.75	jj
Male	11	0.62 ± 0.21	0.15 ± 0.04	7.29 ± 1.90	13.70 ± 1.44	
Female	13	0.47 ± 0.23	0.08 ± 0.03	5.17 ± 1.58	11.68 ± 2.69	
Total	24	0.54 ± 0.23	0.11 ± 0.05	6.14 ± 2.03	12.60 ± 2.42	haha/++,j+
Male	36	0.43 ± 0.17	1.92 ± 0.62	6.89 ± 2.28	13.42 ± 2.35	
Female	39	0.47 ± 0.25	1.60 ± 0.78	4.95 ± 1.69	11.67 ± 2.13	HaHa,Haha/
Total	75	0.45 ± 0.21	1.75 ± 0.72	5.88 ± 2.22	12.51 ± 2.40	++,j+

GT activity is expressed as nmol/min per mg of protein. Each value is the mean ± S.D. Parenthesis indicates the activator(s) used for the enzyme assay. No: number of animals. ND: not detectable. Triton: 0.02% Triton X-100. NEA: 10 mM N-nitrodiethylamine.

Breeding of Gunn-LA Wistar rats with defects in bilirubin and androsterone GT isoenzymes

In order to breed Gunn-LA Wistar rats, male F2 Gunn-LA Wistar rats were crossed with female F2 rats with a single defect in androsterone GT activity (Table 4). There were two types of genetic expression of GT activities in F3 progeny. In Type 1, all the offsprings showed a single defect in androsterone GT activity. In Type 2, defects in bilirubin and androsterone GT activities and a single defect in androsterone GT activity were segregated in the ratio of 1:1. These results indicate that the mother of Type 1 progeny had homozygous genotype (++) in terms of bilirubin GT, whereas the mothers of Type 2 progeny had heterozygous genotype (j+). Thus Gunn-LA Wistar rats can be raised by matings of male Gunn-LA Wistar rats (haha/jj) with female LA Wistar rats with heterozygous genotype in terms of bilirubin GT (haha/j+). Fifty percent of the litters are expected to be Gunn-LA Wistar rats. Hooded and albino Gunn-LA Wistar rats were selected and have been maintained by inbreeding to establish a uniform genetic background. In a manner similar to Gunn rats, Gunn-LA Wistar rats exhibit some nervous symptoms such as wobbly gait and partial paralysis of the hind limbs.

Table 4. Breeding of Gunn-LA Wistar rats (haha/jj) and LA Wistar rats with heterozygous genotype in terms of bilirubin GT (haha/j+)

Animal	No	Bilirubin (Digitonin)	Androsterone (Triton)	4-Nitrophenol (Triton)	4-Nitrophenol (Triton+NEA)	Genotype
Type 1						
F2 Parent						
Father	1	ND	0.17	2.80	11.93	haha/jj
Mother	1	0.37	0.10	7.28	12.60	haha/++
F3 Offspring						
Male	4	0.48 ± 0.13	0.18 ± 0.01	6.29 ± 0.32	13.88 ± 0.94	
Female	5	0.47 ± 0.17	0.12 ± 0.02	6.27 ± 1.38	13.75 ± 1.27	
Total	9	0.47 ± 0.15	0.15 ± 0.04	6.28 ± 0.99	13.81 ± 1.06	haha/j+
Type 2						
F2 Parent						
Father	1	ND	0.08	0.93	10.54	haha/jj
Mother	2	0.12, 0.36	0.09, 0.08	3.54, 3.45	11.71, 12.26	haha/j+
F3 Offspring						
Male	2	ND	0.14, 0.14	1.80, 1.64	12.02, 14.21	
Female	6	ND	0.10 ± 0.02	1.34 ± 0.25	12.88 ± 1.23	
Total	8	ND	0.11 ± 0.02	1.43 ± 0.28	12.94 ± 1.20	haha/jj
Male	5	0.44 ± 0.11	0.15 ± 0.03	5.92 ± 1.36	15.06 ± 1.83	
Female	3	0.50 ± 0.16	0.08 ± 0.01	5.21 ± 1.35	12.66 ± 1.02	
Total	8	0.46 ± 0.12	0.13 ± 0.04	5.66 ± 1.31	14.16 ± 1.94	haha/j+

GT activity is expressed as nmol/min per mg of protein. Each value is the mean ± S.D. For further explanations see Table 3.

This study is the first demonstration of the genetic linkage of GT genes in the rat. Further study is required to elucidate the chromosomal localization of the GT gene family and the molecular mechanism of the deficiency in GT isoenzymes.

ACKNOWLEDGEMENTS

This investigation was supported in part by a grant from the Ministry of Education of Japan. We thank Drs. Tetsuo Hiraoka and Hisao Tanase, Sankyo Company Ltd. for providing Gunn rats.

REFERENCES

Castle, W. E. (1947): The domestication of the rat. Proc. Natl. Acad. Sci. U. S. A. 33, 109-117.
Castle, W. E. & King, H. D. (1940): Linkage studies of the rat (Rattus norvegicus). III. Proc. Natl. Acad. Sci. U. S. A. 26, 578-580.
Corser, R. B., Coughtrie, M. W. H., Jackson, M. R. & Burchell, B. (1987): The molecular basis of the inherited deficiency of androsterone UDP-glucuronyltransferase in Wistar rats. FEBS Lett. 213, 448-452.
Coughtrie, M. W. H., Burchell, B., Shepherd, I. M. & Bend, J. R. (1987): Defective induction of phenol glucuronidation by 3-methylcholanthrene in Gunn rats is due to the absence of a specific UDP-glucuronosyltransferase isoenzyme. Mol. Pharmacol. 31, 585-591.
Dutton, G. J. (1980): The influence of sex, species, and strain on

glucuronidation. In Glucuronidation of Drugs and Other Compounds, pp 123-134. Boca Raton, FL: CRC Press.

Green, M. D., Falany, C. N., Kirkpatrick, R. B. & Tephly, T. R. (1985): Strain difference in purified rat hepatic 3α-hydroxysteroid UDP-glucuronosyltransferase. Biochem. J. 230, 403-409.

Gunn, C. H. (1938): Hereditary acholuric jaundice in a new mutant strain of rats. J. Heredity 29, 137-139.

Heirwegh, K. P. M., Van de Vijver, M. & Fevery, J. (1972): Assay and properties of digitonin-activated bilirubin uridine diphosphate glucuronyltransferase from rat liver. Biochem. J. 129, 605-618.

Lathe, G. H. & Walker, M. (1957): An enzyme defect in human neonatal jaundice and in Gunn's strain of jaundiced rats. Biochem. J. 67, 9P.

Leyten, R., Vroemen, J. P. A. M., Blanckaert, N. & Heirwegh, K. P. M. (1986): The congenic normal R/APfd and jaundiced R/APfd-j/j rat strains: a new animal model of hereditary non-haemolytic unconjugated hyperbilirubinaemia due to defective bilirubin conjugation. Lab. Animals 20, 335-342.

Matsui, M. & Hakozaki, M. (1977): Variations in biliary metabolites of androsterone in female rats. J. Steroid Biochem. 8, 319-322.

Matsui, M. & Hakozaki, M. (1979): Discontinuous variation in hepatic uridine diphosphate glucuronyltransferase toward androsterone in Wistar rats. A regulatory factor for in vivo metabolism of androsterone. Biochem. Pharmacol. 28, 411-415.

Matsui, M. & Nagai, F. (1985): Multiple forms and a deficiency of uridine diphosphate-glucuronosyltransferases in Wistar rats. J. Pharmacobio-Dyn. 8, 679-686.

Matsui, M. & Nagai, F. (1986): Genetic deficiency of androsterone UDP-glucuronosyltransferase activity in Wistar rats is due to the loss of enzyme protein. Biochem. J. 234, 139-144.

Matsui, M. & Watanabe, H. K. (1982a): Classification and genetic expression of Wistar rats with high and low hepatic microsomal UDP-glucuronosyltransferase activity towards androsterone. Biochem. J. 202, 171-174.

Matsui, M. & Watanabe, H. K. (1982b): Developmental alteration of hepatic UDP-glucuronosyltransferase and sulphotransferase towards androsterone and 4-nitrophenol in Wistar rats. Biochem. J. 204, 441-447.

Matsui, M., Nagai, F. & Aoyagi, S. (1979): Strain differences in rat liver UDP-glucuronyltransferase activity towards androsterone. Biochem. J. 179, 483-487.

Matsui, M., Nagai, F., Suzuki, E. & Okada, M. (1984): Structure-activity relationships of nitrosamines and nitramines which stimulate UDP-glucuronosyltransferase activities in vitro. Biochem. Pharmacol. 33, 2647-2651.

Nagai, F., Takahashi, M., Homma, H., Tanase, H. & Matsui, M. (1987): A comparison of uridine diphosphate-glucuronosyltransferase and other drug metabolizing enzyme activities between two mutant strains of Wistar rats with a genetic deficiency in bilirubin or androsterone glucuronidation. J. Pharmacobio-Dyn. 10, 421-426.

Roy Chowdhury, J., Roy Chowdhury, N., Falany, C. N., Tephly, T. R. & Arias, I. M. (1986): Isolation and characterization of multiple forms of rat liver UDP-glucuronate glucuronosyltransferase. Biochem. J. 233, 827-837.

Scragg, I., Celier, C. and Burchell, B. (1985): Congenital jaundice in rats due to the absence of hepatic bilirubin UDP-glucuronyltransferse enzyme protein. FEBS Lett. 183, 37-42.

Siest, G., Antoine, B., Fournel, S., Magdalou, J. & Thomassin, J. (1987): The glucuronosyltransferases: what progress can pharmacologists expect from molecular biology and cellular enzymology? Biochem. Pharmacol. 36, 983-989.

Yeary, R. A. & Grothaus, R. H. (1971): The Gunn rat as an animal model in comparative medicine. Lab. Animal Sci. 21, 362-366.

RESUME

Les rats Wistar LA qui sont génétiquement déficients en androstérone UDP-glucuronosyltransférase (GT) ont été caractérisés et mis en reproduction. Les rats Gunn qui sont déficients en bilirubine GT et qui présentent une faible activité GT envers le 4-nitrophénol ont été croisés avec les rats Wistar LA. Les hybrides de première génération (F1) montrent des activités normales envers la bilirubine, l'androstérone et le 4-nitrophénol. La F2 présente quatre combinaisons différentes concernant les activités GT bilirubine et androstérone. Les combinaisons sont : déficience pour les deux GT activités, déficience pour l'activité GT bilirubine, déficience seule pour l'activité GT androstérone, activité normale pour les deux substrats. La fréquence de ces combinaisons est la suivante 1:3:3:9, ce qui indique que les gènes des GT bilirubine et testostérone sont localisés sur deux chromosomes différents. Les descendants de F2 ne présentent pas une ségrégation concernant les activités GT déficiente pour la conjugaison de la bilirubine et faible par celle du 4-nitrophénol, ce qui indique que ces deux gènes mutants sont situés sur le même chromosome. Les gênes responsables pour les couleurs albinos et "pelage encapuchonné" ne sont pas liés avec ceux codant pour la bilirubine et l'androstérone GT.

Genetic deficiency of rat and human UDP-Glucuronosyltransferases

Michael W.H. Coughtrie, David Harding, Stuart Wilson, Michael R. Jackson, Sylvie Fournel-Gigleux, Robert Hume* and Brian Burchell

*Department of Biochemistry, Medical Sciences Institute, The University, Dundee, DD1 4HN, Scotland and *Department of Child Life and Health, University of Edinburgh, Edinburgh, Scotland, UK*

ABSTRACT

The molecular basis of heritable defects in glucuronidation is discussed. The inherited defect in androsterone glucuronidation in the mutant LA Wistar rats is due to a deletion in the androsterone UDPGT gene, as demonstrated by Southern blot analysis, resulting in the complete absence of corresponding mRNA and enzyme protein. By investigating Gunn rat strains from different sources we have determined that the phenol and bilirubin UDPGT isoenzymes are absent from Gunn rat liver, and that these deficiencies extend to extrahepatic tissues. This loss of enzyme activity, protein and mRNA appears to arise from a transcriptional or post-transcriptional defect. In human Crigler-Najjar syndrome, type I, bilirubin UDPGT activity is completely absent. However, immunoblot analysis of hepatic microsomes from a patient with type I Crigler-Najjar syndrome using the highly sensitive alkaline phosphatase linked detection system, failed to reveal any obvious differences in the UDPGT isoenzyme profile compared with a relevant control sample. Thus, the Gunn rat may not be a good model for the molecular analysis of Crigler-Najjar syndrome.

Key Words. UDP-glucuronosyltransferase/Gunn rat/Crigler-Najjar syndrome/Immunoblotting/ Genetic disease.

INTRODUCTION

Crigler-Najjar syndrome is a heritable severe, non-haemolytic unconjugated hyperbilirubinaemia, resulting in neurological dysfunction attributed to kernicterus (Crigler and Najjar, 1952). Bilirubin UDP-glucuronosyltransferase[1] enzyme activity is not detectable in type I patients who have serum bilirubin levels >20mg/dl (Arias et al, 1969). Type II patients have serum bilirubin levels below 20mg/dl, and in addition respond to phenobarbitone therapy (Arias et al 1969). In the absence of treatment (phototherapy and/or orthotrophic liver transplantation) the type I form of the disease is usually fatal in infancy (see Pett and Mowat, 1987). The Gunn rat, a mutant strain of Wistar rat is genetically deficient in bilirubin conjugation (Gunn, 1938), and has been extensively studied as a model for Crigler-Najjar type I syndrome (Cornelius and Arias, 1972). However, the Gunn rat is also deficient in UDPGT activity towards a number of planar phenolic aglycones such as 1-naphthol, 2-aminophenol (see Coughtrie et al, 1987a for references), and also towards digitoxigenin monodigitoxoside (Watkins and Klaassen, 1982). We have previously shown the defects in UDPGT enzyme activity in Gunn rats to be due to the absence of bilirubin and phenol (and possibly other) UDPGT isoenzyme proteins (Scragg et al, 1985; Coughtrie et al, 1987a).

Recent work in this laboratory has demonstrated the molecular basis of another inherited defect in UDPGT activity - the inability of the LA Wistar rat to form androsterone glucuronide (Corser et al, 1987). This is due to a large deletion in the androsterone UDPGT gene, resulting in the absence of mRNA encoding the androsterone UDPGT isoenzyme (Jackson and Burchell, 1986; Corser et al, 1987). Thus our efforts have been directed towards elucidating the molecular basis of the deficiencies of UDPGT enzyme activities in the Gunn Rat, and of the inability of the Crigler-Najjar infant to form bilirubin glucuronides. We have used specific antibody and cDNA probes to examine these defects at the molecular level.

EXPERIMENTAL PROCEDURES

Wistar and Gunn rat colonies were maintained in the animal unit of this Institute. Congenic R/APfd (normal) and R/APfd-j/j (jaundiced) (Leyten et al, 1986) rats were purchased from the Catholic University of Leuven, Belgium. The production of antibodies against various purified rat UDPGTs, and the immunoblot methods (peroxidase-linked system) have been described elswhere (Coughtrie et al, 1987a). Alkaline phosphatase immunostaining of Western blots was performed with NBT/BCIP as substrate, as described by the manufacturers (Promega Biotech). UDPGT enzyme activities with various aglycone substrates were performed by established procedures (see Coughtrie et al, 1987a for references), in the presence of optimally-activating concentrations of the non-ionic detergent, Lubrol PX, to counteract the latency of UDPGT (Dutton, 1980).

RESULTS AND DISCUSSION

Molecular basis of the deficiency of androsterone glucuronidation in Wistar rats. A mutant Wistar strain, designated LA (low androstrerone) has been identified and characterised (Matsui et al, 1979). The resulting deficiency of androsterone UDPGT enzyme activity has been shown to be due to a lack of the enzyme protein, both from purification studies (Green et al, 1985; Matsui and Nagai, 1986) and by immunoblot analysis (Corser et al, 1987). Analysis of mRNA levels in LA and HA Wistar rat liver by Northern blot hybridisation with a cloned androsterone UDPGT cDNA demonstrated that there was no synthesis of androsterone UDPGT mRNA in rats exhibiting the LA phenotype (Jackson and Burchell, 1986). The lack of mRNA synthesis was shown by Southern blotting to be the result of a deletion in the androsterone UDPGT gene (Corser et al, 1987), and subsequent analysis of a partial genomic clone revealed a deletion of at least 6.5kb in the gene (Corser, 1988).

Defects of UDPGT enzyme activity in the Gunn rat. Microsomes prepared from Wistar and Gunn rat liver, kidney and lung were assayed for UDPGT activity with a variety of aglycones (Table 1). In all Gunn rat tissues, enzyme activity towards bilirubin was not measurable. In the liver, activity towards the planar phenols 1-naphthol and 2-aminophenol was severely depleted (17% and 5% of Wistar levels, respectively). Testosterone UDPGT activity was 50% of that in Wistar liver. The alkyl ketone 3-pentanone was able to activate the glucuronidation of 2-aminophenol to about 50% of the level seen in Wistar liver microsomes.

Table 1. UDPglucuronosyltransferase activities in Wistar and Gunn rat microsomes

SUBSTRATE	UDPGT ACTIVITY (nmol/min/mg)[1]					
	WISTAR			GUNN		
	Liver	Kidney	Lung	Liver	Kidney	Lung
BILIRUBIN	0.66 ± 0.11	0.25 ± 0.2	N.D.[2]	N.D.	N.D.	N.D
TESTOSTERONE	2.95 ± 0.35	N.D.	N.D.	1.99 ±0.27 (68)[3]	N.D.	N.D.
1-NAPHTHOL	52 ± 13	22 ± 4	4.2 ± 0.2	8.81 ± 2.32 (17)	N.D.	N.D.
2-AMINOPHENOL	1.74 ± 0.5	0.45 ± 0.06	0.2 ± 0	0.09 ± 0.01 (5)	N.D.	N.D.
2-AMINOPHENOL +10mM 3-pentanone	3.22 ± 0.34	0.46 ± 0.09	0.2 ± 0	1.45 ± 0.15 (45)	N.D.	N.D.

1. Values represent mean ± S.D. of at least 3 separate pools of tissue assayed in the presence of optimally-activating concentrations of Lubrol PX.
2. Not detectable.
3. Figures in parentheses indicate the percentage of Wistar activity.

In contrast, no phenol UDPGT enzyme activity was measurable in either kidney or lung microsomes prepared from Gunn rats, and bilirubin UDPGT activity was also deficient in the kidney (Wistar lung microsomes possess no bilirubin UDPGT activity). These data demonstrate the defects in glucuronidation reactions in the Gunn rat, and confirm that these defects exist in the extrahepatic tissues.

It is interesting to note the lack of stimulation of 2-aminophenol UDPGT activity by 3-pentanone in microsomes prepared from extrahepatic organs of both Wistar and Gunn rats. We have previously suggested that the residual levels of phenol UDPGT activity observed in Gunn rat liver may reflect the overlapping substrate specificity of UDPGT isoenzymes (Coughtrie et al, 1987a,b). Based on substrate specificity determinations using purified UDPGTs (Falany and Tephly, 1983; Falany et al, 1986), it is possible that in the Gunn rat, the residual phenol UDPGT enzyme activity observed is carried out by 17β-hydroxysteroid (testosterone) UDPGT. Purified testosterone UDPGT catalysed the formation of 4-nitrophenol and 1-naphthol glucuronides at about 25-30% of the rate measured with purified 4-nitrophenol UDPGT (Falany and Tephly, 1986). If the stimulation of hepatic phenol UDPGT enzyme activity in the Gunn rat by alkyl ketones (Lalani and Burchell, 1979; Table 1) resulted from an effect of these compounds on testosterone UDPGT, then the absence of a stimulatory effect of 3-pentanone on extrahepatic 2-aminophenol UDGT enzyme activity could be due to the lack of testosterone UDPGT activity (Table 1) and enzyme protein (Coughtrie, 1986) in Wistar and Gunn rat kidney and lung. The effect of 3-pentanone on the ability of purified Gunn rat testosterone UDPGT to conjugate planar phenols remains to be determined.

Glucuronidation reactions in congenic R/APfd and R/APfd-j/j rat liver. The animals available in this Institute are not in-bred, congenic strains. In order to eliminate the possibility of the phenol UDPGT deficiency in the Gunn rat being the result of an unrelated mutation we obtained congenic R/APfd (normal) and R/APfd-j/j (jaundiced) rats from Leuven, Belgium. The generation of these strains has been described (Leyten, et al, 1987). We determined UDPGT enzyme activities in liver microsomes prepared from these animals, and from first generation heterozygotes, designated R/APfd-j/+ (Table 2). The data obtained agree well with those obtained with our Wistar and Gunn rats, with a complete absence of bilirubin UDPGT enzyme activity, and the depletion of phenol UDPGT activities to 5% (2-aminophenol) and 10% (1-naphthol) of the normal (R/APfd) levels. Heterozygotes showed approximately 50% of normal activity towards bilirubin, 1-naphthol and 2-aminophenol, and normal levels of testosterone UDPGT enzyme activity.

Table 2. Hepatic UDP-glucuronosyltransferase activities in congenic Wistar and Gunn rats

	UDPGT ACTIVITY (nmol/min/mg)		
		STRAIN	
AGLYCONE	R/APfd	R/APfd-j/+	R/APfd-j/j
BILIRUBIN	0.66 ± 0.06	0.33 ± 0.04 (50)	0 (0)
1-NAPHTHOL	18.2 ± 1.3	8.32 ± 0.35 (46)	1.75 ± 0.76 (10)
ANDROSTERONE	0.03 ± 0.01	0.03 ± 0.01 (100)	0.02 ± 0.01 (67)
TESTOSTERONE	1.82 ± 0.01	2.17 ± 0.09 (119)	1.09 ± 0.44 (60)
2-AMINOPHENOL	0.94 ± 0.12	0.43 ± 0.01 (46)	0.05 ± 0.00 (5)
2-AMINOPHENOL + 10mM 3-pentanone	2.05 ± 0.06	1.37 ± 0.14 (67)	0.53 ± 0.25 (26)

Data presented as mean ± S.D. for 3 pools of liver. Assays were perfromed in the presence of optimally-activating concentrations of Lubrol PX, determined for each aglycone and rat strain.

These congenic strains exhibited the LA (low androsterone) UDPGT phenotype (Matsui and Hakozaki, 1979), indicating that the parent strains from which these congenic strains were generated were deficient in androsterone glucuronidation. 2-Aminophenol UDPGT activity in R/APfd-j/j rat liver microsomes was not stimulated to the same extent (11-fold) as in Gunn rat liver microsomes (16 fold - Table 1).

Immunoblot analysis of normal and jaundiced rat liver microsomes. The preparation and characterisation of an anti-UDPGT antibody (RAK1) directed against purified rat kidney bilirubin/1-naphthol UDPGTs has previously been reported (Coughtrie et al, 1987a). This antibody specifically recognised bilirubin (54,000 daltons) and phenol (53,000 daltons) UDPGT isoenzymes on immunoblot analysis of rat microsomes. At least two minor bands (56,000 and 57,000 daltons) were also recognised. When this antibody was used to probe Western blots of Wistar, Gunn, R/APfd; R/APfd-j/+ and R/APfd-j/j rat liver microsomes, it was shown that the immunostaining bands of 54 and 53 kDa were absent from the Gunn and R/APfd-j/j liver microsomes (Fig. 1, lanes G and j/j). The heterozygous R/APfd-j/+ microsomes demonstrated decreased immunostaining of these bands (Fig. 1, lane j/+). A very faint band was visible in the R/APfd-j/j rat liver microsomes (Fig. 1, lane j/j) at approximately 52-53 KDa, and it is not clear whether this represents a UDPGT isoenzyme. These data confirm previous observations that the immunoreactive polypeptides corresponding to bilirubin and phenol UDPGT isoenzymes are absent from jaundiced Gunn rat liver microsomes, and that the congenic R/APfd-j/j rat liver microsomes also appear to be deficient in these isoenzymes.

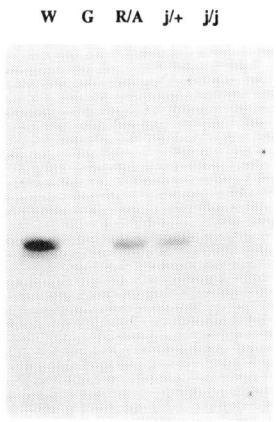

RAK1 - Bilirubin/Phenol- Specific

Fig. 1. Western blot analysis of Wistar and Gunn rat liver microsomes. Microsomes (50µg) were resolved on SDS-PAGE, and electroblotted onto nitrocellulose. Immunostaining with RAK1 (anti-rat kidney bilirubin/phenol UDPGT) was performed using the peroxidase-linked visualisation system. W = Wistar; G = Gunn; RA = R/APfd; j/+ = R/APfd-j/+; j/j = R/APfd-j/j.

We have recently described the loss of a putative mRNA species coding for bilirubin UDPGT in the Gunn rat by Northern blot analysis with a human UDPGT cDNA recognising several UDPGT messages, including a clofibrate-induced species in Wistar rats (Burchell et al, 1987). Similarly, Gunn phenol UDPGT mRNA appears to be synthesised at only 10% of Wistar levels, as detected by Northern blot anaylsis with a rat kidney phenol UDPGT cDNA, and only one intact phenol UDPGT gene appears to be present in the Gunn rat, as determined by Southern blot analysis of

Gunn rat genomic DNA (D. Harding et al, unpublished work).

Immunoprecipitation of ^{125}I-labelled microsomal UDPGTs. Microsomal proteins were labelled with ^{125}I, and UDPGTs precipitated with anti-rat liver testosterone/4-nitrophenol UDPGT (RAL1, Burchell et al, 1984). This antibody displays broad recognition of UDPGT isoenzymes. Following SDS-polyacrylaminde gel electrophoresis of immunoprecipitates, gels were autoradiographed (Figure 2). The antibody failed to precipitate proteins in the molecular weight range 53-54 kDa from Gunn rat liver microsomes, which were present in Wistar microsomes. The induction of a 54kDa polypeptide with 3-methylcholanthrene and a 52kDa protein with phenobarbitone in Wistar rats is clearly visible. These data complement the immunoblot analysis, demonstrating the absence of immunoreactive bilirubin and phenol UDPGTs from Gunn rat liver microsomes. Thus, either these proteins are not synthesised in the Gunn rat, or they are synthesised in such a form as to be non-immunoreactive with two polyclonal anti-UDPGT antibody preparations.

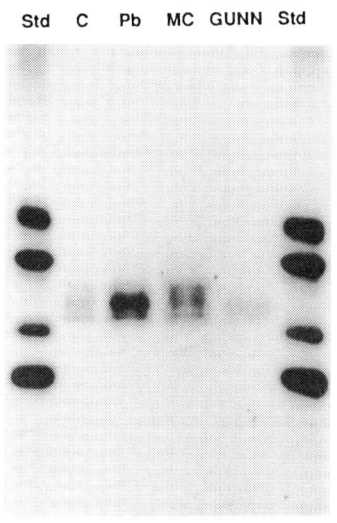

Figure 2. Immunoprecipitation of ^{125}I-labelled microsomal UDP-glucuronosyltransferases. Rat liver microsomes were labelled with ^{125}I, and UDPGTs were immunoprecipitated with RAL1 (anti-rat liver testosterone/phenol UDPGT). Following SDS-PAGE of precipitates, gels were autoradiographed. C = control Wistar; Pb = phenobarbitone-treated Wistar; MC = 3-methylcholanthrene-treated Wistar; G = control Gunn. Labelled molecular weight standards are albumin (68kDa), pyruvate kinase (57kDa), fumarase (44kDa) and aldolase (40kDa).

Roy Chowdhury et al (1987) reported the purification of unreactive bilirubin and phenol UDPGT isoenzymes from detergent-solubilised Gunn rat liver microsomes by chromatofocusing. In our experience, however, individual UDPGT isoenzymes are not completely resolved by chromatofocusing, even using FPLC/Mono P, and the various isoenzyme peaks contain sometimes considerable contamination with other UDPGTs (M. Coughtrie and S. Shepherd, unpublished work). It is quite possible that the 4-nitrophenol UDPGT activity purified from Gunn rat liver microsomes is the result of testosterone UDPGT, as there is significant (15% of total) testosterone UDPGT activity in their broad fraction 1 (pH 8.9-8.4) from chromatofocusing (Roy Chowdhury et al, 1987). The protein which they identified as 4-nitrophenol UDPGT in Wistar and Gunn rats (approx 50kDa) is not the protein which we have determined to be phenol UDPGT [53kDa] (Scragg et al, 1985; Coughtrie et al, 1987), which is absent from Gunn rat liver microsomes as determined by Western blotting (Fig.1). Testosterone UDPGT is the fastest migrating (on SDS-PAGE) UDPGT species yet purified from rat liver, with a subunit molecular weight of 50kDa (Falany and Tephly, 1983). The ability of purified testosterone UDPGT to catalyse the glucuronidation of 1-naphthol and 4-nitrophenol has been demonstrated (Falany and Tephly, 1983) and we have presented some evidence here of the possible contribution of testosterone UDPGT to the glucuronidation of planar phenols in Gunn rat liver.

The genetic defect in Crigler-Najjar syndrome. We have previously described a Crigler-Najjar infant, exhibiting the type I phenotype (Burchell et al, 1987). In this infant, bilirubin UDPGT enzyme activity was not detectable, whereas testosterone UDPGT was 7-fold higher than normal, probably the result of induction due to phenobarbitone therapy. Immunoblot analysis of liver microsomes from this infant using the peroxidase linked method appeared to show the absence of a 54kDa polypeptide. We have since re-analysed this sample by immunoblotting using the 10-fold more sensitive alkaline phosphatase-linked visualisation system (Figure 3). With the broad spectrum RAL1 anti-UDPGT activity, no apparent difference in the profile of immunoreactive polypeptides was observed between the Crigler-Najjar liver microsomes and microsomes from a normal infant of the same postnatal age. Induction of several bands in the Crigler-Najjar microsomes by phenobarbitone therapy is clearly visible. Thus, in contrast to the Gunn rat, no apparent lack of immunoreactive protein(s) was evident in the Crigler-Najjar infant. We have confirmed these findings with liver microsomes from a second Crigler-Najjar type I child and with other anti-UDPGT antibodies (M. Coughtrie and H. van Es, unpublished work).

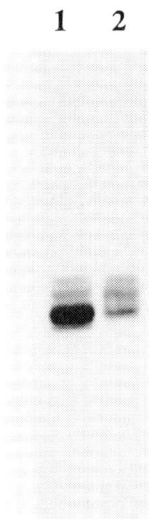

Figure 3. Immunoblot analysis of Crigler-Najjar type I liver microsomes. Liver microsomes (15µg) from a type I Crigler-Najjar infant, 12 weeks *post partum* (1) and a normal infant, 13 weeks *post partum* (2) were electrophoresed on a 7.5% polyacrylamide gel in the presence of 0.1% SDS. Following transfer to nitrocellulose and exposure to anti-UDPGT antibody RAL1, immunoreactive polypeptides were visualised by alkaline phosphatase-conjugated anti-goat IgG, with NBT/BCIP as substrate.

CONCLUDING REMARKS

The data presented here call into question the suitability of the Gunn rat as a good model for studying the molecular basis of the inherited Crigler-Najjar syndrome. In the Gunn rat, the bilirubin and phenol UDPGT proteins appear to be absent, resulting from decreased synthesis of possibly non-translated mRNA species. However, in the Crigler-Najjar syndrome, there appears to be a full complement of immunoreactive UDPGTs, indicating that the putative defective bilirubin UDPGT protein is synthesised in a form that is still immunoreactive. To resolve the differences in these inherited deficiencies of UDPGT in the Gunn rat and Crigler-Najjar child, we must first isolate the genes encoding the deficient enzymes. By analysis of these genes, we will be able to determine the nature of the genetic lesion(s) resulting in these conditions.

Acknowledgements We are grateful to Sheila Smith for technical assistance. Financial support for this work was obtained from the Medical Research Council and the Wellcome Trust. BB is a Wellcome Trust Senior Lecturer.

Footnote.
1. Abbreviations used: UDPGT - UDP-glucuronosyltransferase; RAL1 - sheep anti-rat liver testosterone/phenol UDPGT; RAK1 - goat anti-rat kidney bilirubin/phenol UDPGT; NBT - nitro blue tetrazolium; BCIP - 5-bromo-4-chloro-3-indolyl phosphate; SDS-PAGE - sodium dodecyl sulphate polyacrylamide gel electrophoresis.

REFERENCES

Arias, I.M., Gartner, L.M., Cohen, M., Esser, J.B. and Levi, A.J. (1969). Chronic non-hemolytic unconjugated hyperbilirubinemia with glucuronyltansferase deficiency. *Am.J. Med.* **47**: 395-409.

Burchell, B., Kennedy, S., Jackson, M. and McCarthy, L. (1984). The biosynthesis and induction of microsomal UDP-glucuronyltransferase in avian liver. *Biochem. Soc. Trans.* **12**: 50-53.

Burchell, B., Coughtrie, M.W.H., Jackson, M.R., Shepherd, S.R.P., Harding, D., and Hume, R. (1987).Genetic Deficiency of Bilirubin glucuronidation in rats and humans. *Mol. Aspects Med.* **9**:429-455

Cornelius, E.E. and Arias, I.M. (1972). Animal model of human disease. Crigler-Najjar syndrome animal model: hereditary nonhemolytic hyperbilirubinemia in Gunn rats. *Am.J. Pathol.* **69**:369-372.

Corser, R.B., Coughtrie, M.W.H., Jackson, M.R. and Burchell, B. (1987). The molecular nasis of the inherited deficiency of androsterone glucuronyltransferase in Wistar rats. *FEBS Lett.* **213**:448-452.

Corser, R.B. (1988). *Ph.D. Thesis.* University of Dundee.

Coughtrie, M.W.H. (1986). *Ph.D. Thesis.* University of Dundee.

Coughtrie, M.W.H., Burchell, B., Shepherd, I.M. and Bend, J.R. (1987). Defective induction of phenol glucuronidation by 3-methylcholanthrene in Gunn rats is due to the absence of a specific UDP-glucuronosyltransferase isoenzyme. *Mol. Pharmacol.* **31**: 585-591.

Crigler, J.F. and Najjar, V.A. (1952). Congenital familial non-hemolytic jaundice with kernicterus. *Paediatrics* **10**: 169-180.

Dutton, G.J. (1980). *Glucuronidation of drugs and other compounds.* Boca Raton, FL: CRC Press.

Falany, C.N and Tephly, T.R. (1983). Separation,purification and characterisation of three isoenzymes of UDP-glucuronosyltransferase from rat liver microsomes. *Arch. Biochem.*

Biophys. **227**: 248-258.

Falany, C.N., Green, M.R., Swain, E. and Tephly, T.R. (1986). Substrate specificity and characterisation of rat liver *p*-nitrophenol, 3α-hydroxysteroid and 17β-hydroxysteroid UDP-glucuronosyltransferases. *Biochem.J.* **238**: 65-73.

Green, M.D., Falany, C.N., Kirkpatrick, R.B. and Tephly, T.R. (1985). Strain differences in purified rat hepatic 3α-hydroxysteroid UDP-glucuronosyltransferase. *Biochem. J.* **230**: 403-409.

Gunn, C.K. (1938). Hereditary alcoholuric jaundice. *J. Hered.* **29**: 137-139.

Jackson, M.R. and Burchell, B. (1986). The full-length coding sequence of androsterone UDP-glucuronosyltransferase and a comparison with other members of this gene family. *Nucl. Acids Res.* **14**: 779-795.

Lalani, El-N.M.A., and Burchell, B. (1979). Stimulation of defective Gunn rat liver uridine diphosphate-glucuronyltransferase activity *in vitro* by alkyl ketones. *Biochem.J.* **177**: 993-995.

Leyten, R., Vroemen, J.P.A.M., Blanckaert, N. and Heirwegh, K.P.M. (1986). The congenic normal R/APfd and jaundiced R/APfd-j/j rat strains: a new animal model of heriditary non-haemolytic unconjugated hyperbilirubinaemia due to defective bilirubin conjugation. *Lab. Animals* **20**: 335-342.

Matsui, M. and Hakozaki, M. (1979). Discontinuous variation in hepatic uridine diphosphate glucuronyltransferase towards androsterone in Wistar rats. *Biochem. Pharmacol.* **28**:411-415.

Matsui, M. and Nagai, F. (1986). Genetic deficiency of androsterone UDP-glucuronyl-transferase activity in Wistar rats is due to the loss of enzyme protein. *Biochem. J.* **234**: 139-144.

Pett, S. and Mowat, A.P. (1987). Crigler-Najjar syndrome types I and II. Clinical experience - King's College Hospital 1972-1978. Phenobarbitone, phototherapy and liver transplantation. *Molec. Aspects Med.* **9**: 473-482.

Roy Chowdhury, N., Gross, F., Moscioni, A.P., Kram, M., Arias, I.M. and Roy Chowdhury, J. (1987). Isolation of multiple normal and functionally defective forms of uridine diphosphate glucuronosyltransferase from inbred Gunn rats. *J. Clin. Invest.* **79**:327-334.

Scragg, I., Celier, C. and Burchell, B. (1985). Congenital jaundice in rats due to the absence of hepatic bilirubin UDP-glucuronosyltransferase enzyme protein. *FEBS Lett.* **183**: 37-42.

Watkins, J.B. and Klaassen, C.D. (1982). Induction of UDP-glucuronosyltransferase activities in Gunn, heterozygous and Wistar rat livers by pregnenolone-16α-carbonitrile. *Drug Metab. Dispos.* **10**: 590-594.

Résumé

Nous avons étudié les bases moléculaires de différents déficits génétiques de la glucuronoconjugaison. Le déficit génétique de la conjugaison de l'androstérone rencontré chez une espèce mutante issue du rat Wistar (LA) est dû à une délétion du gène codant pour l'UDPGT androstérone, apparente par Southern blotting et qui résulte en une absence totale de l'ARNm et de la protéine enzymatique correspondants. Au moyen de rats Gunn provenant de différentes origines, nous avons montré que les isoformes d'UDPGT conjugant la bilirubine et les phénols sont absentes du foie de rat Gunn, et que cette déficience est également observée dans les tissus extra-hépatiques. Cette absence de l'activité catalytique, de la protéine et de l'ARNm proviendrait d'un déficit transcriptionnel ou post-transcriptionnel.

Chez l'homme, dans la maladie de Crigler-Najjar, l'activité UDPGT bilirubine est complètement absente. Cependant l'analyse par immunoblotting des microsomes hépatiques d'un patient atteint de la maladie de Crigler-Najjar de type I, au moyen d'un système de détection hautement sensitif utilisant la phosphatase alkaline, ne révèle aucune différence de profil des isoenzymes d'UDPGT comparée à un échantillon approprié. Il semble donc que le rat Gunn ne soit pas un modèle adéquat pour l'étude des bases moléculaires de la maladie de Crigler-Najjar.

Cellular and subcellular basis of glucuronidation

Bases cellulaires et subcellulaires de la glucuronoconjugaison

Investigation of UDP-Glucuronosyltransferase isoenzymes restricted-specificity in liver microsomes

B. Antoine, J.A. Boutin* and G. Siest

Centre du Médicament, UA CNRS 597, 30 rue Lionnois, 54000 Nancy, France
* Institut de Recherches Servier, 11 rue des Moulineaux, 92150 Suresnes, France

SUMMARY

Several ideas are presented about the study of the pluri-specificity of the UDP-glucuronosyltransferase (UDPGT) isoenzymes towards exogenous substrates. We develop here a simple mathematical theory based on the use of series of alternative substrates and induction. Data illustrated that for each series of substrates, it exists a linear relationship between velocities (and V) before versus after induction. This relationship allows the in situ characterization of a given selectively induced isoenzyme with restricted specificity. We suggest a methodology to better characterize the several isoenzymes involved in the glucuronidation of an exogenous substrate. This procedure, based on the determination of kinetic parameters of each isoenzyme, needs the use of a wide range of substrate concentrations and the plot of the data according to Eadie-Scatchard. 4-nitrophenol glucuronidation was closely investigated: whereas at least two isoenzymes with different affinities were shown to be involved in the rat liver microsomes, only a single one seems to be implicated in the kidney. All these observations show that a better knowledge of the isoenzymes substrate-specificity according to the substrate concentration used is an absolute requisite for purification studies.

KEYWORDS

UDP-glucuronosyltransferase, substrate specificity, kinetic analysis, liver microsomes.

INTRODUCTION

UDP-glucuronosyltransferases (UDPGT, E.C 2.4.1.17) are a family of isoenzymes associated with most cellular membranes (Antoine et al., 1983) of many organs. One of the most difficult aspect of their characterization is the determination of each isoenzyme substrate-specificity. From polypeptides or cDNAs isolation, two great clusters of isoenzymes are distinguishable: the first, strictly specific for endogenous aglycones and the other, showing an adaptation for the glucuronidation of exogenous substrates (see Siest et al., 1987).
Our purpose was to focus on "xenobiotic"-specialized isoenzymes (commonly 3-methylcholanthrene or phenobarbital inducible) which possibly developed a broad specificity for various chemical structures and which are those to be considered in relation to prevision of xenobiotics metabolism.
Our present approach is based on kinetic analysis performed _in situ_, on detergent-activated membranes. Such _in situ_ analysis permits i) to avoid the partial lost of activity (or even of specificity) that occurs during enzyme purification procedures (see Boutin, 1987) ii) to analyse the simultaneous interactions of several isoenzymes with a given exogenous substrate ; _in situ_ observations being more representative of reality.

Our aim in this paper was to give the basis of a methodology in order to characterize through measurement of activities towards series of alternative substrates, the active site of an inducible isoenzyme. Furthermore, we suggest a methodology to evaluate, more carefully than usually published, the individual kinetic characteristics of overlapping isoenzymes.

RESULTS AND DISCUSSION

1) Studies on the microsomal glucuronidation of alternative substrates. Influence of induction.

Whenever data obtained after induction are plotted <u>versus</u> control data for glucuronidation of xenobiotics of related structure, it can be observed that the plot is linear in Vind and Vcon.

A simple mathematical model was developed to assess this kinetic behaviour with respect to the overlapping capability of isoenzymes.

$$V_{con} = V_1 + V_2 \quad (V_{con} = V_{control})$$
$$V_{ind} = nV_1 + V_2 \quad (V_{ind} = V_{induced})$$
$$\text{and } V_{con} = 1/n \, V_{ind} + \frac{n-1}{n} V_2$$

where "n" is the induction factor and V2 is a potential overlapping, non-induced, activity. In order to obtain a linear relationship in Vcon and Vind, the second term of the equation, V2, should be negligible in the experimental conditions used, i.e. a single isoenzyme should be involved in a given substrate glucuronidation.

This type of observation can be done with almost all the published works on
UDPGT conjugation. To make any sense, these data should, nevertheless, have
been obtained with at least five to ten chemically related compounds
(Table 1).

Table 1 : Evaluation of the induction level (n) of inducible UDPGT
isoenzymes in relation to their substrate-specificity

Substrates/species	Inducer	r	n	Reference
Phenols (9)/rat	MC	0.90	2.8	Okulicz-Kozarin et al, 1981
Coumarins (7)/rat	MC	0.85	2.7	Thomassin et al, 1985
Terpenoids (20)/ guinea-pig	PB	0.90	4.3	Boutin et al, 1985
Phenols (6)/pig	BNF	0.94	3.4	Boutin et al, 1981
Phenols (18)/Gunn rat	PB	0.81	19.5	Mackenzie and Owens, 1983
Phenols (4)/rat	MC	0.98	3.9	Ullrich and Bock, 1984

Numbers in brackets are the numbers of the chemically-related substrates whose liver microsomal glucuronidation levels were plotted in Vcon and Vind ; "r" being the correlation coefficient of the linear
equation;MC = 3 methylcholanthrene, PB = phenobarbital, BNP = B-naphthoflavone

This method is a simple and complete way to evaluate the nature of the
isoenzyme induced by a given treatment, and the limit of recognition of
this isoenzyme for the various structures of the substrates tested.

*2) About K value in term of substrate-specificity evaluation of an
isoenzyme: practical and theoretical considerations.*

Determination of kinetic parameters consists of one possible characterization of a specific isoenzyme activity. V (Vmax) gives an idea of the amount
of an active enzyme ; K, the dissociation constant, gives an indication of
its affinity for a given chemical structure (the substrate). More important
is V/K, the first-order rate constant, that is related to the efficiency of
the catalysis towards a given substrate. The determination of such kinetic
values is simple enough but does require the use of appropriate range of
substrate concentration (i.e. from 0.3 to 2 K) to be closer to reality
(Segel, 1975). Such theoretical considerations concern the case of one
substrate being transformed by a single enzyme. Considering the particular
case of drug-metabolizing enzymes (either cytochromes P-450 or UDPGT),
their broad specificity is now known to be supported by several overlapping
isoenzymes, mainly in the case of exogenous substrates. In practical terms,
such considerations mean that several isoenzymes are competiting for a
given substrate, relatively to their own K and V, and therefore depending
on the substrate concentration (Miners et al., 1988, Pacifici et al., 1984,
Boobis et al., 1981).

As an example we choose 4-nitrophenol as a typical overlapping substrate because of its flatness (Okulicz-Kozarin et al., 1981) and its exogenic origin. The kinetical characterization of the several isoenzymes involved in 4-nitrophenol glucuronidation required the use of a wide range of substrate concentrations especially in the low values (i.e. from 0.005 to 0.3 mM) and the use of the representation of Eadie-Scatchard.

Figure 1 clearly shows that 4-nitrophenol is glucuronidated by at least two different UDPGT with different K in rat liver microsomes (figure 1A) whereas by a single (or several with similar K) isoenzyme in the kidney (figure 1B).

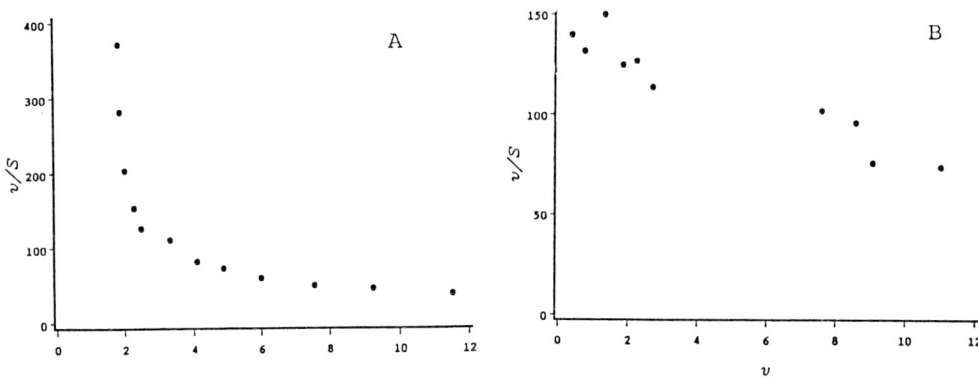

Figure 1 : Eadie-Scatchard plot for 4-nitrophenol glucuronidation of rat A) liver and B) kidney-microsomal fraction

Estimation of the kinetic parameters of each isoenzyme involved :
Liver : V1 = 5   K1 = 0.02   V1/K1 = 250
        V2 = 20   K2 = 0.24   V2/K2 = 85
Kidney V = 24   K = 0.17   V/K = 141

V is in nmol.mn^{-1}.mg^{-1}prot ; K in mM
4-nitrophenol glucuronidation was measured by the method of Mulder and van Doorn (1975) assessed by Colin-Neiger et al. (1984) and Antoine et al. (1988) with a constant UDP-glucuronic acid concentration of 4.5 mM.

In such a case where V1<V2 and K1<K2 and at low substrate concentrations, the relative contributions of the two isoenzymes will depend on their respective V/K ratio (Segel, 1975). In our example, these ratio differ by a factor of 3. Accordingly, the low K-low V isoenzyme is the major contributor to the observed initial velocity <u>at low substrate concentrations</u>. However, considering the published data in which kinetic parameters were evaluated the used range of substrate concentrations (i.e. usually from 0.05 to 0.5 mM, whenever it is mentioned) only permits to characterize the high K-high V isoform. The only examples of use of lower substrate concentrations concern the determination of kinetic parameters of UDPGT isoenzymes specific for endogenous substrates such as steroids and bilirubin.

Then, in conclusion, we strongly point out that kinetic characterization of UDPGT isoenzymes activity require the use of a carefully assessed methodology without which reported data are either partial or meaningless.

ACKNOWLEDGMENTS

The authors are deeply indebted to the continuous excellent secretarial works provided over the 10 last years by Mrs Chantal thirion.

REFERENCES

Antoine, B., Magdalou, J. and Siest, G. (1983): Functional heterogeneity of UDP-glucuronosyltransferases in different membranes of rat liver. <u>Biochem. Pharmacol</u>. 32, 2629-2632.

Antoine, B., Boutin, J.A., and Siest, G. (1988): Further evaluation of the Mulder and van Doorn kinetic procedure for the measurement of the microsomal UDP-glucuronosyltransferase activities. <u>Biochem. J.</u>, 252, 930-931

Boobis, A.R., Kahn, G.C., Whyte, C., Brodie, M.J. and Davies, D.S. (1981) : Biphasic o-deethylation of phenacetin and 7-ethoxycoumarin by human and rat liver microsomal fractions. <u>Biochem. Pharmacol</u>. 30, 2451-2456.

Boutin, J.A., Lepage, C., Batt, A.M. and Siest, G. (1981) : The activity of hepatic UDP-glucuronosyltransferase from control and induced pigs towards 17 hydroxylated aglycones. <u>IRCS Med. Sci</u>. 9, 633-634.

Boutin, J.A., Thomassin, J., Siest, G. and Cartier, A. (1985): Heterogeneity of hepatic microsomal UDP-glucuronosyltransferase(s) activities: conjugations of phenolic and monoterpernoïd aglycones in control and induced rats and guinea-pigs. <u>Biochem. Pharmacol.</u> 34, 2235-2249.

Boutin, J.A. (1987): Indirect evidences of UDP-glucuronosyltransferase heterogeneity: how can it help purification? <u>Drug Metab. Rev.</u> 18, 517-551.

Colin-Neiger, A., Kauffmann, I., Boutin, J.A., Fournel, S., Siest, G., Batt, A.M. and Magdalou, J. (1984): Rapid centrifugal analysis of UDPGT activities. Assessment of the Mulder and van Doorn kinetic assay. J. <u>Biochem. Biophys. Meth.</u> 9, 69-79.

Mackenzie, P.I. and Owens, I.S. (1983) : Differences in UDP-glucuronosyl transferase activities in congenic inbred rats homozygous and heterozygous for the jaundice locus. <u>Biochem. Pharmacol</u>. 32, 3777-3781.

Miners, J.O., Lillywhite, K.J., Matthews, A.P., Jones, M.E. and Birkett, D.J. (1988) : Kinetic and inhibitor studies of 4-methylumbelliferone and 1-naphthol glucuronidation in human liver microsomes. <u>Biochem. Pharmacol</u>. 37, 665-671.

Mulder, G.J. and van Doorn, A.B.D. (1975): A rapid NAD+ linked assay for microsomal UDP-glucuronosyltransferase of rat liver and some observations on substrate specificity of the enzyme. Biochem. J., 151, 131-140.

Okulicz-Kozarin, I., Schaefer, M., Batt, A.M., Siest, G. and Loppinet, V. (1981): Stereochemical heterogeneity of hepatic UDP-glucuronosyl transferase activities in rat liver microsomes. Biochem. Pharmacol. 30, 1457-1461.

Pacifici, G.M., Colizzi, C., Giuliani, L. and Rane A. (1984) : Nuclear and microsomal UDP-glucuronosyltransferase in human liver. In Advance in glucuronoconjugation, Matern S, Bock K.W. and Gerok W. Eds, MTP Press Limited, London, pp 341-350.

Segel, I.H. (1975): in Enzyme kinetics: behaviour and analysis of rapid equilibrium and steady-state enzyme systems, Wiley Interscience, New-York)

Siest, G., Antoine, B. Fournel-Gigleux, S., Magdalou, J. and Thomassin, J. (1987): The glucuronosyltransferases: What progress can pharmaco logists expect from molecular biology and cellular enzymology? Biochem. Pharmacol. 36, 983-989.

Thomassin, J., Boutin, J.A. and Siest, G. (1985): UDP-glucuronosyltrans ferase(s) activities towards natural substrates in rat liver microsomes : kinetic properties and influence of Triton X-100 activation. Pharmacol. Res. Commun. 17, 1005-1015.

Ullrich, D. and Bock, K.W. (1984) : Glucuronide formation of various drugs in liver microsomes and in isolated hepatocytes from phenobarbital- and 3-methylcholanthrene-treated rats. Biochem. Pharmacol. 33, 97-101.

Résumé

Plusieurs schémas d'investigation pour l'étude de la pluri-spécificité des isoenzymes UDP-glucuronosyltransferase (UDPGT) vis-à-vis des substrats exogènes sont proposés.

Une première méthode permet la caractérisation in situ d'une isoenzyme UDPGT donnée, sélectivement induite et de spécificité restreinte. Cette méthode repose sur une théorie mathématique simple et nécessite l'utilisation de séries de substrats alternatifs. Les résultats de la littérature supportent notre théorie, à savoir que pour une même famille de molécules, il existe une relation linéaire entre leurs velocités avant et après induction.

Une seconde méthodologie pour une meilleure caractérisation des multiples isoenzymes impliquées dans la glucuronoconjugaison d'un substrat exogène est suggérée. Cette procédure, basée sur la détermination des paramètres cinétiques de chaque isoenzyme, nécessite l'utilisation d'un grand éventail de concentrations en substrat et la représentation des résultats selon Eadie et Scatchard. C'est ainsi que sont dénombrées au moins à deux les isoenzymes impliquées dans la glucuronoconjugaison du 4-nitrophénol ; l'isoenzyme présentant la meilleure affinité n'étant pas visualisable à forte concentration en substrat.

L'ensemble de ces observations montre qu'une meilleure connaissance de la spécificité de substrat des isoenzymes est une requête absolue dans l'optique de purification.

Modulation of Hepatic Bilirubin Transport and Glucuronidation by the Lipid Microenvironment of Substrate

Dorothy I. Whitmer*, John L. Gollan**

*Section of Gastroenterology and Hepatology, University of Minnesota, School of Medicine Minneapolis, Minnesota, USA
**Harvard Medical School Gastroenterology, Division Brigham and Women's Hospital 75 Francis Street Boston, Massachusetts, USA

ABSTRACT

It has been assumed that hydrophobic substrates such as bilirubin are bound to cytoplasmic proteins for transport to UDP-glucuronyltransferase in hepatocytes. We postulated that lipophilic substrates partition into membranes rather than the aqueous phase, and that this membrane-bound substrate may constitute the immediate pool for biotransformation. We have investigated the intramembrane transport, intermembrane transfer and glucuronidation of bilirubin, a prototype hydrophobic molecule. Bilirubin was incorporated into unilamellar model membranes of natural egg phosphatidylcholine, and rates of glucuronidation were measured in rat liver microsomes using a radiochemical assay. Membrane-bound bilirubin underwent microsomal glucuronidation more rapidly than bilirubin bound to the high-affinity binding sites on hepatic cytosolic proteins. [^{3}H]- and [^{14}C]bilirubin were shown to exchange freely between membrane and cytosolic pools, but, with higher molar ratios of bilirubin:protein, the membrane pool provided a higher proportion of substrate for glucuronidation. Next, bilirubin was incorporated into model membranes of native phospholipid purified from hepatic microsomes; rates of glucuronidation were much more rapid than for bilirubin in egg phosphatidylcholine membranes, and the proportion of bilirubin diglucuronide versus monoglucuronide formed was significantly greater. A new technique to study model membrane-microsome interaction demonstrated that membrane fusion was not the mechanism responsible for enhanced substrate delivery to UDP-glucuronyltransferase. Thus, hydrophobic substrates may undergo intra-membrane transport and membrane-membrane transfer to the site of glucuronidation within hepatocytes; characteristics of the lipid microenvironment of bilirubin substratte may govern rates of glucuronidation and the proportion of diglucuronide formed.

KEY WORDS: glucuronidation, bilirubin, membrane, liposome, vesicle, UDP-glucuronyltransferase, liver microsomes

Hydrophobic molecules such as unconjugated bilirubin that are taken up from plasma by hepatocytes are thought to bind solely to cytosolic proteins for transport to the sites of glucuronidation in endoplasmic reticulum. However, there is evidence to suggest that both xenobiotic and endogenous lipophilic substrates entering the hepatocyte may partition between binding proteins and the lipid milieu of intracellular membranes, and that the intramembranous substrate constitutes the immediate precursor pool for biotransformation (1). We postulated that bilirubin may be transported to UDP-glucuronyltransferase within the lipid phase of hepatocyte intracellular membranes, and that the lipid composition and physical characteristics of the membrane influence the rates of bilirubin glucuronide formation. To examine this hypothesis, bilirubin was incorporated into model membranes comprised of native phospholipid purified from rat liver microsomes or natural lipids of defined composition. We then evaluated the exchange of substrate in vitro between membrane and cytosolic protein pools, and compared the relative efficiency of transfer of bilirubin from the two pools to microsomal UDP-glucuronyltransferase for conjugation. Finally, we investigated the relationship between model membrane (liposomal) lipid composition and rates of mono- and diglucuronide synthesis, and examined the mechanism of substrate transfer from model membranes to microsomes.

INCORPORATION OF BILIRUBIN INTO MODEL MEMBRANES AND DETERMINATION OF ITS PHYSICAL STATE AND LOCATION WITHIN THE MEMBRANE BILAYER

We elected to use small, unilamellar model membranes for these studies in order to take advantage of particular features of these membrane preparations. The single bilayer permits study of direct transfer of bilirubin from the membrane phase directly to microsomes, rather than diffusion of substrate through multiple membrane lamallae and interposed aqueous layers. In addition, small vesicles can be eluted from a Sepharose column, separated from microsomes on centrifugation, and they disperse light minimally, thus enabling study of spectral characteristics of the incorporated bilirubin.

Unconjugated bilirubin and phospholipids were combined in organic solvent, desiccated, sonicated in Tris buffer and centrifuged at high speed. The supernatant, a clear yellow liquid, contained vesicles of 240-330 Å diameter by quasielastic light scattering. Using Sepharose 4B chromatography (Fig. 1), it was evident that bilirubin eluted only with phospholipid, and therefore was associated with the lipid bilayer, rather than the internal or external aqueous phase of the vesicles (1). The spectral characteristics of the model membranes showed that

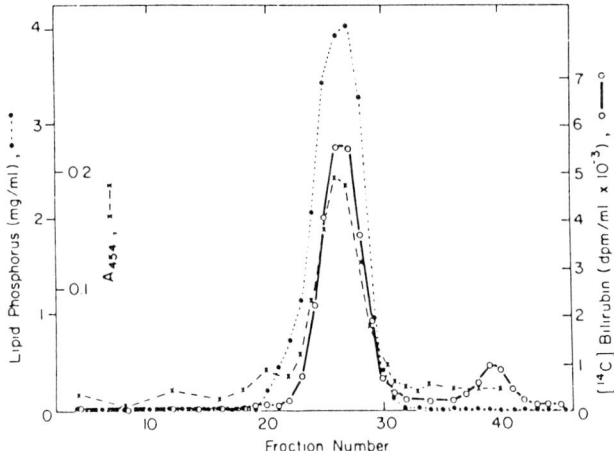

FIG. 1. **Chromatography of [^{14}C]bilirubin liposomes on Sepharose 4B.** Liposomes (1.25 ml) containing 81 mg of lipid phosphorus and 53 μg of [^{14}C]bilirubin (2045 dpm/μg) were applied to a column (60 × 1.4 cm) of Sepharose 4B, equilibrated and eluted at 4 °C with 0.1 M KCl, 10 mM Tris-HCl buffer, pH 7.4. Fraction volumes were 2.8 ml and recoveries of lipid phosphorus and radioactivity in the liposome peak were 71 and 65%, respectively.

the incorporated bilirubin IX-α was internally hydrogen-bonded and not aggregated (1). Thus, native unconjugated bilirubin IX-α can be readily incorporated into phospholipid membrane bilayers. The results of subsequent studies (see below) suggest that the bilirubin is associated with phospholipid headgroups rather than the hydrophobic core region of the bilayer.

TRANSFER OF BILIRUBIN FROM MODEL MEMBRANES OR BINDING PROTEINS TO HEPATIC MICROSOMES FOR GLUCURONIDATION

Experimental design. Velocities of bilirubin glucuronide formation from membrane-bound or protein-bound substrate were measured to determine the relative contribution of these pools to the supply of substrate for glucuronidation, and to examine the mechanism of bilirubin transfer from model membranes to microsomes. The rates of bilirubin mono- and diglucuronide synthesis were determined by radiochemical assay, using radiolabeled bilirubin substrate in the presence of the presumed physiologic allosteric effector, UDP-N-acetylglucosamine. Separation and analysis of the conjugates formed was achieved by alkaline methanolysis, thin-layer chromatography and scintillation counting.

Movement of substrate within the bilayer. We had considered that if bilirubin were incorporated into the hydrophobic core region of the bilayer, there may be an initial "lag phase" before product formation is detectable, corresponding to diffusion of bilirubin to the vesicle surface. However, no such lag phase was observed (1), suggesting that bilirubin is associated with the phospholipid head groups or that substrate in the membrane core region exchanges freely with that on the surface.

Substrate affinity for the membrane bilayer and binding proteins. The initial velocity of total glucuronide formation, using a physiologic concentration (15 μM) of bilirubin in natural (egg) phosphatidylcholine vesicles, was more rapid than for bilirubin bound to the high affinity sites of bovine serum albumin (i.e., in a bilirubin:albumin molar ratio of 1:2) ($p<0.001$), or for bilirubin bound to liver cytosol or purified glutathione S-transferases (representing in vivo hepatic cytosolic binding proteins) in a 1:1 molar ratio ($p<0.05$) (1). These and other similar experiments emphasize the principle that rates of glucuronidation are enhanced by increasing the concentration of bilirubin relative to that of binding proteins, thereby increasing the concentration of "free" or dissociated substrate. Moreover, it is apparent that bilirubin exhibits an avidity for the natural phosphatidylcholine bilayer that is comparable to its association with "low affinity" sites on serum albumin. These conclusions were confirmed by the observation on Sepharose-4B chromatography, that [^{3}H]bilirubin bound to albumin or to glutathione S-transferases and [^{14}C]bilirubin in model membranes exhange freely according to the relative availability of protein binding sites (1). Although the comparative in vivo affinities of intracellular membranes and cytosolic proteins have not been measured directly in hepatocytes, it has been estimated (1) that concentrations of bilirubin in the two pools are comparable under physiologic conditions, and that the relative proportion of bilirubin in membranes is enhanced as the total intracellular concentration of pigment increases.

Mechanism(s) of substrate transfer:Kinetic analysis. To address the mechanism(s) of bilirubin transfer from model membranes to microsomes, detailed kinetic studies were performed over a range of concentrations (2.5-50 μM) of bilirubin that was either bound to purified glutathione S-transferases or incorporated into liposomal membranes. The data for total glucuronide synthesis from both substrates obeyed Michaelis-Menten kinetics; the observed values for apparent Km and Vmax were not significantly different (Fig. 2). Scatchard analysis revealed a single component in each instance (1). The proposed mechanism for substrate transfer from binding proteins to microsomes must account for the inverse

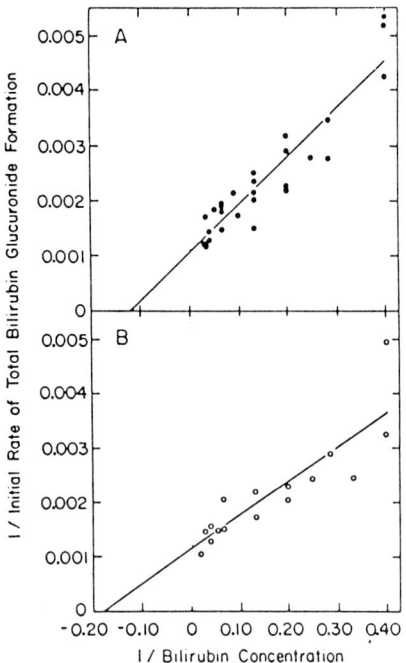

Fig. 2. Kinetics of total bilirubin glucuronide formation from [^{14}C]bilirubin liposomes and from bilirubin bound to glutathione S-transferases. Each *point* represents the initial velocity of total glucuronide synthesis, determined by linear regression analysis using at least 6 time points obtained during the radioassay. Bilirubin substrate concentrations were 2.5–50 μM. *A*, [^{14}C]bilirubin liposomes. *B*, [^{14}C]bilirubin bound to purified glutathione S-transferases in a 1:1 ratio.

relationship between binding affinity and glucuronidation rate (see above) and the aqueous insolubility of unconjugated bilirubin. Thus, protein-bound bilirubin is likely to be transferred to microsomes by collision rather than by dissociation and diffusion through the aqueous phase with reassociation. The mechanism for bilirubin transfer from model membranes to microsomes may be similar. On the basis of the kinetic data, it appears that relative to binding proteins, the membrane microenvironment of bilirubin in phosphatidylcholine vesicles does not promote enhanced substrate access or delivery to the active site of UDP-glucuronyltransferase, as might occur with membrane fusion.

EFFECT OF MODEL MEMBRANE LIPID COMPOSITION ON TRANSFER AND GLUCURONIDATION OF BILIRUBIN

The experimental results above suggest that membrane-bound substrates may constitute a significant pool in vivo for glucuronidation. We postulated that the lipid composition of membranes incorporating bilirubin may influence intracellular movement of substrate (i.e. selectivity for specific hepatocyte organelle membranes) as well as rates of mono- and diglucuronide synthesis. To examine this hypothesis, bilirubin was incorporated into vesicles prepared from phospholipid that had been purified from native rat liver microsomes by Folch extraction, and Sephadex G-25 and silicic acid chromatography. Bilirubin in these native microsomal phospholipid vesicles was glucuronidated more than twice

TABLE

Glucuronidation of liposomal bilirubin; effect of liposomal membrane lipid composition

[^{14}C]Bilirubin (7.2×10^3–1.2×10^4 dpm/μg) was incorporated into liposomes prepared from purified microsomal phospholipid or egg phosphatidylcholine (PC), with or without one other lipid. The bilirubin liposomes were then added as substrate (15 μM bilirubin) to microsomal UDP-glucuronyltransferase assay mixtures for determination of the initial velocity (0–3 min) of total bilirubin glucuronide formation (monoglucuronides plus diglucuronide formation, mean ± S.E.).

Lipid composition of bilirubin liposomes	n	Total bilirubin glucuronide formation	Bilirubin diglucuronide/ monoglucuronide ratio
		pmol/mg protein/min	
Phosphatidylcholine, 100%	12	534 ± 16	0.40 ± 0.05
Purified microsomal phospholipid	7	1168 ± 144[a]	0.84 ± 0.18[b]
PC, 75%; phosphatidylethanolamine, 25%	3	856 ± 81[a]	0.51 ± 0.14
PC, 90%; phosphatidylinositol, 10%	3	971 ± 53[a]	0.39 ± 0.07
PC, 90%; phosphatidylserine, 10%	3	801 ± 41[a]	0.33 ± 0.03
PC, 95%; sphingomyelin, 5%	3	536 ± 21	0.26 ± 0.02
PC, 95%; cholesterol, 5%	3	361 ± 36[a]	0.42 ± 0.08

[a] $p < 0.001$.
[b] $p < 0.01$.

as rapidly ($p<0.001$) as bilirubin in model membranes of egg phosphatidylcholine (Table). Native phospholipid was then subjected to quantitative thin-layer chromatography to determine phospholipid composition, and model membranes of different composition were designed to determine the relationship between membrane phospholipid head group composition and the rate of glucuronidation of incorporated substrate. Bilirubin in model membranes incorporating phosphatidylethanolamine, phosphatidylserine or phosphtidylinositol was glucuronidated more rapidly than bilirubin in model membranes of phosphatidylcholine alone (Table). The incorporation of sphingomyelin resulted in no change in the glucuronidation rate of membrane-bound bilirubin, whereas cholesterol-containing vesicles were associated with a reduced rate of glucuronidation ($p<0.001$).

Glucuronidation rates and physical characteristics of membranes. The failure of sphingomyelin and cholesterol to increase glucuronidation rates suggested that decreased fluidity of the membrane bilayer may be an important factor in the biotransformation of membrane-bound substrate. Fluidity of model membrane core regions (i.e. that portion of the bilayer formed by the hydrocarbon tail of phospholipids) was monitored by measurement of fluorescence anisotropy of incorporated 1,6-diphenylhexatriene. Although decreased glucuronidation rates were associated with less fluid cholesterol-containing model membranes, there was no relationship between fluidity of model membranes of varying phospholipid head group composition and conjugation rates for incorporated substrate ($r=0.41$) (2). Moreover, hydrodynamic diameter (a reflection of membrane curvature) of liposomes of varying lipid composition did not correlate with the rates of glucuronidation of membrane-bound bilirubin (2).

Effect of model membrane lipid composition on synthesis of mono- and diglucuronides. The ratio of the rates of synthesis of bilirubin diglucuronide (BDG) and monoglucuronide (BMG) (i.e. BDG/BMG) was calculated for each model membrane preparation, as an index of the in vitro synthesis of bilirubin diglucuronide (which is the predominant bilirubin conjugate in rat bile) from a physiologic concentration of bilirubin (15 μM). The mean BDG/BMG ratio for bilirubin substrate incorporated into liposomal membranes of purified hepatic microsomal phospholipid (0.84) was significantly greater than that observed for substrate in egg phosphatidylcholine vesicles (0.4, $p<0.01$) (Table). A detailed kinetic study of glucuronidation of protein-bound bilirubin in primate liver has shown that BDG formation is a high affinity, low capacity process compared to BMG formation, and hence the BDG/BMG ratio is greatest at low substrate concentrations and decreases progressively from 0–20 μM bilirubin (3).

In the present study the substrate concentration was identical, but the glucuronidation rate for bilirubin in the microsomal phospholipid vesicles was markedly increased, suggesting that under these conditions the membrane-bound enzyme may encounter an increased effective substrate concentration. If the mechanism of diglucuronide formation in rat hepatocytes is similar to that in primates, it may be inferred that the microenvironment of membrane-bound bilirubin influences substrate delivery to UDP-glucuronyltransferase, presumably by factors that affect the access of bilirubin or of the cosubstrate, UDP-glucuronic acid, to the enzyme.

MECHANISMS OF BILIRUBIN AND PHOSPHOLIPID TRANSFER FROM MODEL MEMBRANES TO HEPATIC MICROSOMES: DUAL-LABEL STUDIES USING THE AIRFUGE

Our next objective was to determine the nature of membrane-membrane interactions associated with the transfer of bilirubin from unilamellar vesicles to microsomes. A method was devised for incorporation of defined quantities of [^{3}H]bilirubin into vesicle membranes labeled with tracer amounts of [^{14}C]dipalmitoylphosphatidylcholine. The liposomes employed consisted of egg phosphatidylcholine or a mixture of natural phospholipids in the proportions present in native rat liver microsomes (4). The amount of vesicle lipid and microsomal protein was held constant. The vesicles were mixed with microsomes, rapidly layered over silicone oil and immediately centrifuged at 100,000g for one minute in a Beckman Airfuge to separate small vesicles (supernatant) from microsomes (pellet). Timed experiments demonstrated that an equilibrium distribution of bilirubin and phospholipid had been achieved in the time required for separation.

<u>Membrane-membrane interactions in the absence of calcium</u>. In all experiments, as the quantity of [^{3}H]bilirubin initially incorporated into the vesicles increased

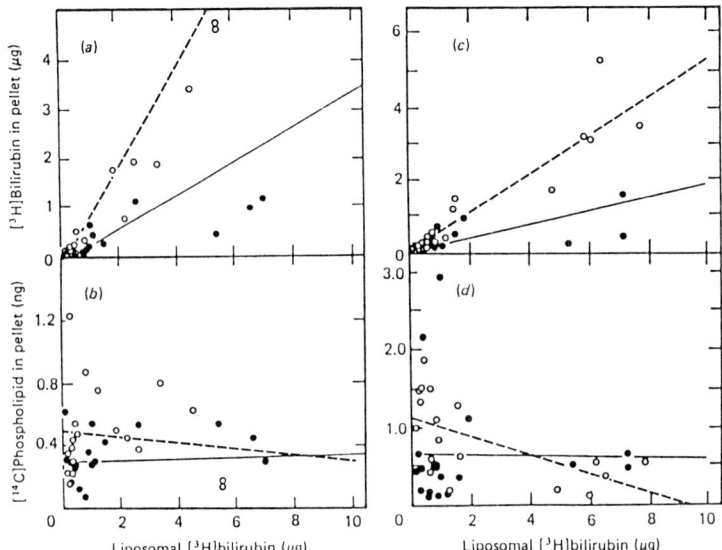

Fig. 3.

Influence of Ca^{2+} on transfer of [^{3}H]bilirubin and [^{14}C]phospholipid from unilamellar liposomes to hepatic microsomes

Increasing amounts of [^{3}H]bilirubin (0.1–12 µg, 2.3–2.8 nCi) were incorporated into liposomes, containing a fixed quantity of lipid P, that were prepared from egg phosphatidylcholine (*a* and *b*) or from model microsomal phospholipid (*c* and *d*) labelled with tracer [^{14}C]dipalmitoyl phosphatidylcholine (112 mCi/mmol). The dual-labelled liposomes were mixed with a constant amount of microsomes, in the presence (O--O) or absence (●—●) of $CaCl_2$ (2 mM), layered over silicone oil and immediately centrifuged at 148 000 g for 1 min in a Beckman Airfuge. The liposomes remained in the supernatant, whereas the microsomes were pelleted below the oil layer; the three phases were then separated and the ^{3}H and ^{14}C radioactivities measured. Each point, the mean of two determinations, represents the quantity of [^{3}H]bilirubin or [^{14}C]phospholipid in the microsomal pellet plotted against the quantity of [^{3}H]bilirubin initially incorporated into the liposomes.

(abscissa range, 0.1-12 µg), so did the amount of [^{3}H]bilirubin appearing in the pellet (solid lines, Fig. 3a and c). The ratio of these quantitites (slope of the linear regression) was not significantly different for phosphatidylcholine vesicles (0.284) and for mixed lipid vesicles (0.190), i.e. approximately 20% of the bilirubin in vesicle membranes was transferred to microsomes (4). Considering that glucuronidation of bilirubin in the mixed lipid vesicles is more rapid (Table), it is apparent that the equilibrium distribution of bilirubin between the membrane populations is unrelated to rates of biotransformation. Of additional interest, however, was the observation that [^{14}C]phospholipid movement to microsomes was constant (0.4% of total for phosphatidylcholine vesicles), irrespective of the quantity of bilirubin transferred (solid lines, Fig. 3b and d). Thus, movement of bilirubin between membranes is not associated with concomitant movement of membrane lipid, suggesting that, in the absence of calcium, substrate is unlikely to be transferred by membrane fusion or adhesion.

Membrane-membrane interactions in the presence of calcium. In the presence of calcium (2mM), a significantly greater proportion of the [^{3}H]bilirubin was transferred from vesicles of both phospholipid compositions to microsomes ($p < 0.001$, dotted lines in Fig. 3a and c). However, phospholipid transfer did not increased (dotted lines in Fig. 3b and d). Therefore, although calcium promotes the transfer of bilirubin substrate from vesicles to microsomes, the data for phospholipid transfer reinforce the observation the neither membrane fusion nor adhesion is involved in the calcium-enhanced intermembrane movement of bilirubin.

IMPLICATIONS OF MEMBRANE TRANSPORT OF SUBSTRATE FOR BIOTRANSFORMATION IN THE HEPATOCYTE

We postulated that as lipid-soluble substrates enter hepatocytes via the sinusoidal surface membrane, they partition between cytosolic binding proteins and intracellular membranes, depending upon the relative magnitude and affinities of the pools. The proportion of bilirubin transported within membranes also is dependent on the rates of lateral diffusion of binding proteins through cytosol and on the relative velocity of glucuronidation and elimination from the membrane pool. The diffusion coefficients for spin-labeled fatty acids in native rat liver microsomal membranes and for ligandin in cytosol are comparable (1), implying that the lateral movement of hydrophobic molecules in the membrane bilayer is as rapid as the three-dimensional diffusion of cytosolic proteins. Moreover, our data suggests that bilirubin in the membrane pool is more efficiently glucuronidated. Thus, the intramembrane pool of bilirubin, which appears to increase as the total intracellular concentration of substrate increases, may assume even greater importance in disorders associated with hyperbilirubinemia or when the mass of intracellular membranes, particularly the endoplasmic reticulum, is enhanced in response to drug administration. Moreover, membrane lipid composition has been shown to be a critical determinant of the rates of mono- and diglucuronide formation from incorporated bilirubin substrate.

REFERENCES

1. Whitmer, D.I., Ziurys, J.C., and Gollan J.L. (1984): Hepatic microsomal glucuronidation of bilirubin in unilamellar liposomal membranes. J. Biol. Chem. 259, 11969-11975.
2. Whitmer, D.I., Russell, P.E., Ziurys, J.C., and Gollan, J.L. (1986): Hepatic microsomal glucuronidation of bilirubin is modulated by the lipid microenvironment of membrane-bound substrate. J. Biol. Chem. 261, 7170-7177.

3. Hauser, S.C., Ziurys, J.C., and Gollan, J.L. (1986): Regulation of bilirubin glucuronide synthesis in primate (Macaca fascicularis) liver. Gastroenterology 91, 287-296.
4. Whitmer, D.I., Russell, P.E., and Gollan, J.L. (1987): Membrane-membrane interactions associated with rapid transfer of liposomal bilirubin to microsomal UDP-glucuronyltransferase. Biochem. J. 244, 41-47.

Résumé

Il est admis que les substrats hydrophobes tels que la bilirubine se fixent aux protéines cytoplasmiques pour être transportés jusqu'à l'UDP-glucuronosyltransférase des hépatocytes. Nous avons postulé que les substrats lipophiles se partagent dans les membranes plutôt que dans la phase aqueuse, et que ce complexe membrane/substrat peut constituer un milieu immédiat de biotransformation. Nous avons étudié le transport intramembranaire, le transfert intermembranaire et la glucuronoconjugaison de la bilirubine, prototype de molécule hydrophobe. La bilirubine est incorporée dans un modèle membranaire unilamellaire de phosphatidylcholine naturelle d'œuf, et les taux de glucuronoconjugaison sont mesurés dans les microsomes de foie de rat par essai radiochimique. La bilirubine fixée à la membrane est conjuguée plus rapidement que celle associée aux sites de fixation à haute affinité des protéines cytosoliques hépatiques. Le marquage de la bilirubine au (^{3}H) et (^{14}C) a montré que ces molécules s'échangent librement entre deux compartiments membranaire et cytosolique, sauf, avec un rapport molaire élevé de bilirubine/protéine ; le compartiment membranaire fournit une forte proportion de substrats pour la glucuronoconjugaison. D'autre part, quand la bilirubine est incorporée dans des modèles membranaires constitués de phospholipides natifs purifiés à partir des microsomes hépatiques, sa glucuronoconjugaison est meilleure que dans le cas de l'incorporation précédente et la proportion de diglucuronide/monoglucuronide de bilirubine formée est significativement élevée. Une nouvelle technique pour étudier le modèle intéraction membrane-microsome a démontré que la fusion membranaire n'est pas le mécanisme responsable de la distribution accrue de substrat à l'UDPGT. Ainsi, les substrats hydrophobes peuvent suivre un transport intramembranaire et un transfert membrane/membrane jusqu'au site de glucuronoconjugaison dans les hépatocytes ; les caractéristiques du microenvironnement lipidique qui entoure la bilirubine peuvent gouverner le taux de glucuronoconjugaison et la proportion du diglucuronide formé.

Is there cytosolic glucuronyl transferase in human liver?

G.M. Pacifici[1], M. Franchi[1] and L. Giuliani[2]

Departments of General Pathology 1 and Surgery 2, Medical School, University of Pisa, 56100 Pisa, Italy

SUMMARY

The activity of the glucuronyl transferase (GT) was measured with 2-naphthol as substrate in the cytosolic and microsomal fractions of human liver. Liver specimens were homogenized in 0.25 M sucrose and the homogenates were subjected to differential centrifugation to isolate the microsomal and cytosolic fractions. The cytosolic fraction was recentrifuged at 105,000xg for 4 hr to sediment eventual light membrane particles. The GT activity (average ±SEM) of 25 liver specimens was 8.98±0.53 nmol/min/mg (microsomes) and 0.17±0.07 nmol/min/mg (cytosol). The kinetics of the GT were studied in 4 liver specimens at varying concentration of 2-naphthol or UDPGA. When 2-naphthol was the variable substrate, the microsomal enzyme obeyed non-Michaelis-Menten kinetics. The K_m (mean±SEM) of the high and low affinity phases were 0.134±0.020 mM and 0.637±0.251 mM, respectively. In contrast, the cytosolic enzyme followed Michaelian kinetics, the K_m was 0.138±0.007 mM. The cytosolic and microsomal GT obeyed Michaelis-Menten kinetics when UDPGA was the variable substrate. The K_m (mean±SEM) was 0.616±0.057 mM (cytosol) and 0.806±0.035 mM (microsomes) (P<0.01). Experiments of inhibition have shown that 4,4'-hydroxy-biphenyl, ethinyloestradiol and oxazepam had different inhibitory effects on the microsomal and cytosolic GT; whereas 2-hydroxy-biphenyl, p-nitrophenol and salicylic acid had similar effect on the two enzymes. The activity of GT was also measured towards ethinyloestradiol. The average of the cytosolic to microsomal ratios was 10 times higher when ethinyloestradiol instead of 2-naphthol was the substrate. Some differences have been observed in the GT assayed in the cytosolic and microsomal fractions. The origin of the cytosolic GT is unknown. We have to take into account that membrane-bound enzymes might be solubilized during liver homogenization. More work has to be done to ascertain whether the authentic cytosolic GT exists or alternatively, the glucuronidation catalyzed by the cytosolic fraction reflects the presence of the enzyme of non-cytosolic origin.

INTRODUCTION

Detoxification includes a number of reactions many of which are conjugation pathways. Among the phase II enzymes, glucuronyl transferase (GT) efficiently removes different molecules from the body. The enzyme catalyzes the conjugation of glucuronic acid with different exogenous and endogenous compounds. This enzyme was thought to be present in the microsomal fraction only. Then, it has been demonstrated that the GT has an ubiquitous distribution in the cell being present in different subcellular organelles of animal (Antoine et al. 1983, 1984; Elmamlouk et al. 1981; Wishart and Fry; 1980a,b; Zalesky and Gessner, 1982; Zalesky et al. 1982) and human (Pacifici et al. 1984, 1986a,b) tissues. Up to now, no information was available on the existence of a non-membrane bound enzyme. The human liver has been found an appropriate source of the nuclear and microsomal GT. We thus used this tissue in our experiments. It was observed that human liver cytosol catalyzes the conjugation of 2-naphthol and ethinyloestradiol with glucuronic acid.

MATERIALS AND METHODS

Patients. Wedge liver biopsies were obtained at laparotomy from patients undergoing colecystectomy. Surplus of the material required for histological analysis was made available for our studies. All liver samples had normal cell architecture.

Subcellular isolation. Liver specimens were homogenized in 4 volumes of 0.25 M sucrose. The homogenates were centrifuged at 12,000xg for 15 min. The supernatants were centrifuged again at 105,000xg for 1 hr. The pellets were resuspended in 0.1 M Tris-HCl (pH 7.4) containing 30% glycerol and investigated as the microsomal fraction. The supernatants were recentrifuged at 105,000xg for 4 hr. The ensuing supernatants were investigated as the cytosolic fraction.

Chemicals. 2-(1,(4,5,8)-^{14}C)-Naphthol with specific activity of 51 mCi/mmol was purchased from the Radiochemical Center (Amersham, England). 17α-(6,7-(^{3}H)N)-Ethinyloestradiol (59.2 Ci/mmol) was from NEN Research Products (Boston, MA, USA). Both compounds were purified by TLC prior to use, and their final radiochemical purity was higher than 99%.

Assays. The activity of the GT was assayed with 2-naphthol as substrate as described by Bock et al (1978) for 1-naphthol. In standard assays, the final concentration of 2-naphthol and UDPGA were 0.5 and 5 mM, respectively. Incubations were carried out at 37 C for 20 min. When the kinetics of the GT were studied at varying concentration of 2-naphthol (0.032, 0.064, 0.125, 0.250, 0.5, 1.0 mM) the concentration of UDPGA was kept constant at 5 mM. At varying concentrations of UDPGA (0.625, 1.25, 2.5, 5.0, 10 mM) the concentration of 2-naphthol was kept constant at 0.5 mM. The glucuronidation of ethinyloestradiol was studied as described by Pacifici and Bock (1988). The mixture of incubation (final volume 0.2 ml) consisted of 0.1 M Tris-HCl (pH 7.4), 5 mM $MgCl_2$, 0.2 mM tritiated Ethinyloestradiol (500,000 cpm), and an aliquot of microsomal or cytosolic protein. Incubations were carried out as described before and were stopped by addition of 0.8 ml of a solution containing 0.4 M TCA and 0.6 M glycine. Samples were extracted in 5 ml of water-saturated ether. The radioactivity of the glucuronide was measured in the water-phase. The enzyme activity measured with both the substrates was computed after correction for blanks. Each sample was assayed in duplicate. The given data were obtained under conditions of linearity with respect to the incubation time and protein concentration.

RESULTS

The effects of incubation time, protein concentration and pH on the cytosolic GT activity are shown in figure 1.

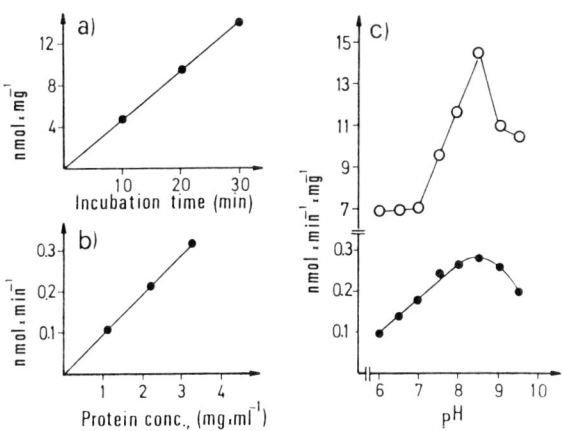

Figure 1. Effects of (a) incubation time, (b) protein concentration and (c) pH on the activity of the GT. Filled and unfilled circles refer to cytosolic and microsomal GT, respectively.

Figure 2 shows the activity of the GT measured in the cytosolic and microsomal fractions of 25 human livers. The activity (mean ±SEM; nmol/min/mg) was 0.17±0.07 (cytosol) and 8.98+0.53 (microsomes). The average (±SEM) of the cytosol to microsomal ratio of the GT activity was 1.85%±0.35. No correlation was observed between the cytosolic and microsomal activities.

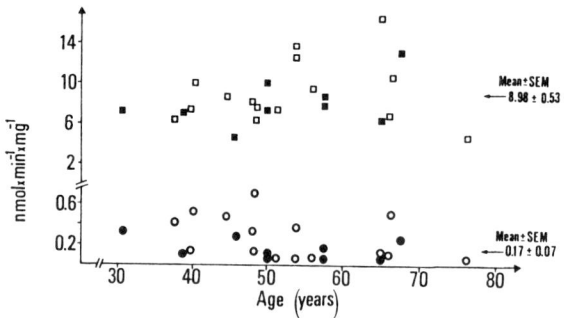

Figure 2. Activity of the GT in the cytosolic (circles) and microsomal (squares) fractions. Filled and unfilled symbols refer to men and women, respectively.

The rate of glucuronidation (mean ±SEM; pmol/min/mg) of EE2 was measured in 10 liver specimens. It was 88.61±22.07 (microsomes) and 18.59±5.05 (cytosol). The cytosolic to microsomal ratio (mean ±SEM) was 23.16±5.41. This ratio did not correlate with that obtained with 2-naphthol. The kinetics of the cytosolic and microsomal GT were studied in 4 livers. The kinetic parameters measured at varying concentrations of 2-naphthol or UDPGA are summarized in tables 1 and 2, respectively. Figure 3 shows the enzyme activity, and the conversion into Eadie-Hofstee plot, of a representative experiment. At varying concentrations of UDPGA, both cytosolic and microsomal GT obeyed Michaelis-Menten kinetics with slight, but significantly different ($p<0.02$), values of Km, whereas at varying concentrations of 2-naphthol, the cytosolic enzyme only obeyed Michaelian kinetics. The microsomal enzyme showed a more complex kinetic pattern constituted by 2 phases: one with higher and the other with lower affinity for 2-naphthol.

Table 1. Kinetic parameters of the cytosolic and microsomal GT measured at varying concentrations of 2-naphthol. The subscripts 1 and 2 denote the first and second phase of the curve. The first phase was obtained at concentrations of 2-naphthol ranging between 0.032 and 0.125 mM, whereas the second phase was obtained at concentrations between 0.125 and 1 mM.

Patients		Cytosolic GT		Microsomal GT			
Age	Sex	Km^a	$Vmax^b$	Km^a_1	$Vmax^b_1$	Km^a_2	$Vmax^b_2$
65	F	0.120	0.31	0.150	15.5	1.433	82.8
50	M	0.150	0.16	0.181	20.7	0.712	55.9
31	M	0.131	0.47	0.072	12.6	0.205	21.1
66	M	0.152	0.20	0.132	9.1	0.201	12.8
Mean		0.138	0.28	0.134	14.5	0.637	43.1
±SEM		0.007	0.06	0.020	2.1	0.025	14.0

^{a} mM, ^{b} nmol/min/mg.

Table 2. Kinetic parameters of the cytosolic and microsomal glucuronyl transferases obtained at varying concentrations of UDPGA.

Patients		Cytosolic GT		Microsomal GT	
Age	Sex	Km^a	$Vmax^b$	Km^a	$Vmax^b$
65	F	0.500	0.052	0.756	16.90
50	M	0.505	0.113	0.736	9.97
31	M	0.723	0.296	0.818	10.60
66	M	0.736	0.092	0.917	11.70
Mean		0.616	0.138	0.806	12.29
±SEM		0.057	0.047	0.035	1.36
		A	B	C	D

^{a} mM, ^{b} nmol/min/mg
Student's t test for paired data. A is different from C ($p < 0.02$). B is different from D ($p < 0.001$).

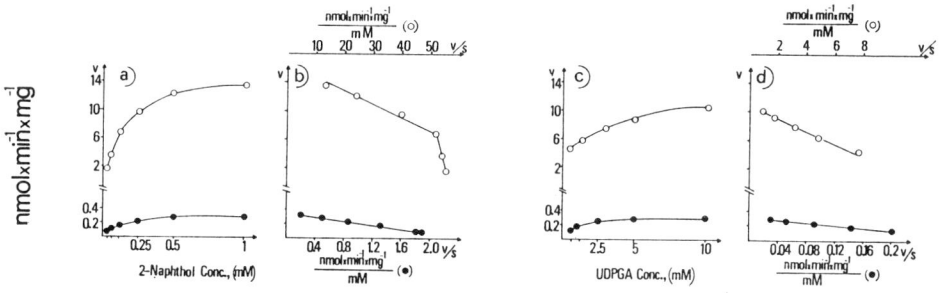

Figure 3. Effect of the concentration of 2-naphthol (a) and UDPGA (c) on the activity of the GT measured in the cytosolic (filled) and microsomal (unfilled circles) fractions. Panels b and d show the transformation into Eadie-Hofstee plot of the activities shown in a and d, respectively. The liver donors were a man 68 years old (a and b) and a man 31 years old (c and d).

The inhibition of 2-naphthol glucuronidation was studied as well. The compounds 2-OH-biphenyl, p-nitrophenol and salicylic acid had inhibitory effect on both the cytosolic and microsomal GT. In contrast, 4,4'-OH-biphenyl, ethinyloestradiol and oxazepam inhibited the cytosolic GT only. The results from a liver specimen are depicted in figure 4. The effect of a single concentration of each inhibitor was studied on 4 livers and the results are shown in figure 5.

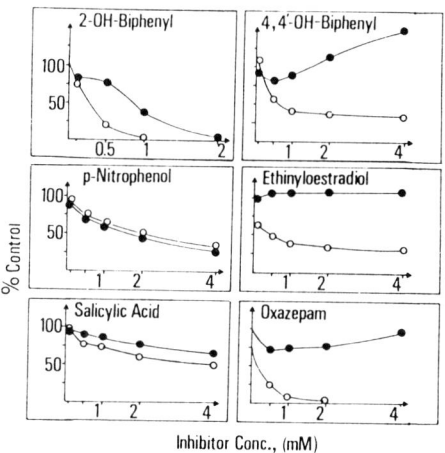

Figure 4. Effect of different concentrations of six compounds on the rate of glucuronidation of 2-naphthol. Unfilled circles (cytosolic fraction) filled circles (microsomal fraction)

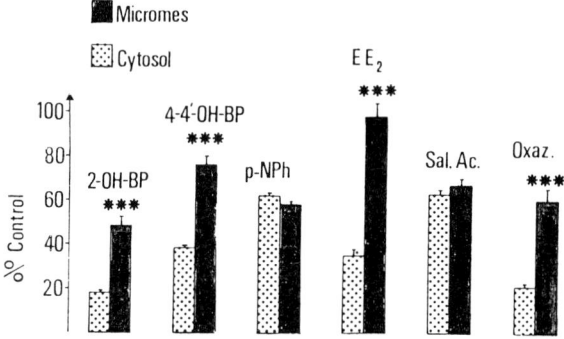

Figure 5. Effect of a single concentration of different compounds on the rate of 2-naphthol glucuronidation in the cytosolic and microsomal fractions of the human liver. Columns refer to the mean from 4 livers. Vertical bars are the SD of the mean. 0.5 mM 2-OH-biphenyl (2-OH-BP); 1 mM 4-4'-OH-biphenyl (4-4'-OH-BP); 1 mM p-nitrophenol (p-NPh); 0.5 mM ethinyloestradiol (EE2), 2 mM salicylic acid (Sal. Ac.); 0.5 mM oxazepam (Oxaz).

The effect of Triton-X100 (0.1%) were investigated as well. Triton X-100 had different effect on the cytosolic and microsomal GT. The activity of the microsomal enzyme was increased up to 140% of the control whereas that of the cytosolic enzyme was lowered to 70% of the control.

DISCUSSION

Homogenization and the procedures required for the isolation of subcellular fractions may solubilize membrane bound enzymes with consequent alteration of the compartmentation of cell enzymes. The activity of the glucuronyl transferase measured in the cytosolic fraction might reflect the presence of a solubilized enzyme of membrane origin. Keeping this in mind, we performed a number of parallel experiments with the microsomal and cytosolic fractions in order to ascertain whether differences may be detected in the glucuronidation of 2-naphthol.

At varying concentrations of 2-naphthol, the enzyme obeys Michaelis-Menten kinetics in the cytosolic fraction whereas non-Michaelian kinetics were observed with the microsomal fraction. Interestingly, the Km of the high affinity phase of the microsomal enzyme was almost identical to that of the soluble enzyme. Non michaelian kinetics observed with the microsomal GT are in agreement with those observed with 1-naphthol (Miners et al. 1988; Pacifici et al. 1984). At varying concentrations of UDPGA, the enzyme present in the soluble and microsomal fractions obeys Michaelis-Menten kinetics, the Km values were slightly, but siglificantly, different.

The inhibition pattern of the GT is different when it is studied in the cytosolic and microsomal fractions. Ethinyloestradiol, oxazepam and 4,4'-hydroxy-biphenyl are powerful inhibitors of the cytosolic GT whereas they do not inhibit the microsomal enzyme. Among these three molecules, oxazepam was the most powerful inhibitor. Interestingly, this compound does not inhibit the glucuronidation of 2-naphthol and 1-naphthol (Pacifici et al. 1984) catalyzed by the human liver microsomal GT.

Finally, the cytosolic fraction catalyzed the glucuronidation of ethinyloestradiol. The cytosolic to microsomal activity ratio does not correlate with that for 2-naphthol. In addition, the ratio average is over 10 times higher for ethinyloestradiol than 2-naphthol.

Several differences were observed in the glucuronidation of 2-naphthol catalyzed by the cytosolic and microsomal fractions. More work has to be done to ascertain whether the presence of the GT in the cytosolic fraction is an artefact or alternatively, an authentic soluble enzyme is present in human liver.

REFERENCES

Antoine, B., Magdalou, J. and Siest, G (1983): Functional heterogeneity of UDP-glucuronyltransferases in different membranes of rat liver. Biochem. Pharmacol. 32 , 2629-2632

Antoine, B., Magdalou, J. and Siest, G. (1984): Kinetic properties of UDP-glucuronosyltransferase(S) in different membranes of rat liver cells. Xenobiotica 14 , 575-579

Bock, K.W., Brunner, G., Hoensch, H., Huber, E. and Josting, D. (1978). Determination of microsomal UDP-glucuronyltransferase in needle-biopsy specimens of human liver. Eur. J. Clin. Pharmacol. 14 , 367-373

Elmamlouk, T.H., Mukhtar, H. and Bend, J.R. (1981): The nuclear envelope as a site of glucuronyltransferase in rat liver, properties and effect of inducers on enzyme activity. J. Pharmacol. Exp. Ther. 219 , 27-34

Miners, J.O., Lillywhite, K.J., Matthews, A.P., Jones, M.E. and Birkett, D.J. (1988): Kinetic and inhibitor studies of 4-methylumbelliferone and 1-naphthol glucuronidation in human liver microsomes. Biochem. Pharmacol. 37 , 665-671

Pacifici, G.M., Colizzi, C., Giuliani, L. and Rane, A. (1984): Nuclear and microsomal glucuronyl transferase in human liver: In Advances in glucuronide conjugation (Matern, S, Bock, K.W., Gerok, W. eds) MTP Press, Lancaster, pp 341-350

Pacifici, G.M., Giuliani, L. and Calcaprina, R. (1986a): Glucuronidation of 1-naphthol in nuclear and microsomal fractions of the human intestine. Pharmacology 33 , 103-107

Pacifici, G.M., Bencini, C. and Rane, A. (1986b): Presystemic glucuronidation of morphine in humans and rhesus monkeys: subcellular distribution of the UDP-glucuronyltransferase in the liver and intestine. Xenobiotica 16 , 123-126

Pacifici, G.M. and Back D.J. (1988) Sulphation and glucuronidation of ethinyloestradiol in human liver in vitro. J. Steroid Biochem. In Press

Wishart, G.J. and Fry, J.(1980a): Uridine diphosphate glucuronyltransferase activity in nuclei and nuclear envelope of rat liver and its apparent induction by phenobarbital. Biochem. Soc. Trans. 5, 705-706

Wishart, G.J. and Fry, D.J. (1980b): Evidence from rat liver nuclear preparations that latency of microsomal UDP-glucuronyltransferase is associated with vesiculation. Biochem. J.: 186, 687-691

Zalesky J. and Gessner, T (1982): Re-investigation of the presence of UDP-glucuronosyltransferase in rat liver mitochondria. Res. Comm. Chem. Pathol. Pharmacol. 73, 279-292

Zalesky, J., Bansal, S.K. and Gessner, T. (1982): Nuclear membrane-bound UDPglucuronosyltransferase of rat liver. Can. J. Biochem. 60, 972-979

Résumé

Nous avons mesuré l'activité glucuronyltransférase (GT) dans les fractions cytosolique et microsomale hépatiques humaines, en présence de 2-napthol comme substrat. Les échantillons de foies sont homogénéisés dans du saccharose 0,25 M et les homogénats sont soumis à des centrifugations différentielles pour isoler les fractions cytosolique et microsomale. La fraction cytosolique est recentrifugée à 105 000 x g pendant 4 heures pour sédimenter d'éventuelles particules membranaires légères. L'activité GT (moyenne $\pm$ SEM) des 25 fragments hépatiques est 8,95 $\pm$ 0,53 nmol/min/mg (microsomes) et 0,17 $\pm$ 0,07 nmol/min/mg (cytosol). La cinétique de la GT est étudiée sur 4 fragments hépatiques en présence de concentrations variables en 2-naphtol et UDPGA. Si le 2-naphtol est le substrat variable, l'enzyme microsomale n'obéit pas à des cinétiques de type Michaelis-Menten. Le Km (moyenne $\pm$ SEM) pour les sites à haute et basse affinités sont 0,134 $\pm$ 0,020 mM et 0,637 $\pm$ 0,251 mM, respectivement. Au contraire, l'enzyme cytosolique suit une cinétique de type Michaelien, le Km est 0,138 $\pm$ 0,007 mM. Les Gt cytosolique et microsomale suivent la cinétique de Michaelis-Menten lorsque l'UDPGA est le substrat variable. Le Km (moyenne $\pm$ SEM) est 0,616 $\pm$ 0,057 mM (cytosol) et 0,806 $\pm$ 0,035 mM (microsomes) ($P < 0,01$). Des expériences d'inhibition montrent que le 4,4'-hydroxy-biphényle, l'éthinyloestradiol et l'oxazépam provoquent des effets inhibiteurs différents sur les GT microsomale et cytosolique, tandis que les 2-hydroxy-biphényle, p-nitrophénol et l'acide salicylique ont des effets similaires sur les deux enzymes. L'activité GT est aussi mesurée avec l'éthinyloestradiol. La moyenne des rapports d'activité enzyme cytosolique/enzyme microsomale est 10 fois supérieure pour la conjugaison de l'éthinyloestradiol que celle du 2-naphtol. Quelques différences ont été observées également entre les GT cytosolique et microsomale. L'origine de l'enzyme cytosolique est inconnue. Nous devons considérer que les enzymes membranaires peuvent être solubilisées pendant l'homogénéisation du foie. Beaucoup de travail reste à faire pour confirmer ou non l'existence d'une GT cytosolique authentique ou, au contraire, déterminer que la glucuronoconjugaison catalysée par la fraction cytosolique reflète la présence d'une enzyme d'origine non cytosolique.

Evidence that bilirubin UDP-Glucuronosyltransferase faces the lumen of the endoplasmic reticulum in rat liver

F. Van Stapel* and N. Blanckaert**

Katholieke Universiteit Leuven
*Biomedical NMR Unit, Campus Gasthuisberg O/N 08, 3000 Leuven, Belgium
**Clinical Pathology, UZ-KUL Medical Centre, 3000 Leuven, Belgium

ACKNOWLEDGEMENTS

This research was supported by grants of the National Institutes of Health, U.S.A. and the National Lottery, Belgium.

ABSTRACT

Knowledge of the topology of the UDP-glycosyltransferases in the endoplasmic reticulum (ER) is of key importance for understanding the regulation of expression of hepatic transferase activities. In this paper we present evidence for the presence within the microsomal lumen of a pool of endogenous intact UDP-glucose (UDPGlc) that has direct access to the active centre of the bilirubin UDP-glycosyltransferase system. This observation implies a lumenal orientation of the UDP-sugar-binding site of the microsomal enzyme. A pool of endogenous UDP-glucuronic acid (UDPGlcUA) could not be demonstrated. A lumenal orientation of bilirubin UDP-glucuronyltransferase is indirectly postulated on the basis of the evidence that a single enzyme may be responsible for microsomal glucosidation and glucuronidation of bilirubin and on the basis of the observation that the glucuronyltransferase is inactivated by membrane-impermeant proteases in disrupted microsomes, but not in native microsomal vesicles with an intact membrane permeability barrier.

KEYWORDS

Bilirubin, UDP-glycosyltransferase, Mannose-6-phosphatase, Microsomes, Topology, Latency, Proteases

INTRODUCTION

The hepatic glycosidation of numerous xenobiotics and endogenous compounds (e.g. bilirubin) is mediated by a family of microsomal UDP-glycosyltransferase isoenzymes. A number of these isoenzymes have been purified and the primary cDNA sequences of several glucuronyltransferases have been deciphered (Mackenzie, 1986 a&b; Jackson & Burchell, 1986; Iyanagi et al., 1986; Jackson et al., 1987).

Microsomal UDP-glucuronyltransferase activity is only fully expressed after disruption of the native membrane vesicles. Some investigators (Hallinan & de Brito, 1981) have suggested that the latency of microsomal transferase activity reflects compartmentation of the enzyme within the lumen of the vesicle, whereby the intact ER membrane constitutes a permeability barrier between substrates (especially the negatively charged UDP-sugars) and the catalytic site. Therefore a transport mechanism for UDP-sugars has been postulated. The latency of the transferases would reflect rate-limiting translocation of the co-substrates well below the potential glycosidation rate of the lumenal transferases. Disruption of the membrane would eliminate the need to translocate the substrates across the membrane and thereby the postulated rate-limiting substrate translocation step. Others (Vessey & Zakim, 1978) have suggested that there is no need for invoking a compartmental model. They explain the submaximal activity in native microsomes by conformational constraints imposed by the specific unperturbed lipid environment. Perturbation of the membrane would induce more active enzyme conformers.

The compartmental hypothesis is supported by the following experimental evidence: The cDNA sequences, identified sofar for a number of UDP-glucuronyltransferase isoforms, suggest that these enzymes are integral membrane proteins, anchored in the membrane by a hydrophobic transmembrane segment located close to the C-terminus while most of the protein including the N-terminus may protrude within the lumen of the ER. It remains to be established, however, that the catalytic domain has a lumenal orientation in intact microsomal vesicles. Such topology would be consistent with the following experimental results. (1) The cysternal orientation of the glucuronyltransferase is consistent with the fact that inactivation of transferase activities by membrane-impermeant reagents requires disruption of the membrane barrier (Hallinan & de Brito, 1981). (2) The existence of a lumenal compartment in which UDPGlcUA can accumulate may explain why efficient transfer of GlcUA from p-nitrophenolglucuronide to o-aminophenol in the presence of UDP is observed only in intact microsomes (Berry & Hallinan, 1974). This phenomenon would involve coupling of glucuronyltransferase-catalyzed formation of UDPGlcUA from p-nitrophenolglucuronide and UDP with transfer of GlcUA to o-aminophenol by a forward reaction. The "coupled reaction" is efficient only in native microsomes, possibly because UDPGlcUA formed by the reverse reaction needs to accumulate within the microsomal lumen in order to drive the coupled forward glucuronyltransferase-catalyzed reaction.

We demonstrated directly the existence of such an intramicrosomal UDP-sugar pool, which is accessible to the bilirubin conjugating transferase isoform. This enzyme is responsible for UDP-sugar dependent bilirubin glycosidation with either glucuronic acid (GlcUA), glucose (Glc) or xylose (Xyl). Our results support the hypothesis that the UDP-sugar binding site of microsomal bilirubin UDP-glycosyltransferase is lumenally oriented.

METHODS

The preparation of microsomes has been described in detail elsewhere (Vanstapel, Pua & Blanckaert, 1986). The integrity of the microsomal membrane permeability barrier was assessed by measurement of the latency of mannose 6-phosphatase (Arion et al., 1976; Vanstapel, Pua & Blanckaert, 1986). Throughout this paper "intact microsomes" refers to microsomes with higher than 95% latency of the mannose-6-phosphatase. Enzymatic activities expressed by intact microsomes are referred to as "basal activities". The fully revealed activity in optimally detergent disrupted vesicles is called "total activity".

Permeabilisation of the microsomal membrane barrier was achieved by one of several procedures. The sonication procedure has been described elsewhere (Vanstapel & Blanckaert, 1987). Detergent treatment involved the pre-incubation of microsomes (2 mg protein/ml) with the indicated concentrations (0-4 mM) of the detergent Chapso for 60 min at 0 °C (Vanstapel & Blanckaert, 1988a). Treatment with Staphylococcal α-toxin involved exposure of microsomes (2mg protein/ml) to 50-500 µg toxin/mg protein at pH 7.0 for 10 min at 37 °C (Vanstapel & Blanckaert, 1988a). Treatment with protease consisted of incubating the microsomes (10-14 mg protein/ml) at 20 °C with subtilisin (Nagarse^R; 200 µg/mg protein). The reaction was interrupted by 5-fold dilution of the mixture with incubation buffer containing 250 µM phenylmethylsulfonyl fluoride.

Microsomal bilirubin glucuronidation (Vermeir, Vanstapel & Blanckaert, 1984) was assayed with the ethyl anthranilate method, using 100 µM bilirubin substrate (with 50 µM albumin) and 5 mM UDPGlcUA. For measurement of endogenous esterification of bilirubin, in the absence of added UDP-sugar donor-substrate, we used a sensitive radioassay with 1 µM bilirubin substrate. The method is based on the separation of unreacted pigment substrate and the bilirubin mono- and di-esters by t.l.c., after conversion of the glycosidic reaction products to mono- and dimethyl esters. Identification of the conjugating sugar moieties was performed by analysis of the azopyrromethene derivatives prepared by diazo-cleavage of parent tetrapyrrolic bilirubin glycosides, using the ethyl anthranilate diazoreagent (Blanckaert & Heirwegh, 1986).

RESULTS

1. Endogenous esterification of bilirubin by liver microsomes

1.a. Endogenous esterification: the phenomenon

When native rat liver microsomes were incubated with [^{14}C]bilirubin without added UDP-sugar, bilirubin esters were formed despite the absence of added UDP-sugar (Fig. 1.A). Because esterification appeared to depend upon an endogenous source of sugar-donor substrate the reaction was called "endogenous" esterification. The nature of the conjugating sugar in these endogenously formed bilirubin esters was investigated after conversion of the [^{14}C]-bilirubins in the incubation medium to o-ethyl anthranilate azoderivatives. Radioactivity co-chromatographed with azopyrromethene monoglucoside; also after additional acetylation of the pigment and the reference compound (Blanckaert & Heirwegh, 1986). These findings demonstrated that the endogenously formed bilirubin mono-esters were predominantly glucosides.

1.b. Endogenous esterification is catalyzed by UDP-glycosyltransferase and therefore depends upon intact UDP-sugar

The endogenous glucosidation reaction appeared to be catalyzed exclusively by bilirubin UDP-glycosyltransferase. The endogenous esterification reaction was undetectable in microsomes from liver of homozygous Gunn rats (Fig. 1.A), which are characterized by a complete lack of bilirubin UDP-glycosyltransferase activity with UDPGlcUA, UDPGlc and UDPXyl (Carbone & Grodsky, 1957; Schmid et al., 1958; Fevery, Leroy & Heirwegh, 1972).

The interpretation that endogenous glucosidation is catalyzed by bilirubin UDP-glycosyltransferase implies that intact UDPGlc was present in the microsomal vesicles.

Fig. 1. Endogenous esterification of bilirubin by rat liver microsomes

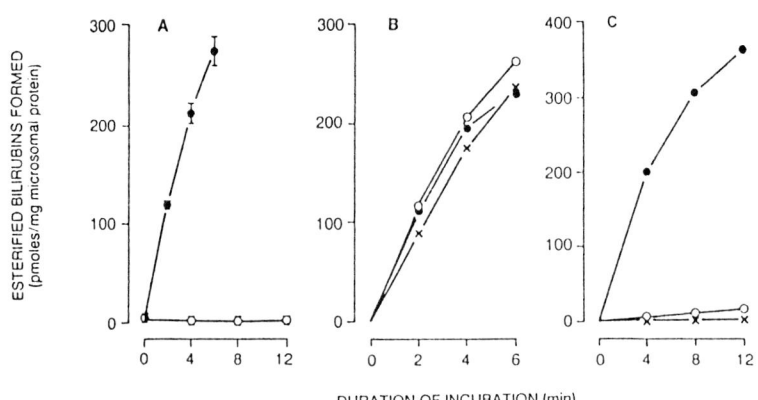

DURATION OF INCUBATION (min)

We show esterification of bilirubin by microsomes in the absence of added UDP-sugar in the incubation mixture. The microsomal protein concentration was 1 mg/ml. The enzymic assays were started by the addition of 1:1 µM bilirubin:albumin. Panel A shows the time dependent formation of bilirubin esters by native microsomes from normal rats (●; mean values ± 1 S.D.; n=9) or homozygous mutant Gunn rats (o; n=5). Panel B depicts endogenous esterification by normal rat liver microsomes that had been washed once (o), twice (●), or three times (x). Panel C depicts bilirubin esterification by normal microsomes (●), and microsomes disrupted by Chapso treatment (o), or sonication (x).

1.c. Endogenous esterification depends on a pool of UDP-sugar present within the lumen of the microsomal vesicles

In our standard preparation, microsomes (Vanstapel, Fua, Blanckaert, 1986) are isolated from a 4-fold diluted total liver homogenate, followed by a wash cycle comprising resuspension of the microsomes in ice-cold fresh homogenisation buffer and repelleting of the vesicles. Subjecting the microsomes to additional wash cycles did not lead to a substantial decrease of the endogenous esterification rate (Fig. 1.B), suggesting that extramicrosomal UDP-sugar was a negligible source of the reaction's cosubstrate.

The inefficacy of additional washings to abolish the endogenous esterification suggested that UDP-sugars trapped inside the microsomal vesicles served as the direct glycosyl donor-substrate, and therefore that the UDP-sugar binding site of the transferase faced the lumen of the microsomes. This hypothesis was consistent with the observation that the endogenous esterification reaction was almost completely abolished, when the vesicles were disrupted by either detergent treatment or sonication (Fig. 1.C). The loss of endogenous esterification activity coincided with the loss of the capability of the membrane to exclude small hydrophilic molecules such as mannose 6-phosphate (as assessed by assaying the latency of mannose-6-phosphatase).

A comprehensive explanation for the effect of elimination of the membrane permeability barrier on endogenous esterification of bilirubin is that opening the microsomal vesicle causes dissipation of an intravesicular pool of UDPGlc into the total incubation medium and thereby dramatically reduces the effective concentration of sugar donor-substrate available to bilirubin UDP-glycosyltransferase.

1.d. Uptake of UDPGlc and UDPXyl by intact microsomes

Orientation of the UDP-glycosyltransferase system toward the microsomal lumen also implies the necessity to translocate UDP-sugar from the cytoplasmic to the lumenal side of the endoplasmic reticulum.

We tested whether preincubation of the microsomes with the known UDP-sugar cosubstrates of the bilirubin-conjugating transferase, would result in expansion of the microsomal UDP-sugar pool and hence in increased rates of endogenous esterification of bilirubin. Preincubation of intact microsomes with 5 mM UDPGlc or 5 mM UDPXyl added to the incubation medium resulted in significant enhancement of the rate of esterification by the pre-loaded microsomes (Fig. 2). Analysis of the bilirubin esters after conversion to the ethyl anthranilate azoderivatives, revealed that after loading the vesicles with UDPXyl predominantly xylosides were formed (Xyl/Glc ratio: 5.7). Preloading of intact microsomes from homozygous Gunn rat liver did not result in any detectable esterification.

Fig. 2. Effect of pre-loading microsomes with UDP-sugar on endogenous esterification of bilirubin

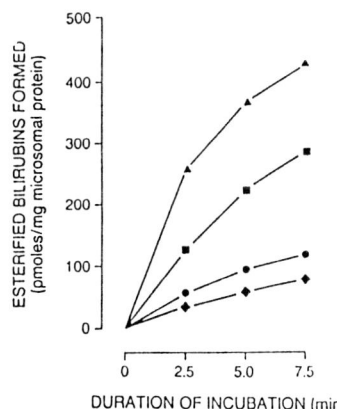

Intact rat liver microsomes (10 mg protein/ml) were incubated for 10 min at 37 °C in the regular bilirubin UDP-glycosyltransferase assay buffer (Vermeir, Vanstapel & Blanckaert, 1984) without added UDP-sugar (●) or with 5 mM UDP-GlcUA (◆), UDPGlc (■), or UDPXyl (▲). Then, the microsomes were pelleted by centrifugation at 4 °C to separate them from the external medium, and washed a second time. The endogenous esterification reaction in the washed microsomes was assayed as described under Fig. 1.

Bilirubin conjugation was markedly reduced (to <5% of the activity in intact vesicles) when the pre-loaded microsomes were disrupted with Chapso prior to assessing endogenous esterification. While disruption stimulates bilirubin UDP-glycosyltransferase activity toward exogenously provided cosubstrate, loss of endogenous activity by disruption therefore served as a control on the completeness of removal of external cosubstrate, that might have been carried through the wash and reisolation cycle, to which the pre-treated microsomes were subjected before endogenous esterification was assayed. Thus, the enhancement of endogenous esterification by the pretreatment corresponded to expansion of the intramicrosomal UDP-sugar pool.

We were unable to demonstrate endogenous glucuronidation. There is no obvious reason why the microsomes would spontaneously and selectively have lost UDPGlcUA. Pre-incubation of the microsomes with 5 mM UDPGlcUA, failed to lead to an enhancement of the endogenous esterification rate. In fact, we consistently observed a slight decrease in endogenous esterification rates in microsomes that had been pre-incubated with exogenous UDPGlcUA. Moreover, after pre-incubation with UDPGlcUA the vesicles still produced predominantly bilirubin glucosides (GlcUA/Glc ratio: 0.03), as found in control microsomes (GlcUA/Glc ratio: 0.07) incubated in the absence of added UDP-sugar.

1.e. Temperature-dependent uptake of UDPGlc and UDPXyl by intact microsomes

Preloading the microsomes with 5 mM UDPXyl at 37 °C resulted in a shift from predominant glucosidation (Xyl/Glc ratio: 0.02) to xylosidation (Xyl/Glc ratio: 5.7). The incorporation of Xyl into bilirubin esters proves that intact UDPXyl is taken up by the vesicles. Xylosidation became the dominant event after pre-incubation at 37 °C, while, when pre-loading with UDPXyl was attempted at 0 °C, glucosidation remained the major event (Xyl/Glc ratio: 0.44).

The temperature sensitivity of the pre-loading process suggests that uptake of the nucleotide is carrier-mediated.

2. Probing the topology of microsomal bilirubin UDP-glucuronyltransferase

2.a. Latency of microsomal glucuronyltransferase activity depends on the structural integrity of the vesicles

Collectively, the above findings indicate that the glycosyl- and xylosyltransferase activities depended on a lumenal enzyme domain. However we failed to demonstrate that intact UDPGlcUA is present within the lumen of intact microsomal vesicles, or that this substrate interacts with the transferase at the lumenal side of the microsomal membrane.

To examine whether this compartmentation extended to the UDPGlcUA-binding site, we examined whether the latency of microsomal glucuronyltransferase activity depended on the structural intactness of the microsomal vesicles, as would be predicted by the compartmental model. We determined the effects of variable degrees of disruption of the membrane permeability barrier on transferase activity. Impairment of the membrane barrier was independently assessed from the effects on the latency of lumenal mannose-6-phosphatase, which is widely accepted as a reliable quantitative index of integrity of the microsomal vesicles (Arion et al., 1976).

We produced a full spectrum of degrees of disruption of the microsomal membrane by 3 entirely different approaches (see methods). (1)

Pre-treatment with increasing concentrations of the detergent Chapso. (2) Sonication for variable lengths of time. (3) Permeabilization by pore-forming staphylococcal α-toxin. The degree of loss of latency was assessed by comparing enzymic activities (transferase and phosphatase) in treated vesicles, with the activity in vesicles subjected to additional optimal enzyme activation by subsequent Chapso treatment.

For each of these treatments, conditions resulting in complete release of phosphatase latency coincided with optimal transferase activation. The changes in latency of bilirubin UDP-glucuronyltransferase correlated closely to the response of mannose-6-phosphatase to gradual disruption of the microsomal membrane (r^2 = 0.965, 0.980, 0.960 respectively for Chapso, sonication, and α-toxin treatment). This parallellism, which persisted for each of these qualitatively different membrane-disruptive procedures, appeared to reflect a common mechanism responsible for constraint of catalytic activity in native microsomes. The observed structure-dependent latency for the phosphatase and the transferase may reflect rate-limiting permeation of the hydrophilic mannose 6-phosphate and UDPGlcUA substrates across the intact microsomal membrane.

2.b. An intact membrane protects the transferase against inactivation by proteases

The topology of some glucuronyltransferases (mainly the p-nitrophenol conjugating isoform) has been investigated by comparing the efficacy of membrane-impermeant proteases to inactivate the transferase in intact or disrupted microsomes (Hallinan & de Brito, 1981). We applied this approach to the bilirubin-conjugating isoform.

Only 10% of total transferase activity was lost in intact microsomes treated with subtilisin for 30 min. By contrast, when microsomes, in which the permeability barrier had been eliminated by detergent pretreatment, were exposed to subtilisin the total transferase activity gradually fell. After 30 min the remaining activity was less than 30% of the values in intact microsomes treated with the protease.

These findings indicate that bilirubin UDP-glucuronyltransferase is susceptible to inactivation by subtilisin, but that the intact microsomal membrane restricts access of the protease to the catalytic enzyme.

DISCUSSION

The so-called "endogenous" esterification of bilirubin seems to depend on an intramicrosomal UDP-sugar pool, which after disruption of the native vesicles is dissipated in the incubation medium and thereby diluted and rendered ineffective. This interpretation implies that the catalytic center of the enzyme is oriented towards the lumen of the vesicles. Our conclusion is also supported by the demonstration of accumulation within the microsomal lumen of intact UDPGlc and UDPXyl cosubstrate.

Thus, our results leave little doubt about the lumenal orientation of the UDPGlc- and UDPXyl-binding site of microsomal bilirubin UDP-glycosyltransferase. Conclusions about the UDPGlcUA-binding site need to remain less firm, as we failed to demonstrate the presence of intact UDPGlcUA in native microsomes as well as in microsomes pre-incubated with exogenoulsy added nucleotide. However, in view of the evidence that a single enzyme (Burchell & Blanckaert, 1984) and maybe even a common UDP-sugar-binding site (Chowdhury et al., 1986) is involved in the esterification of bilirubin with GlcUA as well as with Glc or Xyl, it is likely that also the UDPGlcUA binding-site is lumenally oriented. At least such a common lumenal orientation would suffice to explain the observed protection by the intact membrane against protease-mediated inactivation of bilirubin UDP-glucuronyl-transferase.

A lumenal orientation of the transferase necessitates, a mechanism that allows microsomal uptake of UDP-sugar cosubstrate. Using a rapid ultra-filtration method, we recently investigated the kinetics of microsomal uptake of radiolabeled UDPGlc and UDPGlcUA (Vanstapel & Blanckaert, 1988b). Our findings confirmed carrier-mediated uptake of intact UDPGlc inside the microsomal lumen. Microsomes accumulate to a similar extent UDPGlcUA-derived label, but this is not present as the intact nucleotide. Failure to demonstrate microsomal accumulation of intact UDPGlcUA does not exclude the possibilty that intact UDPGlcUA can be translocated across the microsomal membrane. Carrier mediated UDPGlc uptake was inhibited by UDPGlcUA, indicating affinity of the carrier for that nucleotide. Moreover, UDPGlcUA trans-stimulated the efflux of labeled UDPGlc from the microsomes. These observations suggest that UDPGlcUA may be transported across the ER membrane by a carrier-mechanism shared with UDPGlc.

Future kinetic studies of this nature may reveal whether the rate of UDP-sugar uptake indeed is well below the potential glycosidation rate of the microsomal transferase in disrupted vesicles, and thus whether the proposed lumenal topology of the bilirubin UDP-glycosyl-transferase may suffice to explain such properties as the latency of the transferase activities in intact microsomes. Consistent with this hypothesis, the latency of the bilirubin UDP-glucuronyltransferase activity appeared to be structure-dependent. The degree of activation of the transferase by any of the three reported treatments (detergent, sonication, pore-forming toxin) was a direct function of the pre-existing degree of structural intactness of the membrane. Therefore, information on the membrane integrity appears to be essential for the interpretation of effects of any treatment on the kinetic properties of the microsomal glucuronyltransferase system.

REFERENCES

Arion, W.J. et al. (1975): Microsomal membrane permeability and the hepatic glucose-6-phosphatase system. Interactions of the system with D-mannose 6-phosphate and D-mannose. J. Biol. Chem. 251, 4901-4907

Berry, C., Hallinan, T. (1974): 'Coupled transglucuronidation': A new tool for studying the latency of UDP-glucuronyltransferase. FEBS Lett. 42, 73-76

Blanckaert, N., Heirwegh, K.P.M. (1986): pp.31-79: Analysis and preparation of bilirubins. In Bile pigments and Jaundice. Molecular, Metabolic and Medical Aspects. (Ostrow, J.D., Ed.) Marcel Dekker Inc.

Burchell, B., Blanckaert, N. (1984): Bilirubin mono- and diglucuronide formation by purified rat liver microsomal bilirubin UDP-glucuronyltransferase. Biochem. J. 223, 461-465

Carbone, J.V., Grodsky, G.M. (1957): Constitutional nonhemolytic hyperbilirubinemia in the rat: defect of bilirubin esterification. *Proc. Soc. Exptl. Biol. Med. 94*, 461-463

Chowdhury, N.R. et al. (1986): Substrates and products of purified rat liver bilirubin UDP-glucuronosyltransferase. *Hepatology 6*, 123-128

Fevery, J., Leroy, P., Heirwegh, K.P.M. (1972): Enzymic transfer of glucose and xylose from uridine diphosphate glucose and uridine diphosphate xylose to bilirubin by untreated and digitonin-activated preparations from rat liver. *Biochem. J. 129*, 619-633.

Hallinan, T., de Brito, A.E.R. (1981): Topology of endoplasmic reticular enzyme systems and its possible regulatory significance. *Horm. Cell. Regul. 5*, 73-95.

Iyanagi, T. et al. (1986): Cloning and characterization of cDNA encoding 3-methylcholantrene inducible rat mRNA for UDP-glucuronosyltransferase. *J. Biol. Chem. 261*, 15607-15614.

Jackson, R., Burchell, B. (1986): The full length coding sequence of rat liver UDP-glucuronyltransferase cDNA and comparison with other members of this gene family. *Nucleic Acid Res. 14*, 779-795.

Jackson, M.R. et al. (1987): Cloning of a human liver microsomal UDP-glucuronosyltransferase cDNA. *Biochem. J. 242*, 581-588.

Mackenzie, P.I. (1986a): Rat liver UDP-glucuronosyltransferase. Sequence and expression of a form of a cDNA encoding a phenobarbital-inducible form. *J. Biol. Chem. 261*, 6119-6125.

Mackenzie, P.I. (1986b): Rat liver UDP-glucuronosyltransferase. cDNA sequence and expression of a form glucuronidating 3-hydroxyandrogens. *J. Biol. Chem. 261*, 14112-14117.

Schmid, R. et al. (1958): Congenital jaundice in rats, due to a defect in glucuronide formation. *J. Clin. Invest. 37*, 1123-1130.

Vanstapel, F., Pua, K., Blanckaert, N. (1986): Assay of mannose 6-phosphatase in untreated and detergent-disrupted rat liver microsomes for assessment of integrity of microsomal preparations. *Eur. J. Biochem. 156*, 73-77.

Vanstapel, F., Blanckaert, N. (1987): Endogenous esterification of bilirubin by liver microsomes. Evidence for an intramicrosomal pool of UDP-glucose and lumenal orientation of bilirubin UDP-glycosyltransferase. *J. Biol. Chem. 262*, 4616-4623.

Vanstapel, F., Blanckaert, N. (1988a): Topology and regulation of bilirubin UDP-glucuronyltransferase in sealed native microsomes from rat liver. *Archiv. Biochem. Biophys.* in press.

Vanstapel, F., Blanckaert, N. (1988b): Carrier-mediated translocation of uridine diphosphate glucose into the lumen of rough endoplasmic reticulum-derived vesicles from rat liver. *J. Clin. Invest.* in press.

Vermeir, M., Vanstapel, F., Blanckaert, N. (1984): Radioassay of UDP-glucuronyltransferase catalysed formation of bilirubin monoglucuronides and bilirubin diglucuronide in liver microsomes. *Biochem. J. 223*, 455-459.

Vessey, D.A., Zakim, D. (1978): pp. 247-255: Are Glucuronidation reactions compartmented? In: *Conjugation reactions in drug biotransformations* (Aitio, A., Ed.) Elsevier/North-Holland Biomedical Press.

Résumé

La connaissance de la topologie des UDP-glucuronosyltransférases dans les membranes du réticulum endoplasmique est d'une importance capitale pour la compréhension de la régulation de leur expression. Dans cet article, nous présentons des arguments en faveur de la présence dans la membrane luminale d'un pool endogène d'UDP-glucose qui a un accès direct au site actif de la bilirubine UDP-glycosyltransférase. Cette observation implique une orientation luminale du site de fixation de l'UDP-sucre de l'enzyme microsomale. Un pool d'acide UDP-glucuronique n'a pas pu être mis en évidence.
L'orientation luminale de la bilirubine UDP-glucuronosyltransférase est postulée indirectement sur la base évidente qu'une seule enzyme doit être responsable de la glucosidation et glucuronoconjugaison de la bilirubine, et sur le fait que la glucuronyltransférase est inactivée par des perméases ne passant pas la membrane, dans des microsomes dissociés, mais pas dans des vésicules intactes possédant une barrière de perméabilité membranaire intacte.

Glucuronidation in human hepatoma cell lines and liver microsomes

Sylviane Dragacci, Jacques Magdalou, Denyse Bagrel, Marina Roques, Sylvie Fournel-Gigleux and Gérard Siest

Centre du Médicament, U.A. CNRS n° 597, 30 rue Lionnois, 54000 Nancy, France

ABSTRACT

Glucuronidation of various drugs and endogenous compounds was investigated in human samples, using hepatoma cell lines and fresh liver biopsies as biological models. The activity of different UDP-glucuronosyltransferases measured with 1-naphthol, bilirubin, testosterone and androsterone as substrates was determined in human hepatoma cell lines Hep G2, Hep 3B, SK-HEP-1 and Mz-Hep-1. For comparison purpose, glucuronidation reactions were also determined in rat hepatoma cell lines Fao and H5-6. The human cells were characterized by a low level in glucuronidation of 1-naphthol. The highest activity was obtained with Mz-Hep-1 (2.40 $\pm$ 0.94 nmol/min/mg); the formation of 1-naphthol glucuronide, which proceeded at a rate of 0.015 nmol/min/mg in Hep G2 cells was absent in SK-HEP-1 cells. Bilirubin UDP-glucuronosyltransferase could not be detected in all the human hepatoma cell lines tested. By contrast, the rat cells conjugated, although at different extents, 1-napthtol, bilirubin and testosterone quite efficiently. Only androsterone glucuronidation was not observed.
In human liver biopsies, the activity of UDP-glucuronosyltransferase toward 4-nitrophenol, nopol (a monoterpenoid alcohol), bilirubin or clofibric acid was easily detected but presented a wide range of variations in the population studied. This was the consequence of drug intake or alcohol and cigarette consumption. Smoking increased glucuronidation of 4-nitrophenol and bilirubin by 30 and 18%, respectively, whereas alcohol stimulated bilirubin UDP-glucuronosyltransferase. This enzyme form was significantly enhanced in patients treated with the hypolipidaemic drugs clofibrate and fenofibrate. The imidazole-containing structures cimetidine and albendazole presented opposite effects. Cimetidine decreased bilirubin glucuronidation by 44%, whereas albendazole increased all the activities tested, especially 1-naphthol glucuronidation.

KEYWORDS

Human and rat hepatoma cells - human liver biopsies - isoenzymes - drug intake

INTRODUCTION

In man, glucuronidation reactions play a major role in the elimination of drugs, bilirubin or steroid hormones (1). Because of the difficulty in the availability of human samples such as biopsies or post-mortem fragments, determination of UDP-glucuronosyltransferases properties has been limited to few studies untill now (Bock et al., 1984. Dragacci et al., 1987).
Species differences with respect to absorption, distribution or metabolism cannot allow extrapolation of drug properties and action from animal to man. Therefore, in order to investigate drug biotransformation in man, alternate biological models such as human cell cultures can be used for this approach.
Indeed hepatoma cell lines are good candidate to follow and characterize UDP-glucuronosyltransferases. They are generally easy to handle, and the expression of the enzyme activity, the substrate specificity or the response to inducers can be reproduced to mimic the situation *in vivo*. Some of human established cell lines have been found to retain many of the liver specific functions including secretion of lipoproteins, bile acids, plasma proteins ... This is particularly the case of hepatoma cell line Hep G2 .
This work was carried out to determine the activity of UDP-glucuronosyltransferase (1-naphthol) in the human hepatoma cell lines. The results were compared with those found using rat liver hepatoma cells and hepatic microsomes prepared from human biopsies.

MATERIALS AND METHODS

Cell culture and treatments. Hepatoma cells (Hep G2, Hep 3B, SK-HEP-1, Mz-Hep-1, from man, Fao and H5-6 from rat) were grown at 37°C in a humidified atmosphere of 5% CO_2 in air. The cells were maintained in Dulbecco's minimun essential medium (Gibco, Cergy-Pontoise, France) supplemented with 10% v/v Nu-serum (Collaborative Research, Bedford, MA), except for Mz-Hep-1, whose medium was supplemented with 10% v/v fetal calf serum (Flow, Puteaux, France). Penicillin (100 IU/ml), streptomycin (100 g/ml) and fungizone (0.25 g/ml, Gibco) were added to the different media. Cells (1.0 to $1.5.10^6$) were seeded in 100 mm- plastic dishes. The medium was changed each 48 hr.
 The cells were harvested and washed twice with phosphate-buffered saline, pH 7.4 (Eurobio, Paris, France), scraped and suspended again in the buffer. After centrifugation (300 x g for 10 min), cells were stored at -80°C. Cell viability and growth were monitored during all the time course of the experiment.
Human liver biopsies. Liver biopsies were collected from 65 patients undergoing laparotomy for cholecystectomy (Service de Chirurgie Digestive, Pr. P.Boissel, CHU Nancy, France). Age, sex, preoperative and anesthetic drugs were documented. The biosies were immediately stored in liquid nitrogen. Microsomes were prepared by differential ultracentrifugations, as previously described (Dragacci et al., 1987a). The conditions used allowed maximal conservation of human liver UDP-glucuronosyltransferases.
Glucuronidation assays. The activity in liver biosies was determined on fully activated microsomes with Triton X-100 (Sigma, St. Louis, MO) by the method of Colin-Neijer et al. (1984), with 4-nitrophenol, 1-naphthol (Merck, Darmstadt, FRG) and a monoterpenoid alcohol nopol (Fluka, Buchs, Switzerland) as substrates. Glucuronidation of bilirubin was monitored on microsomes activated with digitonin (Merck, Darmstadt, FRG), using the method of Heirwegh et al (1972). Clofibric acid (Ega-Chemie, Steinheim, FRG) glucuronidation was measured according to Hamar-Hansen et al. (1986) with ($U-^{14}C$) UDP-glucuronic acid (Amersham, Les Ulis, France).
Glucuronidation of 1-naphthol in cell lines was followed on crude homogenate without any activation by detergent. We previously determined

that addition of detergent completely inhibited the transferase reaction. The technique of Bock et al. (1974) with (1-^{14}C)naphthol (Amersham, Les Ulis, France) and that of Rao et al. (1976) for tritiated testosterone and androsterone were used. Bilirubin glucuronidation was measured by the method mentioned above.

RESULTS AND DISCUSSION

UDP-glucuronosyltransferase in human hepatoma cell lines. The enzyme activity toward various substrates in different types of human hepatoma cells, in comparison with that measured in rat hepatoma cells, is presented in Table 1. The results show that, among the two rat cell lines tested which derived both from line H4 II EC3 of Pitot et al. (1964) adapted to growth *in vitro* from the Reuber H 35 hepatoma (1961), Fao was the most active in glucuronidation of substrates. This cell line could be a suitable model to follow drug metabolism, since it also expresses different monooxygenase systems (Wiebel et al., 1984). By contrast, glucuronidation was generally low in human cell lines (Table 1). Only conjugation of 1-naphthol could be detected under our assay conditions in Mz-Hep-1 and Hep G2 cells, but not in SK-HEP-1 and Hep 3B cells. Mz-Hep-1 cells presented the highest activity for 1-naphthol glucuronidation. The specific activity in Hep G2 was 200 times lower. As refered to Hep G2, our results were in good accordance with those of Bock and Bock-Hennig (1987)). However they differed greatly from those of Grant et al., (this book). These discrepancies could be due to differences in growth medium composition, which interfers greatly in the expression of enzyme activities (Grant, personal communication). Glucuronidation of 1-naphthol in Mz-Hep-1 cell, which is a recently established cell line (Dippold et al., 1985), was quite similar to that measured in H5-6 cells (Table 1). Bilirubin glucuronidation could not be detected in all the human cell lines tested. It will be interesting to determine if UDP-glucuronosyltransferase could be induced in these cells after treatment with phenobarbital, 3-methylcholanthrene or clofibrate, which are known to enhance selectively different isozymes.

On the other hand, human hepatoma cell lines were found to display different ranges of monooxygenase activities (Siest et al., 1988). For example, Hep G2 and Hep G3 were able to metabolize benzo(a)pyrene more efficiently than aldrin; but SK-HEP-1 did not present such activity (Limbosch, 1983). It was interesting to notice that cells, which express essentially cytochrome P-448 type- monooxygenase activity contain mainly the transferase form involved in glucuronidation of planar substrates, such as 1-naphthol, inducible by polycyclic hydrocarbons.

Table 1: UDP-glucuronosyltransferase activity in hepatoma cell lines.

Substrates	Rat		Man			
	Fa O	H 5-6	Hep G2	SK-HEP-1	Hep3B	Mz-Hep-1
1-Naphthol	6.88 ± 0.24	4.23 ± 0.52	0.015 ± 0.002	ND	ND	2.40 ± 0.94
Bilirubin	0.120 ± 0.012	0.060 ± 0.001	ND	-	ND	ND
Testosterone	0.166 ± 0.110	0.012 ± 0.005	ND	-	-	-
Androsterone	ND	ND	ND	-	-	-

The enzyme activity was expressed in nmol/min/mg protein. ND: not detectable ; -: not determined

UDP-glucuronosyltransferase in human liver samples. Table 2 indicates the activity of UDP-glucuronosyltransferase measured with 4-nitrophenol, nopol, bilirubin and clofibric acid as substrates in a human population consisting in 34 to 65 liver biopsies. The age of the patients (both sexes) ranged from 19 to 85 years old. Compared to other mammals, specific activity for glucuronidation of 4-nitrophenol or nopol in man was similar to that found in Sprague-Dawley rat, but was two to five times lower than that of Wistar rat, monkey or pig (Boutin et al., 1981, 1984). By contrast, the rates of glucuronidation of bilirubin and clofibric acid were similar, when compared to rat (Hamar-Hansen et al., 1986, Fournel et al., 1987). However the data showed considerable inter-individual variations, as revealed by the values of the standard coefficients. No correlation could be established between the enzyme activity or the age and sex of the patients (Dragacci et al., 1987a). On the other hand, these different activities were not related each other, which suggested that different isozymes independently regulated were present in human microsomes. Finally no correlation could be drawn between conjugation of bilirubin and that of clofibric acid (Fig.1), thus indicating, that, like in rat (Dragacci et al., 1987b), the two aglycones were glucuronidated by separate forms.

Table 2: UDP-glucuronosyltransferase activity in human liver microsomes

Substrates	Specific activity	Number of biopsies
4-Nitrophenol	19.0 ± 13.1	65
Nopol	6.6 ± 5.4	60
Bilirubin	0.5 ± 0.4	63
Clofibric acid	1.2 ± 0.6	34

Values are the mean (nmol/min/mg microsomal protein) ± SD for the indicated number of biopsies.

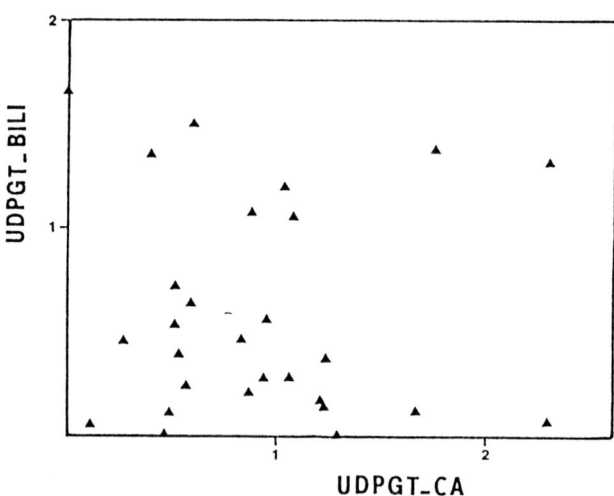

Fig 1: Absence of correlation between glucuronidation of clofibric acid (UDPGT CA) and bilirubin (UDPGT Bili) in human liver microsomes.

In order to determine the variation factors, which influence the activity of UDP-glucuronosyltransferases, different groups of patients were constituted in function of habits (alcohol, tobacco consumptions) or drug intake (Table 3). Smoking more than 10 cigarettes a day slightly increased glucuronidation of 4-nitrophenol and bilirubin by 30 and 18%, respectively. This result indicates that benzo(a)pyrene or related compounds present in cigarette smoke could also induce the enzyme in man. Alcohol drinking enhanced glucuronidation of bilirubin, only (Table 3). However more data should be collected on many other human samples in order to definitively prove the action of alcohol or smoke on UDP-glucuronosyltransferases.

Diazepam (Valium^R), preoperatory administered, increased by 30% conjugation of 4-nitrophenol. Induction was more striking when drugs were given over a large period. For example, in one patient taking clofibrate 500 mg/day for one year, bilirubin UDP-glucuronosyltransferase was 300% increased. In a patient taking an another hypolipidaemic drug fenofibrate, the increase was 200% (Table 3). Similar results could be found with rats treated with fibrates, where a selective increase (2 to 3 times) in glucuronidation of bilirubin was observed (Fournel et al., 1987).

On the other hand, despite their common imidazole structure, cimetidine (an antihistaminic compound) and albendazole (an antihelmentic drug) had oppposite effect on UDP-glucuronosyltransferase. Cimetidine, which is known to inhibit cytochrome P-450 upon binding (Rendic et al., 1983), strongly depleted bilirubin glucuronidation by 44%. By contrast, albendazole markedly increased 4-nitrophenol glucuronidation and, at a lower extent, conjugation of nopol in one patient (Table 3). This result could be favorably compared to that recently described in rats found that imidazole induced mainly glucuronidation of planar substrates in rat (Souhaili-El Amri et al., 1988).

Table 3: UDP-glucuronosyltransferases in the human population
Effect of drugs

Drugs	Substrates		
	4-Nitrophenol	Nopol	Bilirubine
Controls (16)	17.6 ± 5.7	6.9 ± 3.6	0.50 ± 0.20
Tobacco (14)	23.6 ± 7.6	7.2 ± 3.7	0.59 ± 0.24
Chronic alcoholism (7)	21.1 ± 6.8	8.5 ± 4.0	0.94 ± 0.37
Diazepam (8)	24.1 ± 7.7	10.6 ± 4.5	0.71 ± 0.28
Clofibrate (1)	43.8	9.9	1.90
Fenofibrate (1)	22.8	7.0	0.91
Cimetidine (7)	11.8 ± 3.2	6.6 ± 3.5	0.28 ± 0.11
Albendazole (1)	118	29.5	0.84

The activity was expressed in nmol substrate conjugated /min/mg microsomal protein. The values are the means ± SD for the number of patients indicated between brackets.

ACKNOWLEDGEMENTS

The expert technical assistance of Chantal Lafaurie and Haline Bodaud was greatly appreciated.

REFERENCES

Bock, K. W., White, I. N. H. (1974): UDP-glucuronosyltransferase in perfused rat liver and in microsomes: influence of phenobarbital and 3-methylcholanthrene. Eur. J. Biochem., 46, 451-459.
Bock, K. W., Lilienblum W. and Von Bahr, C. (1984): Studies of UDP-glucuronosyltransferase in human liver microsomes. Drug Met. Dispos., 12, 93-97.
Bock, K. W. and Bock-Hennig, B. S. (1987): Differential induction of human liver UDP-glucuronosyltransferase activities by phenobarbital-type inducers. Biochem. Pharmacol., 36, 4137-4143.
Boutin, J. A., Jacquier, A., Batt, A. M., Marlière, P. and Siest. G. (1981): UDP-glucuronosyltransferase activities in human liver microsomes and in some laboratory animal species. Biochem. Pharmacol., 30, 2507-2510.
Boutin, J. A., Antoine, B., Batt, A. M. and Siest G. (1984): Heterogeneity of hepatic microsomal UDP-glucuronosyltransferase (s): comparison between human and mammalian species activities. Chem. Biol. Interac., 52, 173-184.
Colin-Neiger, A., Kauffman, I., Boutin, J., Fournel, S., Siest, G., Batt, A.M. and Magdalou, J. (1984): Assessment of the Mulder and Van Doorn kinetic procedure and rapid centrifugal analysis of UDP-glucuronosyltransferase activities. J. Biochem. Biophys. Methods, 9, 69-79.
Dippold, W. G., Dienes, H. P., Knuth, A., Sachsse, W., Prellwitz, W., Bitter-Suerman, K. H. Meyer, zum Büschenfelde, K. H. (1985): Hepatocellular carcinoma after thorotrast exposure: establishment of a new cell line (Mz-Hep-1). Hepatology, 5, 1112-1119.
Dragacci, S., Thomassin, J., Magdalou, J., Souhaili El Amri, H. and Siest, G. (1987a): Properties of human liver UDP-glucuronosyltransferases. Relationship to other inducible enzymes in patients with cholestasis. Eur. J. Clin. Pharmacol., 32, 485-491.
Dragacci, S., Hamar-Hansen C., Fournel-Gigleux, S., Lafaurie, C., Magdalou, J. and Siest, G. (1987b): Comparative study of clofibric acid and bilirubin glucuronidation in human liver microsomes. Biochem. Pharmacol., 36, 3923-3927.
Fournel, S., Magdalou, J., Pinon, P. and Siest, G. (1987): Differential induction profile of drug-metabolizing enzymes after treatment with hypolipidaemic agents. Xenobiotica, 17, 445-457.
Hamar-Hansen, C., Fournel, S., Magdalou, J., Boutin, J. A. and Siest, G. (1986): Liquid chromatographic assay for the measurement of glucuronidation of arylcarboxylic acids using uridine diphospho-(U-^{14}C) glucuronic acid. J. Chrom., 383, 51-60.
Heirwegh, K. P. M., Van der Vijver, M. and Fevery, J. (1972): Assay and properties of digitonin-activated bilirubin uridine diphosphate glucuronosyltransferase from rat liver. Biochem. J., 129, 605-618.
Limbosch, S. (1983): Benzo(a)pyrene and aldrin metabolizing activities in cultured human and rat hepatoma cell lines. J. Natl. Cancer Inst., 71, 281-286.
Pitot, J. C., Peraino, C., Moore, P. A. and Potter, V. R. (1964): Hepatomas in tissue culture compared with adapting liver in vivo. Natl. Cancer Inst. Monograph., 13, 229-241.

Rao, G. S., Haueter, G., Rao M. L. and Breuer, H. (1976): An improved assay for steroid glucuronyltransferase in rat liver microsomes. Anal. Biochem., 74, 35-40.

Rendic, S., Kajfez, F. and Ruf, H. H. (1983): Characterization of cimetidine, ranitidine and related structures interaction with cytochrome P-450. Drug Met. Dispos., 11, 137-142.

Reuber, M. D. (1961): A transplantable bile-secreting hepatocellular carcinoma in the rat. J. Natl. Cancer Inst., 26, 891-897.

Siest, G., Bagrel, D., Levy, M., Febvre, N., Fournel-Gigleux, S., Rolin, S., Sabolovic', N., Wellman-Bednawska, M., Galteau, M. M., and Toyoda, Y. (1988): The use of hepatoma cells in culture as an alternative for the study of drug metabolizing enzymes. In "metabolism of Xenobiotics", Gorrod, J. W., Oelschläger, H. and Caldwell, J., Eds, Taylor and Francis Publ., pp 285-293.

Souhaili-El Amri, H., Fargetton, X., Benoit, E., Totis, M. and Batt, A. M. (1988): Inducing effect of albendazole on rat liver drug-metabolizing enzymes and metabolite pharmacokinetics. Tox. Appl. Pharmacol., 92, 141-149.

Wiebel, F. J., Park, S. S., Kiefer, F., Gelboin, H. V. (1984): Expression of cytochromes P-450 in rat hepatoma cells. Eur. J. Biochem., 145, 455-462.

Résumé

Nous avons étudié la glucuronoconjugaison de xénobiotiques et de substances endogènes dans des échantillons d'origine humaine : des lignées cellulaires d'hépatomes en culture et des microsomes de biopsies hépatiques. L'activité UDP-glucuronosyltransférase a été mesurée avec le 1-naphtol, la bilirubine, la testostérone et l'androstérone comme substrats dans les cellules d'hépatomes humains Hep G2, Hep 3B, SK-HEP-1 et Mz-Hep-1. La glucuronoconjugaison de ces molécules a été également suivie dans des cellules d'hépatomes de rat Fao et H5-6, à titre de comparaison. D'une façon générale les cellules humaines considérées dans cette étude conjuguent le 1-naphtol plus faiblement que celles de rat. La plus forte activité mesurée dans les cellules humaines a été obtenue avec la lignée Mz-Hep-1 (2.40 $\pm$ 0.94 nmol/min/mg); la formation du glucuronoconjugué de naphtol est 100 fois plus faible dans les cellules Hep G2 (0.015 nmol/min/mg), et absente dans les cellules SK-HEP-1. L'UDP-glucuronosyltransférase (bilirubine) n'a été détectée dans aucune des cellules humaines. Au contraire les hépatomes de rats présentent des activités appréciables de glucuronoconjugaison du 1-naphtol, bilirubine et testostérone, quoiqu'à des degrés divers. Nous n'avons pas pu mettre en évidence la conjugaison de l'androstérone.

Les biopsies hépatiques humaines sont capables de glucuronoconjuguer le 4-nitrophénol, le nopol (un terpène hydroxylé), la bilirubine et l'acide clofibrique; cependant les variations inter-individuelles sont très importantes. Ceci peut être en partie la conséquence de la consommation d'alcool et de tabac ainsi que de la prise de médicaments. Le tabac augmente la conjugaison du 4-nitrophénol et de la bilirubine de 30 et 18%, respectivement, alors que l'alcool stimule la bilirubine UDP-glucuronosyltransférase. Cette isoforme est significativement augmentée chez des patients prenant les hypolipémiants clofibrate et fénofibrate. Le traitement par des substances médicamenteuses contenant un noyau imidazole cimétidine et albendazole conduit à des effets opposés. La cimétidine diminue la glucuronoconjugaison de la bilirubine tandis que l'albendazole augmente toutes les activité testées, surtout vis à vis du 1-naphtol.

Conjugation of Chemical Carcinogens in Cultured Hepatocytes

Charlene A. McQueen and Gary M. Williams

American Health Foundation, Valhalla, NY, USA

ABSTRACT

Cultured hepatocytes provide a valuable in vitro model in which to investigate xenobiotic biotransformation. In cultured hepatocytes from rats, conjugation enzymes, including those catalyzing glucuronidation, sulfation and acetylation, were retained at high levels, and in fact, UDP glucuronyltransferase activities actually slightly increased in culture over hepatic levels. Importantly, the sex, age and strain differences in conjugation observed in vivo were maintained in cultured rat hepatocytes. Comparison of 2-acetylaminofluorene (2-AAF) metabolism in hepatocytes from male and female F344 rats revealed that male hepatocytes formed more sulfates and female hepatocytes more glucuronides. This reflects in vivo observations that female rats excrete predominately glucuronides of 2-AAF metabolites. Hepatocytes from 10 week old Long-Evans rats formed more glucuronides of 2-AAF metabolites than did those from 4 week old animals. More glucuronides were also recovered from cultured hepatocytes isolated from adult male Long-Evans rats than from Fischer F344 or Sprague Dawley derived hepatocytes. These studies demonstrate the utility of cultured hepatocytes for the study of glucuronidation of carcinogens.

KEY WORDS

Hepatocytes, 2-Acetylaminofluorene, Sulfates, Glucuronides

INTRODUCTION

Isolated hepatocytes are widely used to investigate xenobiotic biotransformation. Both phase I and phase II biotransformation pathways are well represented in intact hepatocytes isolated from a number of species. Nevertheless, hepatocytes differ in many respects from the whole organ. Isolation techniques are by their nature traumatic and result in cellular alterations. For example, uridine diphosphate (UDP) -D-glucuronic acid is depleted in freshly isolated rat cells (Croci and Williams,1985). When hepatocytes are manintained in monolayer cultures, P-450 content declines with duration of culture, but the decrease is not the same for all species (Maslansky and Williams, 1985). Moreover, changes occur that are specific for particular enzymes. Although aryl hydrocarbon hydroxylase activity declined, UDP-glucuronyltransferase activities were found to increase slightly at 24 hrs. of culture to levels that were higher than those in the intact liver (Croci and Williams, 1985). It was also found that the initially reduced UDP-glucuronic acid levels were restored during the culture period.

Despite changes in specific enzymes, the overall capacity for biotransformation remains intact. Study of the biotransformation of the carcinogens 2-acetylaminofluorene (2-AAF) and 2-aminofluorene (2-AF) in monolayer cultures of rat or rabbit hepatocytes revealed that acetylated, glulcuronidated and sulfated products were formed (McQueen et al., 1985,1988; Diez Ibanez et al., 1987). Biotransformation, including conjugation systems, can be increased by pretreatment with enzyme inducers, such as 3-methylcholanthrene (Schmeltz et al, 1978). This paper describes studies on the contribution of various factors to carcinogen conjugation in cultured hepatocytes.

Conjugation has been shown to play an important role in the carcinogenicity of aromatic amines such as 2-AAF, both through detoxification and activation. 2-AAF is detoxified by ring hydroxylation and conjuguation. In contrast, conjugates of N-hydroxy-2-AAF may be more harmful than the parent compound, as proposed by the Millers almost 20 years ago (Miller and Miller, 1969). The sulfate of N-hydroxy-2-AAF has been implicated in 2-AAF hepatocarcinogenesis in rats (DeBaun et al., 1970; Weisburger et al, 1972). It has been proposed that N-glucuronides of N-hydroxy-2-AAF formed in liver are transported to bladder where the conjugate is hydrolyzed and the free N-hydroxy-2-AAF activated to DNA damaging products (Kadlubar et al, 1979).

METHODS

In the studies reviewed in this report, hepatocytes were isolated by a two step in situ perfusion of the liver (Williams et al., 1982; McQueen and Williams, 1985). Monolayer cultures were initiated by allowing the freshly isolated hepatocytes to attach to tissue culture dishes for two hours.

Biotransformation of 2-AAF was investigated by incubating the cultures with $0.05\mu Ci$ ^{14}C-2AAF/ml. Aliquots of media were analyzed for aqueous and organic soluble products by the method of Smith and Thorgeirrson (1981) as described by McQueen et al. (1985). An aliquot of medium was extracted with ethyl acetate:methanol (90:10). The aqueous layer, containing total water soluble conjugates, was acidified (pH 5.5), incubated with sulfatase, extracted again, and the resulting aqueous layer with sulfates. This fraction was further incubated with β-glucuronidase and following extraction, assayed for loss of glucuronides. All the organic fractions containing 2-AAF and its free metabolites were pooled, evaporated to dryness and resuspended in methanol. Products were separated by HPLC on a Zorbax C_8 column with isopropanol: acetic acid (72:28).

RESULTS AND DISCUSSION

A series of studies was conducted to investigate 2-AAF biotransformation in hepatocytes. It was observed that differences occured in conjugation that were dependent on the sex, age or strain of rats that were used as a source of hepatocytes.

Female rats in vivo excrete predominately glucuronides of 2-AAF metabolites (Weisburger and Weisburger, 1963; Weisberger et al, 1964). When hepatocytes isolated from female F-344 rats were exposed to 2-AAF, 23% of the dose was found to be converted to glucuronides and 6% to sulfates, giving a glucuronide to sulfate ratio of 3.7 (Table 1). Hepatocytes from male rats showed the opposite pattern with almost seven times more sulfates than

Table 1. Conjugation of 2-acetylaminofluorene in F344 rat hepatocytes[a]

Concentration (M)	Glucuronide:Sulfate ratio	
	Male	Female
5×10^{-6}	0.15	3.73
10^{-5}	0.18	3.74
10^{-4}	0.24	1.36

[a] Cultures were incubated 20 hrs.
Data from McQueen et al., 1986.

glucuronides. This predominence of sulfation in males is one basis for the in greater susceptibility to the liver carcinogenicity of 2-AAF through formation of the sulfate ester.

A difference in glucuronide: sulfate ratio was found when biotransformation of 2-AAF was compared in four and ten week old Long Evans rats (Table 2). At each concentration of 2-AAF, the hepatocytes from the younger animals

Table 2. Effect of age on 2-acetylaminofluorene conjugated in hepatocytes from Long Evans rats[a]

Concentration	Age Weeks	Glucuronide:Sulfate ratio
5×10^{-6}	4	0.20
	10	0.87
10^{-5}	4	0.30
	10	0.91
10^{-4}	4	0.17
	10	0.33

[a] Cultures were exposed for 20 hrs.
Data from McQueen and Williams, 1987.

produced more sulfates than glucuronides. With cells from the older animals, the ratio of glucuronides to sulfates was nearly one. These observations correspond with others indicating that sulfation is more important fetally and perinatally than glucuronidation (see Dutton, 1980). In all, 2-AAF biotransformation has been investigated in hepatocytes from adult males of three rat strains (Table 3). More glucuronides were recovered from Long Evans hepatocytes at every concentration of 2-AAF. This strain also had the highest overall conjugation. In contrast, Sprague

Table 3. Strain differences in conjugation of 2-acetylaminofluorene

Intial Concentration (M)	Strain[a]	Percent[b] Sulfates	Glucuronides	Total
5×10^{-6}	F344	37	6	43
	SD	26	14	40
	LE	50	43	93
10^{-5}	F344	16	3	19
	SD	13	6	19
	LE	28	25	53
10^{-4}	F344	3	1	4
	SD	2	1	3
	LE	9	3	12

[a] Adult male F344, Sprague-Dawley (SD) and Long-Evans (LE) rats were used. Cultures were incubated for 20 hrs.
[b] Average of 2 to 4 animals.
Data from McQueen et al., 1986,1987.

Dawley hepatocytes formed twice as many sulfates as glucuronides while hepatocytes from F344 had three to five times more sulfates.

This system also offers the advantage that carcinogen induced DNA damage can be readily assessed by measurement of DNA repair synthesis (Williams, 1977) or of carcinogen binding (Leffert et al, 1977; Poirier et al, 1980). Thus, carcinogen biotransformation can be related to genotoxicity. For the conjugation reaction of acetylation, we have shown that genetically determined differences in the rate of N-acetylation affects susceptibility to the genotoxicity of aromatic amines (McQueen et al, 1982). Hepatocytes isolated from rapid acetylator rabbits were more sensitive to 2-AF or benzidine genotoxicity than hepatocytes from slow acetylators. The overall rate of biotransformation of 2-AF and the types of products formed was similar in the two phenotypes although the quantity of specific products differed (McQueen et al, 1988). Of particular interest is the observation that the major products formed by slow acetylator hepatocytes was a conjugate that migrated with 2-AF on HPLC. It is possible that this product is excreted into urinary bladder where it is hydrolyzed then further metabolized to DNA damaging products.

These examples illustrate that cultured hepatocytes provide a useful _in vitro_ model for conjugation.

REFERENCES

Croci, T. and Williams, G.M. (1985): Activities of several phase I and phase II xenobiotic biotransformation enzymes in cultured hepatocytes from male and femal rats. Biochemical Pharmacology, 34:3029-3035.

DeBaun, J.R., Miller, E.C. and Miller, J.A. (1970): N-hydroxy-2-acetylaminofluorene sulfutransferase: Its probable role in carcinogenesis and protein-(methion-s-yl) binding in rat liver. Cancer Res. 30:577-595.

Diez Ibanez, M.A., Chassebeuf-Padieu, M., Nordman, P. and Padieu, P. (1987: Gas Chromatography-mass spectrometry analysis of tert-butyldimethylsilyl derivatives of 2-acetylaminofluorene and metabolites in isolated rat hepatocytes. Cell Bio. Toxicol. 3:327-340.

Dutton, G.J. (1980): In: Glucuronidation of Drugs and Other Compounds. CRC Press, p.175.

Kadlubar, F.F., Miller, J.A. and Miller, E.C (1977): Hepatic microsomal N-glucuronidation and nucleic acid binding of N-hydroxy arylamines in relation to urinary bladder cancer. Cancer Res. 37:805-814.

Leffert, H.L., Moran, T., Boorstein, R., and Koch, K.S. (1977): Procarcinogen activation and hormonal control of cell proliferation in differentiated primary adult rat liver cell cultures. Nature 267: 58-61.

Maslansky, C.J. and Williams, G.M. (1982): Primary cultures and the levels of cytochrome P-450 in hepatocytes from mouse, rat, hamster and rabbit liver. In Vitro, 18:683-693.

McQueen, C.A., Maslansky, C.J., Glowinski, I.B., Crescenzi, S.B., Weber, W.W. and Williams, G.M. (1982): Relationship between the genetically determined acetylator phenotype and DNA damage induced by hydralozine and 2-aminofluorene in cultured rabbit hepatocytes. Proc. Natl. Acad. Sci., USA 79: 1269-1272.

McQueen, C.A., Miller, M.J., and Williams, G.M. (1986): Sex differences in the biotransformation of 2-acetylaminofluorene in cultured rat hepatocytes. Cell Biology and Toxicology, 2:271-281.

McQueen, C.A., Miller, M.J., Way, B.M. and Williams, G.M. (1988): Extracellular metabolites of 2-aminofluorene in cultures of rapid and slow acetylator rabbit hepatocytes as a model for urinary and biliary metabolites. Chemico-Biological Interactions. In Press.

Miller, J.A. and Miller, E.C. (1969): The metabolic activation of carcinogenic aromatic amines and amides. Prog. Exp. Tumor Res. 11:273-301.

Poirier, M.C., Williams, G.M. and Yuspa, S.H. (1980): Effect of culture conditions, cell type, and species of origin on the distribution of acetylated and deacetylated deoxyguanosine C-8 adducts of N-acetoxy-2-acetylaminofluorene. Mol. Pharmacol. 18: 581-587.

Poupko, J.M., Hearn, W.L. and Radomski, J.L. (1979): N-Glucuronidation of N-hydroxy aromatic amines: A mechanism for their transport and bladder specific carcinogenicity. Toxicol. Appl. Pharmacol. 50:479-484.

Schmeltz, I., Tosk, J., and Williams, G.M. (1978): Comparison of the metabolic profiles of benzo(a)pyrene obtained from primary cell cultures and subcellular fractions derived from normal and methyl-cholanthrene-induced rat liver. Cancer Letter, 5:81-89.

Smith, C.L. and Thorgeirsson, S.S. (1981): An improved high-pressure liquid chromatographic assay for 2-acetylaminofluorene and eight of its metabolites. Anal. Biochem. 133:62-67.

Weisburger, E.K., Grantham, P.H. and Weisburger, J.H. (1964): Differences in metabolism of N-hydroxy-2-fluorenylacetamide in male and female rats. Biochem. 3:808-812.

Weisburger, J.H., Yamamoto, R.S., Williams, G.M., Grantham, P.H., Matsushima, T., and Weisburger, E.K. (1972): On the sulfate ester of N-hydroxy-N-2-fluorenylacetamide as a key ultimate hepatocarcinogen in the rat. <u>Experimental Cell Research.</u> 69:106-112.

Weisburger, J.H. and Weisburger, E.K. (1963): Endogenous and exogenous factors in chemical carcinogenesis by N-2-fluorenylacetamide. <u>Unio. Intern. Contra Cancrum</u>, 19:513-518.

Résumé

Les hépatocytes en culture constituent un modèle fort utile pour suivre la biotransformation des xénobiotiques. Dans les cultures d'hépatocytes de rats, les enzymes de conjugaison dont celles catalysant la glucuronoconjugaison, la sulfoconjugaison et l'acétylation, sont maintenues à de hauts niveaux, et même les activités UDP glucuronosyltransférases sont augmentées légèrement dans les cultures pour atteindre des niveaux supérieurs à ceux du foie. De même les différences liées au sexe, à l'âge et à l'espèce, observées *in vivo*, peuvent être retrouvées dans les hépatocytes de rats en culture.
La comparaison du métabolisme du 2-acétylaminofluorène (2-AAF) dans les hépatocytes de rats F344 mâles et femelles indique que les hépatocytes obtenus à partir de rats mâles forment plus de sulfates alors que les hépatocytes de rats femelles forment plus de glucuronides. Ceci reflète les observations *in vivo* indiquant que les femelles excrètent de façon prédominante les glucuronides du 2-AAF. Les hépatocytes de rats Long-Evans âgés de dix semaines forment plus de glucuronides de 2-AAF que ceux de rats âgés de quatre semaines. On trouve également une quantité plus grande de glucuronides à partir d'hépatocytes en culture isolée de rats mâles Long-Evans adultes que d'hépatocytes obtenus de rats Fischer F344 ou Sprague-Dawley. Ces études démontrent l'utilité des cultures d'hépatocytes pour l'étude de la glucuronoconjugaison des carcinogènes.

Glucuronidation in rat and human hepatocyte cultures and in human HEP G2 hepatoma cells

M.H. Grant, H. Doostdar, M. Maley, W.T. Melvin, J. Engeset and M.D. Burke

Clinical Pharmacology Unit, Departments of Medicine and Therapeutics, Pharmacology, Biochemistry and Surgery, University of Aberdeen, Polwarth Building, Foresterhill, Aberdeen AB9 2ZD, Scotland, UK

ABSTRACT

In human hepatocyte cultures substantial loss of UDP-glucuronyltransferase (GT) activities occurs by 96h, accompanied by a change in the detergent activation characteristics of the enzyme. The activities of the isoenzymes of GT show differential stability in rat hepatocyte cultures. Human Hep G2 hepatoma cells express GT activities towards 1-naphthol and phenolphthalein to a similar extent as freshly isolated human hepatocytes, but show lower activities towards bilirubin morphine and testosterone. GT activities in Hep G2 cells and human hepatocytes show differential induction by phenobarbitone and 1,2-benzanthracene. Bilirubin GT activity is stimulated by dimethylsulfoxide and 5-aminolaevulinic acid in Hep G2 cells.

KEYWORDS

Glucuronidation, cultured hepatocytes, Hep G2 hepatoma cells.

INTRODUCTION

Information about the carcinogenic and cytotoxic potential of xenobiotics in man is usually obtained through extrapolation from animal studies. However, there is increasing evidence that the metabolism of xenobiotics in human tissues is different from that in animals, so it is essential to develop systems that can be used to measure the metabolism and predict the toxicity of xenobiotics directly in man. Cell cultures from human tissues provide a system for studying human xenobiotic metabolism and mechanisms of cytotoxicity and carcinogenesis under defined conditions in vitro.

Primary cultures of hepatic parenchymal cells isolated from experimental animals have become an established method for such studies. However, a major problem inherent with cultured hepatocytes is the instability of a number of specific functions. For example, cytochrome P-450 dependent mixed function oxidase (MFO) activities decline to low levels within the first 24-48h of rat hepatocyte culture (Holme et al., 1983; Grant et al., 1985). We have previously shown that the activities of UDP-glucuronyltransferase (GT) towards 1-naphthol and phenolphthalein are unstable in primary cultures of rat hepatocytes (Grant and Hawksworth, 1986). These GT activities decreased to approximately 50% of those in freshly isolated cells at 24h in culture, followed by an increase between 24 and 72h. Cycloheximide prevented this increase in GT activities suggesting that de novo protein synthesis was involved. In contrast 1-naphthol GT activity in human hepatocyte cultures is stable for 24h and then declines slowly between 24 and 96h (Grant et al., 1987). At present the reason for the decrease in GT activities observed in rat and human hepatocyte cultures is not known, but other research groups have also reported that GT activities towards several substrates decrease during culture of rat hepatocytes (Holme et al., 1983; Driscoll et al., 1982). The experiments in our laboratory on the maintenance of GT activities during culture have been carried out in intact cells and a deficiency in the intracellular supply of UDP-glucuronic acid and/or altered membrane constraint on the transferase may, therefore, be responsible for the decrease in activities.

The supply of human liver suitable for preparing hepatocytes is unpredictable and infrequent and the lifespan of the isolated cells is limited since they do not divide in culture. As a consequence of these problems and of the instability of drug metabolising enzymes during culture, cultured human hepatocytes may not be a practical model in which to investigate human drug metabolism. For this reason we recently turned our attention towards the human Hep G2 hepatoma cell line, which is readily available and immortal in culture. Initial studies indicated that, if cultured in William's E medium instead of the usually used Dulbecco's medium, Hep G2 cells contained certain MFO and GT activities (towards 1-naphthol and phenolphthalein) similar to those found in freshly isolated human hepatocytes (Grant et al., 1988). This cell line may, therefore, provide a more practical system for investigating human hepatic drug metabolism.

In this paper we present data on the maintenance of GT activities in cell homogenates from rat and human hepatocyte cultures, which may help to elucidate the reason for the loss of GT activities. The comparison of GT activities in human adult hepatocytes and in Hep G2 cells has been extended to include 1-naphthol testosterone, morphine and bilirubin. The effect of inducing agents, including, 1,2-benzanthracene (BA) and phenobarbitone (PB), on human GT activities in both hepatocytes and in Hep G2 cells was investigated, to find out if these culture systems provide a suitable model in which to investigate the induction of human GT isoenzymes.

METHODS

1. Cell culture
Hepatocytes from male Sprague-Dawley rats were prepared and cultured on collagen coated plates as described previously (Grant et al., 1985). Human liver samples were obtained from renal transplant donors. Within 30-45 minutes of removal from the body a section of the liver (approximately 50g) was cut off, such that it had only one cut surface and hepatocytes prepared as described previously (Grant et al., 1987). Hep G2 cells were grown in mono-/multi- layer culture and subcultured every 7 days at a 1:3 split ratio. William's E medium was used for all culture experiments, supplemented with 5% (v/v) foetal calf serum (FCS) for hepatocytes and 10% (v/v) FCS for Hep G2 cells. For measurement of GT activities freshly isolated and cultured cells were homogenised in 0.1 M sodium phosphate buffer, pH 7.6, as described previously (Grant et al., 1985).

2. Induction studies
For induction with BA or PB the inducers were added 24h after initiation of hepatocyte cultures or on day 7 after subculture (at confluence) for Hep G2 cells. Cells were exposed to 2mM PB or 25µM BA (in 0.625% (v/v) dimethylsulfoxide (DMSO)

for 3 days, with fresh medium being supplied every day. The effect of 5-aminolaevulinic acid (ALA) and DMSO on Hep G2 cell GT activities was measured by allowing the cells to grow in medium containing 100µM ALA and/or 2% (v/v) DMSO for 7 days before measuring GT activities.

3. Measurement of glucuronidation
The glucuronidation of 50µM 1-naphthol, 0.4mM bilirubin, 2.4mM morphine and 1mM testosterone was measured in homogenates of freshly isolated hepatocytes and cultured cells. 1-Naphthol GT activity was quantified in the presence of 0.5mM UDP-glucuronic acid and 5mM $MgCl_2$ by continuous fluorescence detection of the glucuronide formed (Mackenzie and Hanninan, 1980). Activation of this reaction was carried out using Brij 35 at the indicated ratios of detergent to cell protein. Bilirubin, testosterone and morphine activities were measured in the presence of 4mM UDP-glucuronic acid and 10mM $MgCl_2$, the former using the diazotization procedure and the latter two using ^{14}C-labelled substrates as described previously (Dutton, 1980).

RESULTS AND DISCUSSION

1. Maintenance of GT activities in cultured rat and human hepatocytes
In rat hepatocytes cultured for 24h the activities towards 1-naphthol and morphine had declined to approximately 50% of those in freshly isolated cell homogenates, while activities towards bilirubin and testosterone were maintained at fresh cell values (Table 1). This indicates that the isoenzymes of GT may be differentially stable during culture of rodent hepatocytes as described previously for cytochrome P-450 isoenzymes (Steward et al., 1985). In contrast, in human hepatocytes GT activity towards 1-naphthol did not decrease during 24h culture, whereas after 96h the activity towards all four substrates had decreased markedly.

Table 1. Maintenance of 'native' GT activities in cultured hepatocytes.

	24h rat hepatocyte cultures	96h human hepatocyte cultures	
		A	B
	% fresh cell activities		
1-naphthol	63 ± 7 (3)	43	60
testosterone	60, 53	15	29
morphine	102 ± 16 (3)	18	23
bilirubin	144 ± 13 (3)	19	25

GT was measured in 'native' rat and human hepatocyte cultures (2 human liver samples, A and B) as detailed in Methods. Where n is 3 the mean ± SEM are shown.

Since these experiments on the maintenance of GT in culture were carried out using cell homogenates in the presence of excess added UDP-glucuronic acid, the decrease in GT activities could not have been due to a deficiency in intracellular UDP-glucuronic acid. Activation of 1-naphthol glucuronidation by Brij 35 did not restore the GT activity in 24h cultured rat hepatocytes to that in freshly isolated rat hepatocytes (42 ± 4% (n=3) of the maximally activated GT activity present in freshly isolated cells was measured after Brij activation of 24h cultured cells). Figure 1 shows the response of 1-naphthol GT to activation by

Brij 35 in homogenates of freshly isolated and cultured human hepatocytes. These data indicate that the transferase enzyme is more susceptible to Brij activation in freshly isolated than in cultured isolated cells. In freshly isolated human hepatocyte homogenate 1-naphthol GT activity can be activated approximately 15-fold by Brij; in contrast after 96h in culture maximal activation by the detergent increases GT activity only 3-fold. This suggests that loss of the transferase protein has occurred by this time in cultured human hepatocytes and this may account for the low activities towards the four substrates. A similar but less marked effect was seen with rat hepatocytes.

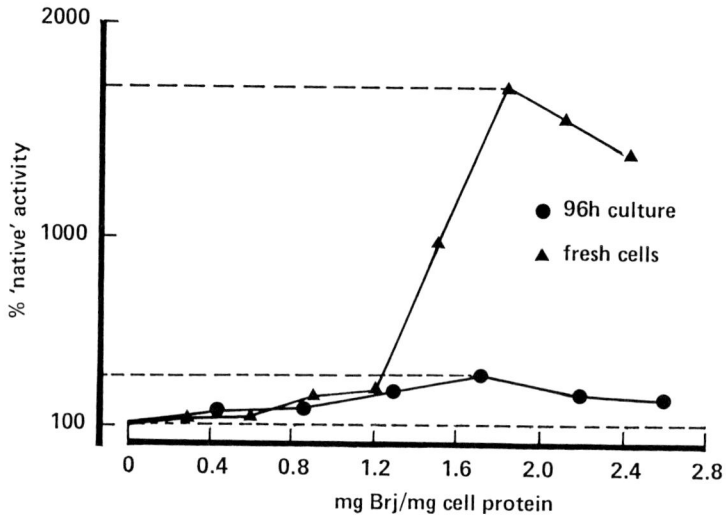

Fig 1. Detergent activation of 1-naphthol GT in human hepatocyte cultures. GT activities are shown as a percentage of the untreated 'native' activity for each sample. Results are from one culture experiment with liver A, a similar effect being observed with liver B.

2. Comparison of GT activities in freshly isolated human hepatocytes and Hep G2 cells.

Initial experiments indicated that the activities of GT towards 1-naphthol and phenolphthalein respectively were similar in intact cell preparations of Hep G2 cells and freshly isolated human hepatocytes (Grant et al., 1988). We have extended this comparison, using 'native' homogenates and the data show that GT activities towards morphine, bilirubin and testosterone are lower in Hep G2 cells than in hepatocytes (Table 2).

GT activities were not activated by detergent in Hep G2 cells and, in fact, 1-naphthol glucuronidation was inhibited at detergent concentrations above 0.1 mg Brij/mg protein. The MFO activities of Hep G2 cells are readily manipulated by altering medium composition (Doostdar et al., 1988), and it may, therefore, be possible to define conditions under which Hep G2 cells express a range of GT activities similar to those in freshly isolated human hepatocytes. We have shown that MFO and GT activities in Hep G2 cells increase during the growth cycle, with GT activity reaching a plateau between days 7 and 10 after subculture (Doostdar et al., 1988). These results indicate that experiments using Hep G2 cells as an in vitro model system for metabolism and cytotoxicity studies should be carefully timed within the cell growth cycle.

Table 2. GT activities in human hepatocyte and Hep G2 cell homogenates.

	Human hepatocytes	Hep G2 cells
	nmol/min/mg cell protein	
1-Naphthol	0.97, 0.61	1.18 ± 0.26 (3)
Bilirubin	11.76, 7.21	1.94 ± 0.14 (3)
	pmol/min/mg cell protein	
Testosterone	258.6, 189.7	14.8 ± 1.8 (3)
Morphine	591.5, 898.0	41.9 ± 7.9 (3)

The GT activities were measured in 'native' cell homogenates as detailed in the methods. The hepatocyte samples are from 2 separate liver samples (A and B). Means ± SEM are shown for Hep G2 cells. The Hep G2 cell GT measurements were carried out 7 days after subculture.

3. Induction of GT activities in Hep G2 cells and in human hepatocytes.
Figure 2 shows the induction of GT activities in human hepatocytes and in Hep G2 cells after exposure to PB or BA. In the hepatocytes bilirubin and testosterone GT activities were induced by PB, whereas morphine and, to a lesser extent, 1-naphthol activities were induced by BA. In Hep G2 cells bilirubin GT was also induced by PB, whereas the activities towards the other three substrates were preferentially induced by BA. The main difference between the pattern of induction

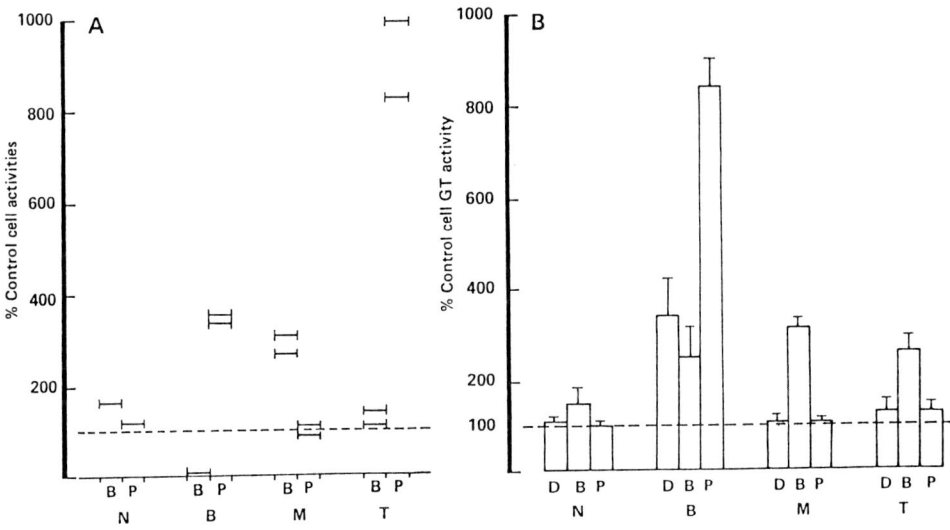

Fig 2. Induction of GT in human hepatocytes (A) and Hep G2 cells (B). The GT activities towards 1-naphthol (N), bilirubin (B), morphine (M) and testosterone (T) were measured in cells treated with dimethylsulfoxide (D), 1,2-benzanthracene (B) and phenobarbitone (P) and the results shown as a percentage of the GT activities present in control untreated cells at the same time in culture. Results for Hep G2 cells are mean ± SEM (n=3) and for hepatocytes the results for the individual livers A and B are shown as horizontal bars on the figure.

in the two cell types is that the marked induction of testosterone by PB (8-9-fold) observed in hepatocytes was not seen in Hep G2 cells and this may reflect the absence of an isoenzyme of GT in the latter cells. It is important to note that in the human hepatocytes the effect of the inducing agents was seen against a background of decreasing GT activities (see Table 1). For this reason Hep G2 cells may provide a more stable system for investigating induction of human hepatic GT. Studies in human microsomes from a 'liver bank' have shown that induction of bilirubin GT (3-fold) occurs in vivo in patients treated with barbiturates (Bock and Bock-Hennig, 1987). This group have also shown that 1-naphthol GT activity was induced 2-fold by 3-methylcholanthrene treatment of Hep G2 cells.

During the course of the induction experiments described above bilirubin GT activity in Hep G2 cells was found to be increased 3-4 fold by 0.625% (v/v) DMSO. This effect did not occur in hepatocytes. Table 3 shows that 2% (v/v) DMSO did not increase the bilirubin GT activity further, but produced an additive effect with ALA. DMSO and ALA had only slight effects on the GT activities towards 1-naphthol and testosterone. The effects of both agents on bilirubin GT activity are thought to be mediated through an increase in haem synthesis (Galbraith et al, 1986), though DMSO and ALA may act at different points in the pathway.

Table 3. The effect of dimethylsulfoxide and 5-aminolaevulinic acid on bilirubin GT activity in Hep G2 cells.

Control	DMSO	ALA	DMSO + ALA
	nmol/min/mg cell protein		
1.94 ± 0.14	6.78 ± 0.43	8.56 ± 0.29	15.94 ± 0.71

Cells were pretreated with DMSO and ALA and GT activity measured as described in the methods. Results are means $\pm$ SEM of 3 experiments.

The responses to the inducing agents PB and BA have been used to classify the isoenzymes of GT present in rodent liver (Bock et al., 1979). However, very little is known about the induction of human liver GT isoenzymes because the induction of drug metabolism is difficult to study in man. Increased GT activities have been described in microsomal liver samples obtained from kidney donors who had been treated previously with inducing drugs such as barbiturates (Bock et al., 1984; Bock and Bock-Hennig, 1987), but such material is only available opportunistically. The type of in vitro cell culture approach used in this study will therefore provide valuable information on the ability of inducing agents to induce human hepatic drug metabolism.

ACKNOWLEDGEMENT

This work was supported by the Wellcome Trust and the Aberdeen University Advisory Committee on Research. MHG was in receipt of a Wellcome Trust Travel Grant.

REFERENCES

Bock, K.W., Josting, D., Lilienblum, W. and Pfeil, H. (1979): Purification of rat-liver microsomal UDP-glucuronyltransferase, separation of two enzyme forms by 3-methylcholanthrene and phenobarbital. Eur. J. Biochem. 98 19-26.
Bock, K.W., Lilienblum, W. and von Bahr, C. (1984): Studies of UDP-glucuronyltransferase activities in human microsomes. Drug Metab. Disp. 12 93-97.

Bock, K.W. and Bock-Hennig, B.S. (1987): Differential induction of human liver UDP-glucuronosyltransferase activities by phenobarbital-type inducers. Biochem. Pharmac. 36 4137-4143.

Doostdar, H., Melvin, W.T., Burke, M.D. and Grant, M.H. (1988): Mixed function oxidation in human Hep G2 hepatoma cells. Biochem. Soc. Trans. In Press.

Driscoll, J.L., Hayner, N.T., Williams-Holland, R., Spies-Karotkin, G., Galetti, P.M. and Jauregui, H.D. (1982): Phenolsulfonphthalein (phenol red) metabolism in primary monolayer cultures of adult rat hepatocytes. In Vitro 18 835-842.

Dutton, G.J. (1980): Principles of assay of glucuronidation in biological tissues or fluids and selected practical procedures. in Glucuronidation of drugs and other compounds p183-204 CRC Press, Florida.

Galbraith, R., Sassa, S. and Kappas, A. (1986): Induction of haem synthesis in Hep G2 human hepatoma cells by dimethylsulfoxide. Biochem. J. 237 597-600.

Grant, M.H., Melvin, M.A.L., Shaw, P., Melvin, W.T. and Burke, M.D. (1985): Studies on the maintenance of cytochromes P-450 and b_5, monooxygenases and cytochrome reductases in primary cultures of rat hepatocytes. FEBS Lett. 190 99-103.

Grant, M.H. and Hawksworth, G.M. (1986): The activity of UDP-glucuronyltransferase sulphotransferase and glutathione-S-transferase in primary cultures of rat hepatocytes. Biochem. Pharmac. 35 2979-2982.

Grant, M.H., Burke, M.D., Hawksworth, G.M., Duthie, S.J., Engeset, J. and Petrie, J.C. (1987): Human adult hepatocytes in primary monolayer culture. Biochem. Pharmac. 36 3211-2316.

Grant, M.H., Duthie, S.J., Gray, A.G. and Burke, M.D. (1988): Mixed function oxidase and UDP-glucuronyltransferase activities in the human Hep G2 hepatoma cell line. Biochem. Pharmac. In Press.

Holme, J.A., Soderlund, E. and Dybing, E. (1983): Drug metabolism activities of isolated rat hepatocytes in monolayer culture. Acta Pharmacol. Toxicol. 52 348-356.

Mackenzie, P.I. and Hanninen, O. (1980): Sensitive kinetic assay for UDP-glucuronyl transferase using 1-naphthol as substrate. Anal. Biochem 109 362-368.

Steward, A.R., Dannan, G.A., Guzelian, P.S. and Guengerich, F.P. (1985): Changes in the concentration of seven forms of cytochrome P-450 in primary culture of adult rat hepatocytes. Mol. Pharmacol. 27 125-132.

Résumé

L'activité UDP-glucuronyltransférase (GT) mesurée avec le 1-naphtol et la morphine diminue au cours des premières 24 heures de culture d'hépatocytes de rats, mais cette activité reste constante avec la testostérone et la bilirubine. L'activité GT envers les quatre composés précédents est nettement diminuée au cours de 96 heures de culture d'hépatocytes humains. Ces diminutions sont observées pour des homogénats cellulaires en présence d'un excès d'acide UDP-glucuronique. Elles s'accompagnent d'une modification des caractéristiques d'activation par les détergents. Comme le montrent des études d'activation avec le 1-naphtol, des pertes de la protéine-enzyme GT peuvent intervenir dans des hépatocytes humains au cours de 96 heures de culture. Des cellules d'hépatomes humains (Hep G2) présentent une activité GT avec le 1-naphtol et la phénolphtaléine, comparable à celle obtenue avec des hépatocytes humains fraîchement isolés, mais ces cellules présentent une activité plus faible avec la bilirubine, la morphine et la testostérone. Avec des cellules Hep G2, l'activité liée à la bilirubine augmente 3 à 4 fois en présence de l'acide 5-aminolaevulinique et/ou du diméthylsulfoxyde. La capacité des activateurs classiques, 1-2 benzanthracène (BA) et phénobarbital (PB) d'augmenter l'activité GT *in vitro* des cellules humaines est étudiée. Pour des cellules Hep G2, l'activité GT liée à la bilirubine est sélectivement augmentée par le PB (8 fois), alors que celle liée à la testostérone, la morphine et le 1-naphtol est activée préférentiellement par le BA. Dans le cas des hépatocytes, les activités GT mesurées avec la bilirubine et la testostérone sont induites par le PB (4 et 8 fois respectivement), alors que celles obtenues avec la morphine et le 1-naphtol sont augmentées par le BA. Il est à noter que les effets inductifs obtenus avec les hépatocytes humains sont évalués en tenant compte de la diminution de l'activité GT. Les cellules Hep G2 semblent donc être un système plus propice pour l'étude de l'induction des isoenzymes hépatiques humaines.

Production of free and glucuroconjugated ring hydroxylated metabolites of 2-acetylaminofluorene in rat liver epithelial cell lines upon cocarcinogen induction

Miguel Diez Ibanez, Martine Chessebeuf-Padieu and Prudent Padieu

Laboratoire de Biochimie Médicale et Centre de Spectrométrie de Masse, Faculté de Médecine, 7 bd Jeanne d'Arc, 21033 Dijon Cedex, France

SUMMARY

Rat liver epithelial cells when selected by trypsin digestion will proliferate into diploid cell lines until immortalization. They possess an epithelial cell cytoskeleton and express liver metabolic function. We report the metabolism of a carcinogen, 2-acetylaminofluorene (2-AAF) into hydroxylated compounds (OH-2-AAF) and glucuronides, and its deacetylation. Cell line cultures from postnatal and adult rats were incubated with 5-100 µmol/l 9-^{14}C-2-AAF. Using 10 µmol 2-AAF/l, OH-2-AAF (in nmol/mg cell protein/24 h, n = 3) were 9-OH (1.28$\pm$0.37), 7-OH (1.08$\pm$0.28) and 5-OH-2-AAF (0.30$\pm$0.08), and 2-aminofluorene (2-AF)$^-$ (1.20$\pm$0.18) from 2-AAF deacetylation. For various doses of 2-AAF (5, 10, 50 and 100 µmol/l) total production and (2-AF/total)% were respectively in nmol/mg cell protein/24 h : 0.86(0 %), 3.86(35 %), 17.8(60 %) and 35.03(89 %). Preincubation of phenobarbital (BP) or 3-methylcholanthrene (3-MC) before incubation of 10 µmol/l 2-AAF increased 1.9 (PB) and 2.5 fold (3-MC) the total synthesis of OH-2-AAF, produced four other OH-2-AAF : 1-OH, 3-OH and two unknown OH-2-AAF and induced glucuronidation of all metabolites : 7-OH>3-OH>5-OH>1-OH>9-OH-2-AAF corresponding to 57 % or 75 % of the total after PB or 3-MC preincubation. Inhibitors of inducers, metyrapone (ME) for PB or α-naphtoflavone (αNF) for 3-MC, affected free and more severely conjugate production, which was reduced by 73 % or 78 % respectively. The synthesis of 2-AF remained totally depressed after 3-MC/αNF preincubation and amounted only 20 % of the total after PB/ME one.

INTRODUCTION

Trypsin dissociation of liver tissue allows to select epithelial cells which are considered as prehepatocytes or stem cells (GRISHAM, 1983 ; SHIOJIRI, 1984 ; WILLIAMS and GUN, 1974). They demonstrate a cytoskeleton of epithelial cells containing keratin which reacts with liver keratin antibodies without any immunological response to vimentin as endothelial cells or cultured hepatocytes and hepatoma cells (FRANKE et al., 1981). Primary proliferative cultures and cell lines were obtained in serum-supplemented medium (SSM) (CHESSEBEUF et al., 1974) or in serum-free medium (SFM) (CHESSEBEUF and PADIEU, 1984). These lines express liver markers : aldolase B in early passages (CHESSEBEUF et al., 1974), synthesis of albumin, transferrin, α-fetoprotein (KAIGHN and PRINCE, 1971 ; BAUSCHER and SCHAEFFER, 1974 ; BORENFREUND et al., 1975 ; TOKIWA et al., 1979) and C_3 component of complement (GUIGUET et al., 1987), tyrosine aminotransferase corticoid induction (CHESSEBEUF et al., 1984), arylhydrocarbon hydroxylase activity

(DIAMOND et al., 1973) and inducibility by benz(a)anthracene (BORENFREUND et al., 1975), epoxide metabolic activation of allylic carcinogens (DELAFORGE et al., 1976), biosynthesis of free and conjugated bile acids (CHESSEBEUF et PADIEU, 1984 ; PADIEU et al., 1985 ; TSACONAS et al., 1986) and hepatic metabolism of progesterone (DESGRES et coll., 1984 ; CHESSEBEUF and PADIEU, 1984).

MATERIAL AND METHODS

The procarcinogen $(9-^{14}C)$-2-acetylaminofluorene $(9-^{14}C$-2-AAF) was purchased from NEN (Du Pont de Nemours, F-75334 Paris), 2-AAF and 2-aminofluorene (2-AF) from Aldrich-Chimie (F-67000 Strasbourg). N-OH, N-acetoxy, 1-OH, 3-OH, 5-OH, 7-OH and 9-OH-2-AAF were given by IIT Research Institute (Chicago, ILL). Solvents were from Merck (Darmstadt, GFR) and tert-butyldimethylsilane, imidazole and dimethylformamide from Applied Science Labs (Deerfield, Il.). Standards were TLC purified and controled by gas chromatography-mass spectrometry (GC-MS). Incubations were carried out in serum-free and protein-free medium (SPFM) (CHESSEBEUF et al., 1986). Incubated 2-AAF was $9-^{14}C$-2-AAF/^{12}C-2-AAF (50:50, w/w) in 2-4 µl ethanol per 5 ml medium. Cells were always preincubated during 10 min in the precursor-free SPFM. Extraction was done with diethylether. The remaining aqueous phases were submitted to glucuronidase and sulfatase and then diethylether extracted. Extracts were evaporated, derivatized into tert-butyldimethylsilyl compounds (tBDMS) and analysed by GC-MS according to DIEZ IBANEZ et al. (1986).

RESULTS AND DISCUSSION

Basal production of free metabolite

The isotopic enrichment $^{14}C/^{12}C$ (50:50) monitored by GC-MS allowed the identification of $9-^{14}C$-2-AAF metabolites by the presence in the mass spectra of pairs of ions exhibiting a 2 mass unit increase and the original isotopic abundance ratio. Incubation in the Fθ12FR15 Fischer rat cultures was done at confluency in SPFM (Ham's F10 containing 50 mg T2000 dextran and 0.76 µmol/l six free fatty acids). Using such a protein-free medium, which sustains normal cell proliferation and growth (CHESSEBEUF-PADIEU et al., 1986), the extraction yield was 94 %. Kinetics of OH-2-AAF production was measured by GC-MS from 1 h to 96 h after incubation of 5 µmol/l of the $9-^{14}C$-2-AAF at 37°C. Up to 100 µmol/l, 2-AAF was not cytotoxic. In addition to hydroxylation, 2-AAF, when above 10 µmol/l, was deacetylated to 2-AF. When incubating 5 µmol 2-AAF/l in the Wistar cell line Wδ95FR8 the time and order of metabolite appearance (in nmol/mg cell protein) was 9-OH at 6 h (0.12), 7-OH at 12 h (0.21) and 5-OH-2-AAF at 36 h (0.03). Conjugates and N-OH-2-AAF, the ultimate carcinogen, were not found.

TABLE I : Production of free metabolites of 2-AAF from different amounts of 2-AAF incubated in the Fischer rat liver epithelial cell line Fθ12FR in confluent cultures at the 15th passage, (n = 3 and two 25 cm^2 flasks per point)

2-AAF (µmol/l)	2-AF	9-OH-2-AAF	5-OH-2-AAF	7-OH-2-AAF	Total	2-AF/Total %
		(nmol/mg cell protein/24 h)				
5	-	0.45 ± 0.12	0.05 ± 0.04	0.36 ± 0.11	0.86 ± 0.10	-
10	1.20 ± 0.18	1.28 ± 0.37	0.30 ± 0.08	1.08 ± 0.28	3.86 ± 0.23	35
50	10.77 ± 0.50	3.89 ± 0.43	0.39 ± 0.19	2.76 ± 0.11	17.81 ± 0.31	60
100	31.32 ± 2.52	0.44 ± 0.31	0.19 ± 0.07	3.08 ± 0.13	35.03 ± 0.76	89

Glucuronide metabolites

The inducer was preincubated at least five days in confluent cultures, either 1 µmol/l 3-methylcholanthrene (3-MC) or 1 mmol/l phenobarbital (PB), the medium being changed every two day. Then 10 µmol/l 2-AAF was incubated for 48 h at 37°C after washing out carefully the effector. The inhibitor, 100 µmol/l metyrapone

(ME) or 50 μmol/l α-naphtoflavone (αNF), was preincubated with its respective inducer PB or 3-MC.

TABLE II : Production of 2-AAF (10 μmol/l) free metabolites and glucuronides in the Wistar rat liver epithelial cell line WAQ7FR at the 13th confluent passage

Incubation mode		2-AF-	9-OH-	1-OH-	3-OH-	5-OH-	7-OH-	Unknown I	Unknown II	Total free or glucuronides	Total free + glucuronides
			(nmol/mg cell protein/24 h)								
Control (free)		1.03 ±0.09	1.94 ±0.15	-	-	0.21 ±0.11	1.37 ±0.33	-		4.55±0.17	-
PB	Free	-	0.37 ±0.11	0.54 ±0.13	1.12 ±0.19	0.55 ±0.01	1.12 ±0.30	-	-	3.70±0.15 FI/C = 81%[a]	8.67±0.12 IR = 1.90[b]
	Glucuronides	-	0.13 ±0.04	0.41 ±0.02	1.21 ±0.26	1.08 ±0.12	1.95 ±0.29	0.16 ±0.08	0.03 ±0.01	4.97±0.12	G/T = 57%[c]
PB + ME	Free	0.39 ±0.05	0.24 ±0.03	0.04 ±0.02	0.14 ±0.04	0.26 ±0.08	0.93 ±0.12	-	-	1.90±0.06 InF = 49%[d]	2.45±0.04 IR = 0.54
	Glucuronides	-	0.02 ±0.01	0.08 ±0.01	0.15 ±0.01	0.12 ±0.03	0.18 ±0.04	0.03 ±0.02	-	0.55±0.22 InG = 89%[e]	G/T = 22% InT = 73%[f]
3-MC	Free	-	0.25 ±0.04	0.40 ±0.03	0.81 ±0.01	0.54 ±0.02	0.84 ±0.18	-	-	2.84±0.07 FI/C = 62%	11.24±0.08 IR = 2.47
	Glucuronides	-	0.49 ±0.06	0.80 ±0.38	2.73 ±0.10	2.30 ±0.03	1.78 ±0.07	0.26 ±0.04	0.04 ±0.01	8.40±0.10	G/T = 75%
3-MC + αNF	Free	-	0.10 ±0.02	0.02 ±0.01	0.25 ±0.03	0.15 ±0.01	0.45 ±0.07	-	-	0.97±0.03 InF = 66%	2.5±0.03 IR = 0.5
	Glucuronides	-	0.07 ±0.02	0.10 ±0.04	0.42 ±0.07	0.27 ±0.02	0.63 ±0.05	0.04 ±0.02	-	1.53±0.04 InG = 82%	G/T = 61% InT = 78%

(a) : FI/C% = (induced free)/control)%, (b) : Induction ratio IR = Total induction/total control, (c) : glucuronidation ratio G/T : glucuronides/total induction, (d), (e) and (f) : inhibition ratio (In) of free (InF), glucuronides (InG) or total (InT) = (control - InX)/control, PB : phenobarbital, 3-MC : 3-methylcholanthrene, ME : metyrapone, α-NF : αnaphtoflavone, (n = 4, 2x25 cm² flasks).

Table II shows that two other free and glucuronidated OH-2-AAF were synthesized after 3-MC or PB preincubation : 3-OH-2-AAF one of the most important metabolite, and 1-OH-2-AAF. Glucuronides of the five OH-2-AAF were more abundant than free metabolites and three were the major products : 7-OH>3-OH>5-OH> after PB preincubation and 3-OH>5-OH>7-OH after 3-MC one. The increase of production of these compounds was more pronounced after 3-MC preincubation, 2.47 fold, than after PB, 1.90 fold. As regard to control, free compound synthesis decreased to 81 % or 62 % after PB or 3-MC preincubation. The inhibitor of either PB (metyrapone ME) or 2-MC (α-naphtoflavone αNF) affected the synthesis of both free and hydroxylated metabolites such that the induction ratio IR was lowered to 0.54 (PB+ME) and 0.55 (3-MC+αNF) as compared to 1.90 (PB) and 2.47 (3-MC). When these cell lines were assayed at different passages, over one year, the same metabolic activity was maintained. When comparing two cell lines adapted to grow in the three different mediums, SSM, SFM and SPFM, all metabolites were found and PB and 3-MC inducibility was similar. However in SPFM, a depleted nutrient medium, the same overall metabolism was found but reduced to 30 % of SSM level. The ultimate carcinogen N-OH-2-AAF was not detected due either to a lack of sensitivity of the method or an extinction of the metabolic step. However N-OH-2-AAF must be produced, because in vivo it is unstable and isomerized into 3-OH-2-AAF, the first or the second metabolite by importance and into 1-OH-2-AAF, as shown by WEISBURGER and WEISBURGER (1973), and SMITH and THORGEIRSSON (1981). In addition N-OH-2-AAF has a low GC-MS response despite that we greatly improved existing techniques of analysis of 2-AAF metabolism. In conclusion we report the first complete study on 2-AAF metabolism by rat liver epithelial cell lines and new developments in mass spectrometry analysis of 2-AAF and metabolites. .

REFERENCES

Bausher, W.H. & Schaeffer, W.I. (1974) : A diploid rat liver cell culture. 1. Characterization and sensitivity to aflatoxine B1. In Vitro 9, 286-293.
Borenfreud, E., Higgins, P.J., Steinglass, M. & Bendich, A. (1975) : Properties and malignant transformation of established rat liver parenchymal cells in culture. J. Nat. Cancer Inst. 55, 43-51.
Chessebeuf, M., Olsson, A., Bournot, P., Desgrès, J., Guiguet, M., Maume, G., Perissel, B. & Padieu, P. (1974) : Long term cell culture of rat liver epithelial cells retaining some hepatic function. Biochimie 56, 1365-1379.
Chessebeuf, M., Fischbach, M. & Padieu, P. (1984) : Time course study of L-tyrosine aminotransferase induction in serum-supplemented and serum-free rat liver cell lines. Cell Biol. Toxicol. 1, 31-40.
Chessebeuf, M. & Padieu, P. (1984) : Rat liver epithelial cell cultures in serum-free medium. Primary cultures and derived cell lines expressing hepatic function. In Vitro 20, 780-795.
Chessebeuf-Padieu, M., Mignot, G., Tsaconas, C., Fischbach, M., Padieu, P. & Mack, G. (1986) : Serum free and protein free medium for the continuous culture of epithelial cell lines, and myeloma and hybridoma strains. In, "Ther. Agents Produced by Gene Engineering.", MEDSI, Paris, pp. 385-397.
Delaforge, M., Janiaud, P., Chessebeuf, M., Padieu, P. & Maume, B.F. (1976) : Possible occurence of the epoxide-diol metabolic pathway for hepatocarcinogenic safrol in cultured rat liver cells, as compared with whole animal, a metabolic study by mass spectrometry. In, "Adv. Mass Spectrom. in Biochem. and Med.", Vol. II; A. Frigerio, Ed., Spectrum Publications, New York, pp. 65-89.
Desgrès, J., Fay, L., JO, D.H., Guiguet, M. & Padieu, P. (1984) : Oxydoreductive and hydroxylating metabolism of progesterone in rat liver epithelial cell lines. I. Metabolic pathways in a chemically defined incubation medium. J. Steroid Biochem. 21, 391-403.
Diamond, L., MacFall, R., Tashiro, Y. & Sabatini, D. (1973) : The WIRL-3 rat liver cells lines and their transformed derivatives. Cancer Res. 33, 2627-2636.
Diez-Ibanez, M.A., Chessebeuf-Padieu, M., Nordmann, P. & Padieu, P. (1987) : Gas chromatography-mass spectrometry analysis of N-tert-butyldimethylsily derivatives of 2-acetylaminofluorene and metabolites in isolated rat hepatocytes. Cell Biol. Toxicol. 3, 327-340.
Franke, W.W., Mayer D., Schmid, E., Denk, H. & Borenfreund, E. (1981) : Differences of expression of cytoskeletal proteins in cultured rat hepatocytes and hepatoma cells. Exp. Cell Res. 134, 345-365.
Grisham, J.W. (1983) : Cell types in rat liver cultures : their identification and isolation. Mol. Cell. Biochem. 53/54, 23-33.
Guiguet, M., Exilie-Frigère, M.F., Dethieux, M.C., Bidan, Y. & Mack, G. (1988) : Biosynthesis of the third component of complement in rat liver epithelial cell lines and its stimulation by effector molecules from cultured human mononuclear cells. In Vitro Cell. Develop. Biol. 23, 821-829.
Kaighn, M.E. & Prince, A.M. (1971) : Production of albumin and other serum proteins by clonal cultures of normal human liver. Proc. Nat. Acad. Sci. U.S., 2396-2400.
Padieu, P., Maume, G., Hussein, N., Chessebeuf, M. & Tsaconas, C. (1985) : Biosynthesis of sterols and bile acids in rat liver epithelial cell lines. Biochim. Biophys. Acta 833, 245-261.
Smith, B.A. & Thorgeirsson, S.S. (1981) : An improved high-pressure liquid chromatographic assay for 2-acetylaminofluorene ang eight of its metabolites. Anal. Biochem. 113, 62-67.
Shiojiri, N. (1984) : Analysis of differentiation of hepatocytes and bile duct cells in developing mouse liver by albumin immunofluorescence. Develop. Growth Differ. 26, 555-561.
Tokiwa, T., Nakabayashi, H., Miyazaki, M. & Sato, J. (1979) : Isolation and characterization of diploid clones from adult rat and newborn rat liver cell lines. Biomed. Mass Spectrom. 12, 19-24.
Tsaconas, C., Padieu, P., Maume, G., Chessebeuf, M., Hussein, N. & Pitoizet, N. (1986) : Gas chromatography-mass spectrometry of isobutyl ester trimethylsilyl ether derivatives of bile acids and application to the study of bile sterol and bile acid biosynthesis in rat liver epithelial cell lines. Anal. Biochem. 157, 300-315.
Weisburger, E.K. & Weisburger, J.H. (1958) : Chemistry, carcinogenity and metabolism of 2-fluorenamine and related compounds. Adv. Cancer Res. 5, 331-431.
Williams, G.M. & Gunn, J.M. (1974) : Long term cell culture of adult rat liver epithelial cells. Exp. Cell Res. 69, 106-112.

KEY WORDS

Carcinogen, 2-acetylaminofluorene, liver cell lines, hydroxylation, glucuronides

Résumé

Des cultures de cellules épithélilales de foie de rat proliférant un milieu contenant du sérum ou dans deux milieux synthétiques dont l'un est sans protéine, hydroxylent le 2-acétylaminoflurène et le désacétylent en 2-AF, en absence de phénobarbital ou de 3-méthylcholanthrène. En présence des inducteurs les glucuronides sont produits en accroissant le métabolisme. Leurs inhibiteurs, la métyrapone et l'α-naphtoflavone dépriment fortement ce métabolisme. L'activité est maintenue dans toutes les lignées durant un an de culture (trente passages).

Glucuronidation and glucosidation of bile acids in normal tissues and carcinoma of man

H. Matern, H.-U. Marschall, H. Wietholtz and S. Matern

Department of Internal Medicine III, Medical Faculty, Aachen University of Technology, 5100 Aachen, FRG

ABSTRACT

Conjugation of bile acids with glucuronic acid and with glucose has been characterized in hepatic and extrahepatic tissues of man and in human tumor tissues. In contrast to major bile acids lacking a 6-hydroxy group the bile acid hyodeoxycholic acid was exclusively glucuronidated at the 6-OH position with microsomes from human liver, kidney or small intestine. Enzymatic formation of 6-glucuronides of hyodeoxycholic acid showed an efficiency which is about 100-fold, 500-fold or 3-fold the efficiency observed for the enzymatic synthesis of glucuronides of the major bile acid chenodeoxycholic acid with microsomes from liver, kidney or intestine, respectively. In contrast to bile acid glucuronidation rates of bile acid glucoside formation in liver, kidney or intestine were similar for the 6α-hydroxylated bile acid hyodeoxycholic acid and for chenodeoxycholic acid lacking a 6-hydroxy group. Major activity of bile acid glucosidation was observed in kidney and small bowel mucosa where the efficiency was 3-6-fold the efficiency observed in liver or 6-13-fold the efficiency estimated for the glucuronidation of chenodeoxycholic acid in kidney or intestine, respectively. In human hepatoma or adenocarcinoma of the kidney glucuronidation of bile acids was deficient or nearly not detectable as was observed for the glucuronidation of other endogenous compounds, whereas bile acid glucosidation was increased in hepatoma and decreased but detectable with high activity in adenocarcinoma of the kidney.

KEYWORDS

Bile acids, glucuronidation, glucosidation, human microsomes, tumor metabolism

INTRODUCTION

In bile acid metabolism two mechanisms of glycoside conjugation are known at present in man: glucuronidation (Back, 1974; Matern et al., 1984b; Irshaid and Tephly, 1987) and glucosidation (Matern et al., 1984a). In order to evaluate the physiological importance of both bile acid conjugation pathways in man glucuronic acid and glucose conjugation of primary and secondary bile acids have been characterized in hepatic and extrahepatic tissues of man as well as in human tumor tissues. Alterations of bile acid conjugating activities in human tumor tissues have been compared with those observed for glucuronic acid conjugation of other endogenous compounds and p-nitrophenol.

MATERIALS AND METHODS

Human liver samples were obtained from organ donors (n = 5) within 30 min after cessation of life support and perfusion with cold 0.9 % NaCl. Intestinal or renal biopsy specimens were obtained from surgical patients who had undergone intestinal resection due to Crohn's disease of the ileum (n = 6) or nephrectomy due to adenocarcinoma of the kidney (n = 3). Kidney samples were restricted to the cortical region. A human hepatoma cell line was derived from a human primary malignant hepatoma after 50 passages in nude mice retaining its original histological appearance. Tumor fragments were frozen in liquid nitrogen after regular growth following subcutaneous transplantation. For the present study hepatomas were excised after 20 days of implantation into female, 8-12-week-old nude mice (NMRI strain).

Tissue specimens were stored, homogenized and microsomes were prepared as described in a previous report (Matern et al., 1984b).

Glucosyltransferase activity towards bile acids was estimated as described previously (Matern et al., 1984a) with 2mM octyl β-D-glucopyranoside as glucose donor and 0.1 mM chenodeoxycholic or 0.05 mM deoxycholic acids, if not stated otherwise, with the modification that 0.1 M sodium acetate, pH 5.0, was used as buffer in the reaction mixtures. Glucosidation of 0.16 mM bilirubin was assayed according to a published procedure (Fevery et al., 1977). Glucuronic acid conjugation of the following aglycone substrates was estimated as described: 0.1 mM concentrations of bile acids (Matern et al., 1984b); 0.16 mM bilirubin (Heirwegh et al., 1972); 30 µM estrone, testosterone or androsterone (Rao et al., 1976) and 0.5 mM p-nitrophenol (Yuasa, 1977) using [C-14]p-nitrophenol (0.1 µCi/µmole) as substrate. All microsomal conjugating activities have been estimated under fully activating conditions which were achieved by the addition of detergents to the following enzyme assays: glucuronic or glucose conjugation of bilirubin (6 mg digitonin/mg protein from all tissues); glucuronidation of: p-nitrophenol (0.6 mg Brij 58/mg protein from hepatoma); estrone, testosterone or androsterone (0.5 mg Brij 58/mg protein from kidney). All other enzyme activities could not be further stimulated by the addition of detergents.

RESULTS AND DISCUSSION

6α-Glucuronidation and 3α-glucuronidation of bile acids in normal tissues of man

Whereas the main bile acids lacking a 6α-hydroxy group have been shown in man to be glucuronidated at C-3 the glucuronides of secondary bile acids containing a 6α-hydroxy group such as hyodeoxycholic acid have been detected as 6-glucuronides in human urine (Almé and Sjövall, 1980). In order to compare the efficiency of 6α-glucuronidation with that of 3α-glucuronidation of bile acids in man the kinetic parameters of UDP-glucuronosyltransferase activity towards chenodeoxycholic and hyodeoxycholic acids have been determined in microsomes from human liver, kidney and small bowel.

Table 1. Kinetic parameters of human microsomal UDP-glucuronosyltransferase activity towards bile acids

Organ	Km		Vmax		Vmax/Km	
	CDCA	HDCA	CDCA	HDCA	CDCA	HDCA
Liver	0.083	0.026	0.23	7.4	2.8	284.6
Kidney	0.081	0.018	0.11	12.2	1.4	677.8
Small bowel	0.100	0.036	0.11	0.13	1.1	3.6

Km, mM; Vmax, nmol/min/mg of protein. CDCA, chenodeoxycholic acid, 3α, 7α-dihydroxy-5β-cholanoic acid; HDCA, hyodeoxycholic acid, 3α, 6α-dihydroxy-5β-cholanoic acid. Bile acid concentrations in the assay mixtures: 0.01-0.5 mM for CDCA; 0.005-0.07 mM for HDCA.

As shown in Table 1 hyodeoxycholic acid is a better substrate of UDP-glucuronosyltransferase than chenodeoxycholic acid not only with regard to Km-values but also with regard to maximal reaction rates. From the ratio of the Vmax to Km values it may be seen that the efficiency of hyodeoxycholic acid glucuronidation is about 100 times, 500 times or 3 times the efficiency of chenodeoxycholic acid glucuronidation in liver, kidney or small bowel mucosa of man, respectively. The glucuronides of hyodeoxycholic acid enzymatically synthesized with microsomes of human liver, kidney or small bowel were shown by gas chromatographic-mass spectrometric analysis to be conjugated exclusively at the 6α-position (Marschall et al., 1987b); Radominska-Pyrek et al., 1987). Thus, glucuronidation of bile acids at the 6α-hydroxy group appears to be a major pathway of bile acid conjugation in man in contrast to bile acid 3α-glucuronidation. The high efficiency of hyodeoxycholic acid glucuronidation observed in liver, kidney and intestine of man (Table 1) may be the reason for the observed rapid clearance of hyodeoxycholic acid and its glycine conjugate into urine (Sacquet et al., 1983; Parquet et al., 1985). Since hyodeoxycholic acid is formed by 6α-hydroxylation of lithocholic acid it has to be clarified whether formation of 6-glucuronides coupled to 6α-hydroxylation plays a role as a detoxication mechanism of the toxic bile acid lithocholic acid.

Glucosidation of bile acids in normal tissues of man
Bile acids have been described to be conjugated not only with glucuronic acid but also with glucose by a sugar nucleotide-independent glucosyltransferase isolated from human liver microsomes (Matern et al., 1984a). The biological significance of bile acid glucosidation in man has been shown by the identification of bile acid glucosides as normal constituents in human urine (Marschall et al., 1987a). Since bile acid glucuronidation had been described to occur not only in the liver, but also in the kidney and intestine of man (Matern et al., 1984b) the ability of these organs to catalyze the formation of bile acid glucosides has been investigated.

As shown in Table 2 glucosyltransferase activity towards bile acids is localized not only in the liver but also in the kidney and intestine of man. As calculated from the ratio of the Vmax to Km values the efficiency of bile acid glucosidation in extrahepatic organs is about 3-6-fold the efficiency observed in liver with chenodeoxycholic or hyodeoxycholic acids as substrates.
In contrast to bile acid glucuronidation (Table 1) these primary and secondary bile acids are glucosidated with similar efficiency in liver, kidney or intestine, respectively (Table 2). With regard to the main bile acid chenodeoxycholic acid the efficiency of glucosidation is comparable to that of glucuronidation in the liver whereas in extrahepatic organs the efficiency of glucosidation is about 6-13-fold the efficiency estimated for glucuronidation of this bile acid.

Table 2. Kinetic parameters of human microsomal bile acid glucosyltransferase

Organ	Km		Vmax		Vmax/Km	
	CDCA	HDCA	CDCA	HDCA	CDCA	HDCA
Liver	0.039	0.033	0.089	0.063	2.3	1.9
Kidney	0.026	0.039	0.213	0.235	8.2	6.0
Small bowel	0.035	0.036	0.500	0.328	14.3	9.1

Km, mM; Vmax, nmol/min/mg of protein. CDCA, chenodeoxycholic acid; HDCA, hyodeoxycholic acid. Bile acid concentrations in the assay mixtures, 0.01-0.1 mM.

Glucuronidation and glucosidation of endogenous compounds and p-nitrophenol in carcinoma of man

In order to clarify the importance of bile acid glycoside formation not only in normal tissues but also in disease glucosidation and glucuronidation of bile acids and other endogenous compounds as well as of p-nitrophenol have been estimated in tumor tissues of man.

As shown in Table 3 glucuronidation of the bile acids chenodeoxycholic and deoxycholic acids, bilirubin, estrone, testosterone and androsterone was not detectable or decreased in a human hepatoma cell line in contrast to normal liver whereas p-nitrophenol glucuronidation was similar in hepatoma and in normal liver. Glucose conjugation of bilirubin was not detectable in hepatoma whereas glucosidation of chenodeoxycholic and deoxycholic acids was increased in hepatoma in comparison to normal cells (Table 3).

A shown in Table 4 glucuronidation of bile acids and steroid hormones was not only impaired or not detectable in a human hepatoma cell line but also in renal carcinoma biopsy specimens

Table 3. Glucuronidation and glucosidation of endogenous compounds and p-nitrophenol in hepatoma and normal liver of man

	Enzyme activity	
	Hepatoma	Liver
Glucuronidation of:		
Chenodeoxycholic acid	0.004 ± 0.001	0.053 ± 0.015
Deoxycholic acid	< 0.001	0.063 ± 0.021
Bilirubin	0.12 ± 0.01	0.84 ± 0.22
Estrone	< 0.005	0.042 ± 0.011
Testosterone	< 0.005	0.059 ± 0.02
Androsterone	< 0.01	1.13 ± 0.25
p-Nitrophenol	37.9 ± 4.5	36.2 ± 7.4
Glucosidation of:		
Chenodeoxycholic acid	0.11 ± 0.01	0.06 ± 0.015
Deoxycholic acid	0.09 ± 0.008	0.05 ± 0.009
Bilirubin	< 0.05	0.37 ± 0.1

Enzyme activity, nmol/min/mg protein. Values represent mean $\pm$ S.D. for microsomal preparations from the following number of different tissues: hepatoma, $n = 7$; liver, $n = 5$.

in comparison to normal cells. In contrast to glucosidation of bile acids in hepatoma, however, glucosyltransferase activity towards chenodeoxycholic and deoxycholic acids was decreased to about half the activity as compared to normal cells.

The results of Tables 3 and 4 show that bile acid glucosidation and glucuronidation exhibit different patterns of alteration in tumor tissues in comparison to normal cells. Whereas bile acid glucuronidation is deficient or nearly not detectable in hepatoma and renal carcinoma as also observed for other endogenous compounds bile acid glucosidation increased in hepatoma and was decreased but still detectable with high activity in renal carcinoma. These results suggest that bile acid glucosidation might fulfil a role in metabolism that differs from that of bile acid glucuronidation. Further studies are needed to clarify the biological importance of bile acid glucosidation in normal tissues and in tumor tissues of man.

Table 4. Glucuronidation and glucosidation of bile acids and steroid hormones in renal carcinoma and normal renal tissue of man

	Enzyme activity	
	Carcinoma	Kidney
Glucuronidation of:		
Chenodeoxycholic acid	0.003 ± 0.001	0.073 ± 0.019
Deoxycholic acid	0.001 ± 0.001	0.066 ± 0.02
Estrone	< 0.005	0.045 ± 0.011
Androsterone	0.01 ± 0.005	1.68 ± 0.42
Glucosidation of:		
Chenodeoxycholic acid	0.084 ± 0.018	0.18 ± 0.04
Deoxycholic acid	0.074 ± 0.02	0.18 ± 0.05

Enzyme activity, nmol/min/mg protein. Values represent mean ± S.D. for microsomal preparations from three different tissues of carcinoma or kidney, respectively.

REFERENCES

Almé, B. and Sjövall, J. (1980): Analysis of bile acid glucuronides in urine. Identification of 3α, 6α, 12α-trihydroxy-5β-cholanoic acid. J. Steroid Biochem. 13, 907-916.
Back, P., Spaczynski, K. and Gerok, W. (1974): Bile-salt glucuronides in urine. Hoppe-Seyler's Z. Physiol. Chem. 355, 749-752.
Fevery, J., Van De Vijver, M., Michiels, R. and Heirwegh, K.P.M. (1977): Comparison in different species of biliary bilirubin-IXα conjugates with the activities of hepatic and renal bilirubin-IXα-uridine diphosphate glycosyltransferases. Biochem. J. 164, 737-746.
Heirwegh, K.P.M., Van De Vijver, M. and Fevery, J. (1972): Assay and properties of digitonin-activated bilirubin uridine diphosphate-glucuronyltransferase from rat liver. Biochem. J. 129, 605-618.
Irshaid, Y.M. and Tephly, T.R. (1987): Isolation and purification of two human liver UDP-glucuronosyltransferases. Mol. Pharmacol. 31, 27-34.
Marschall, H.-U., Egestad, B., Matern, H., Matern, S. and Sjövall, J. (1987a): Evidence for bile acid glucosides as normal constituents in human urine. FEBS Lett. 213, 411-414.
Marschall, H.-U., Matern, H., Egestad, B., Matern, S. and Sjövall, J. (1987b): 6α-Glucuronidation of hyodeoxycholic acid by human liver, kidney and small bowel microsomes. Biochim. Biophys. Acta 921, 392-397.

Matern, H., Matern, S. and Gerok, W. (1984a): Formation of bile acid glucosides by a sugar nucleotide-independent glucosyltransferase isolated from human liver microsomes. Proc. Natl. Acad. Sci. USA 81, 7036-7040.

Matern, S., Matern, H., Farthmann, E.H. and Gerok, W. (1984b): Hepatic and extrahepatic glucuronidation of bile acids in man. Characterization of bile acid uridine 5'-diphosphate-glucuronosyltransferase in hepatic, renal, and intestinal microsomes. J. Clin. Invest. 74, 402-410.

Parquet, M., Pessah, M., Sacquet, E., Salvat, C., Raizman, A. and Infante, R. (1985): Glucuronidation of bile acids in human liver, intestine and kidney. An in vitro study on hyodeoxycholic acid. FEBS Lett. 189, 183-187.

Radominska-Pyrek, A., Zimniak, P., Irshaid, Y.M., Lester, R., Tephly, T.R. and Pyrek, J.St. (1987): Glucuronidation of 6α-hydroxy bile acids by human liver microsomes. J. Clin. Invest. 80, 234-241.

Rao, G.S., Haueter, G., Rao, M.L. and Breuer, H. (1976): An improved assay for steroid glucuronyltransferase in rat liver microsomes. Anal. Biochem. 74, 35-40.

Sacquet, E., Parquet, M., Riottot, M., Raizman, A., Jarrige, P., Huguet, C. and Infante, R. (1983): Intestinal absorption, excretion, and biotransformation of hyodeoxycholic acid in man. J. Lipid Res. 24, 604-613.

Yuasa, A. (1977): Purification and properties of uridine diphosphate glucuronyltransferase from rabbit liver microsomes. J. Coll. Dairying 7 (Suppl.), 103-156.

ACKNOWLEDGEMENT

This work was supported by a Heisenberg award to H.M. from the Deutsche Forschungsgemeinschaft.

Résumé

La conjugaison des acides biliaires avec l'acide glucuronique et le glucose a été caractérisée dans les microsomes des tissus hépatiques et extrahépatiques humains ainsi que dans les tissus tumoraux chez l'homme. Au contraire des acides biliaires principaux qui n'ont pas de groupe 6-hydroxyle, l'acide biliaire hyodeoxycholique est glucuronidé uniquement en position 6-OH dans les microsomes du foie, du rein et de l'intestin grêle. L'efficience de la synthèse enzymatique des 6-glucuronides de l'acide hyodeoxycholique est plus haute que la synthèse enzymatique de l'acide principal chenodeoxycholique: 100 fois supérieure dans le foie, 500 fois dans le rein et 3 fois dans l'intestin grêle. A la différence de la glucuronoconjugaison la vitesse de glucosoconjugaison dans le foie, le rein et l'intestin grêle est similaire pour les acides biliaires avec et sans groupe 6-hydroxyle comme l'acide hyodeoxycholique et chenodeoxycholique. L'efficience de la glucosoconjugaison des acides biliaires est environ de 3 à 6 fois plus haute dans le rein et dans l'intestin grêle que dans le foie. L'efficience de la glucosoconjugaison est 6 à 13 fois plus haute que l'efficience de la glucuronoconjugaison de l'acide chenodeoxycholique dans les tissus extrahépatiques. Dans le carcinome hépato-cellulaire ou dans l'adénocarcinome du rein chez l'homme la glucuronoconjugaison est déficiente ou à peine détectable alors que la glucosoconjugaison des acides biliaires est accélérée dans le carcinome hépato-cellulaire et décélérée dans l'adénocarcinome du rein quoique détectable avec une haute activité.

Formation and transport of glucuronide-conjugates in the isolated perfused rat liver, intestine and kidney

A.Sj. Koster, M.H. de Vries, F.A.M. Redegeld, * R.P.J. Oude Elferink and * P.L.M. Jansen

*Department of Pharmacology, Faculty of Pharmacy, University of Utrecht, Catharijnesingel 60, NL-3511 GH Utrecht and * Division of Gastrointestinal and Liver Diseases, Academic Medical Centre, Meibergdreef 9, NL-1105 AZ Amsterdam, the Netherlands*

ABSTRACT

The metabolism of 1-naphthol (N) and the transport of 1-naphthyl-β,D-glucuronide (NG) was investigated in isolated vascularly perfused organ preparations of the rat liver, intestine and kidney. In the liver and kidney N-clearance was highly efficient and approached the organ perfusate flow. In the intestine only the perfusate flow through the mucosa was completely extracted of N. These results indicate that the *in vivo* clearance of N can largely be explained by metabolism in these three organs. It is demonstrated that NG is transported by carrier-mediated mechanisms across the canalicular membrane of the liver and the basolateral and brush-border membrane of the intestine and kidney. These mechanisms are sensitive to inhibition by phloridzin (in the intestine) or probenecid (in the kidney). Transport in the canalicular membrane of the liver is reduced substantially in the TR⁻ rat, which has a genetic defect for the biliary excretion of organic anions. Transport in the intestine and kidney is normal in these rats. The results suggest that considerable differences exist between the transport-mechanisms for NG in liver, intestine and kidney.

KEY WORDS

1-naphthol, 1-naphthyl-β,D-glucuronide, liver, intestine, kidney, rat, perfused organs, phloridzin, probenecid, active transport

INTRODUCTION

Simple phenolic compounds like phenol (Cassidy and Houston, 1984), p-nitrophenol (Machida et al., 1982), harmol (Mulder et al., 1984) and 1-naphthol (Mistry and Houston, 1985) are conjugated in a number of organs, including the liver, intestine and kidney. Assessment of the contribution of various organs to the systemic metabolism of these compounds is complicated. Isolated cells and subcellular fractions have been used frequently to demonstrate the possibility of extrahepatic glucuronidation and transport of glucuronides (Schwenk, 1985; Koster, 1985), but quantitatively reliable extrapolation from these model systems to the *in vivo* situation is hampered by a number of uncertainties. Even in isolated cells the *in vivo* polarity of the cells is lost and diffusion- or transport-barriers may be altered. Moreover, possible flow-limitation is absent. *In vivo* experiments, on the other hand, require carefully standardized experimental conditions and/or complicated pharmacokinetic analyses to assess the quantitative importance of extrahepatic metabolism (Mistry and Houston, 1985; Klippert and Noordhoek, 1983; Tremaine et al., 1985). We used isolated vascularly perfused organ preparations to clarify the pharmacokinetic details of the metabolism of 1-naphthol in the liver, intestine, and kidney of the rat. We were particularly interested in the possible active transport of preformed and locally formed glucuronide-conjugates. Part of this work has been published in prelimary (Redegeld et al., 1987; de Vries et al., 1987) and final form (Redegeld and Noordhoek, 1986; Redegeld et al., 1988; de Vries et al., 1988).

MATERIALS AND METHODS

In addition to normal Wistar-rats, transport-mutated Wistar-rats (TR^-) were used as organ donors. In the TR^- rat, the biliary excretion of organic anions (bilirubin, di- and tetrabromosulfophthalein) and neutral steroids (ouabain) is impaired, while the hepatic uptake of these compounds and the biliary excretion of cations and bile acids is not altered (Jansen et al., 1985, 1987). Perfusions of the isolated liver, intestine and kidney were carried out with artifical media at a flow rat of approximately 35, 5 and 23 ml/min, respectively according to established procedures (Meijer et al., 1981; Hartmann et al., 1984; Redegeld et al., 1988). Additional *in vivo* experiments were carried out with intact animals under pentobarbital-anaesthesia (de Vries et al., 1985). 1-Naphthol (N), 1-naphthyl-sulfate (NS) and 1-naphthyl-β,D-glucuronide (NG) were quantitated in bile, intestinal luminal fluid, urine and perfusion media by HPLC-separation of the conjugates and fluorimetric detection (Redegeld et al., 1988). Hepatic, intestinal and renal clearances (Cl_h, Cl_i, Cl_r, respectively) and extraction ratio's (E) were calculated from metabolic and/or transport rates, added concentrations and the relevant organ perfusion flows (Q) (Wilkinson, 1987). All data are given *per* organ or *per* animal (of 250-300 g). The following values for *in vivo* blood flows were used in order to calculate *in vivo* clearance: portal vein flow Q_{pv} = 15 ml/min, total hepatic flow Q_h = 20 ml/min, small intestinal flow Q_i = 8 ml/min and renal flow Q_r = 12 ml/min (*per* two kidneys) (Roth and Rubin, 1976).

EXPERIMENTAL RESULTS

Liver perfusion
When N is added to the perfusate of an isolated liver at non-saturating concentrations the Cl_h of N equals the perfusate flow, indicating a very efficient extraction of N by the liver (E_h = 1.00). When N was infused (200 nmol/min) in the ileocolic vein (a contributory of the portal vein) of anaestetized rats no free N could be demonstrated in the hepatic veins, again indicating complete extraction of N by the liver. The total formation rate of NG under these conditions was 119 ± 31 nmol/min, the remainder being metabolized to NS. NG was found both in the urine and the bile in approximately equal amounts. NS and N could not be demonstrated in the bile. Similar results have been observed before in the perfused liver with harmol (de Vries et al., 1985) and N (Schwenk, 1985). When N was added to the liver-perfusate of TR^- rats total metabolism was not altered, but the appearance rate of NG in the bile was substantially reduced. NG appeared largely in the perfusate under these conditions (Fig. 1).

Cl_h and biliary excretion of preformed NG in the perfused liver of control rats was only 0.0273 ± 0.0077 ml/min. In TR^- rats a further reduction to 0.0018 ± 0.0004 ml/min was seen. These data suggest that hepatic uptake of NG was very slow and that biliary excretion of NG, whether preformed or formed during metabolism of N in the liver, was mediated by a carrier-system, which was altered in the TR⁻ rat. No conclusions can be drawn concerning the nature of the transport-mechanism for NG and NS from the liver into the perfusate. Both passive efflux and carrier-mediated transport through the sinusoidal membrane remain possible (Fig. 3). When NG was infused into the jugular vein of an anaesthetized rat, only 3.8 % of the NG was cleared *via* the bile.

Intestinal perfusion

In the isolated vascularly perfused intestine N was extracted from the vascular bed by metabolism to NG. Only trace amounts of NS are formed in the rat intestine (Schwenk, 1985; Koster, 1985). When N was administered in concentrations < 50 nmol/ml an E_i of 0.31 ± 0.02 was observed, independent of the perfusate flow applied. Cl_i was, as a consequence, completely flow-dependent. This apparent conflict between a low E and complete flow-dependency can be explained by the occurrence of two (or more) parallel vascular beds in the intestinal wall. Only a part of the perfusate flow distributes to the mucosal layer (Q_{muc}) and was completely extracted of N (E_{muc} = 1.00; Cl_{muc} = E_{muc}). When Q_{muc} is temporarily decreased by infusion of noradrenalin (at a constant total Q_i), the E_i of N decreased in parallel. This demonstrated that N was completely extracted from the Q_{muc} only (de Vries et al., 1988). The NG formed was appearing in the perfusate (ca. 95%) and the intestinal lumen (ca. 5%).

In order to establish the possible involvements of active transport mechanisms for NG in the intestine various inhibitors were used. Appearance of NG in perfusate and/or intestinal lumen after luminal administration of N (150 nmol/mol) was not influenced by ouabain or probenecid. However, luminal or vascular administration of phloridzin (50-200 nmol/ml) decreased the appearance rate of NG in the lumen by 80-84%, and the appearance rate of NG in the perfusate by 38-44% (glucuronidation of N in intestinal microsomes was not inhibited at phloridzin concentrations below 1 mM) (Fig. 2). This suggests that the luminally directed transport was more sensitive to phloridzin inhibition than the vascularly directed mechanism. The transport-mechanism on the basolateral side appeared to be more efficient that the luminally directed mechanism because preformed NG and

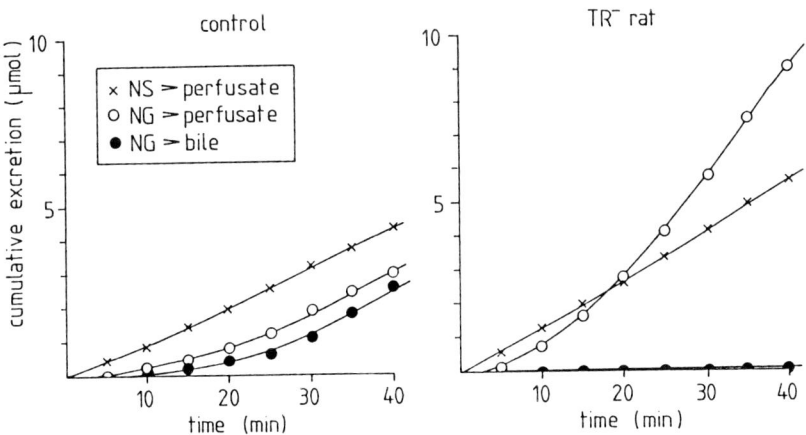

Fig. 1. Appearance of NS and NG in the perfusate and bile of isolated perfused livers of control (left) and transport-mutated (TR⁻) rats (right). N was infused at a rate of 500 nmole/min throughout the experiment. No N or NS could be detected in the bile.

4-methylumbelliferyl-glucuronide (MUG) were transported from lumen to perfusate (Cl = 0.0287 ± 0.0004 ml/min for NG and 0.0144 ± 0.0003 ml/min for MUG), but not in the opposite direction. The net transport of NG from lumen to perfusate was probably the result of NG-uptake from the intestinal lumen, which was partially counteracted by a phloridzin-sensitive luminally directed transport (Fig. 3). This was suggested by the observation that the net transport of NG from lumen to perfusate was increased 2-fold by the addition of phloridzin (200 nmol/ml on the luminal side).

Metabolism of N and appearance of NG in the lumen and perfusate in the perfused intestine of TR^- rats was not different from control rats. This suggests that NG-transport in the intestine was mediated by a carrier-system that is not affected by the mutation.

Kidney perfusion

In the isolated perfused kidney N was metabolized very efficiently. The metabolic Cl at a non-saturating concentration of N (15 nmol/ml) amounts to 5.9 ± 0.9 ml/min (Redegeld et al., 1988). This is 90% of the Cl of p-amino-hippuric acid (PAH). Because the PAH-Cl represents the effective renal perfusate flow, (which was only part of the perfusate flow in the perfused kidney) it is suggested that N is a high-extraction compound in the rat kidney (E = 0.90). Both NS and NG were formed. As in the liver, NS only appears in the perfusate, while NG was distributed in approximately equal amounts over the perfusate and urine. Transport of preformed NG (Redegeld and Noordhoek, 1986), MUG and p-nitrophenolglucuronide in the perfused rat kidney (Cl_r = 2.4 ± 0.3 ml/min for NG, Cl_r = 1.2 ± 0.2 ml/min for MUG, Cl_r = 1.3 ± 0.3 ml/min for p-nitrophenolglucuronide) was probenecid-inhibitable (0.5 mM probenecid). Since these Cl-values exceed the glomerular filtration rate 2- to 4-fold, active transport was indicated. Transport of intracellularly formed NG to the tubular lumen was inhibited by relatively high concentrations of probenecid (5 mM). Taken together, the results indicate that

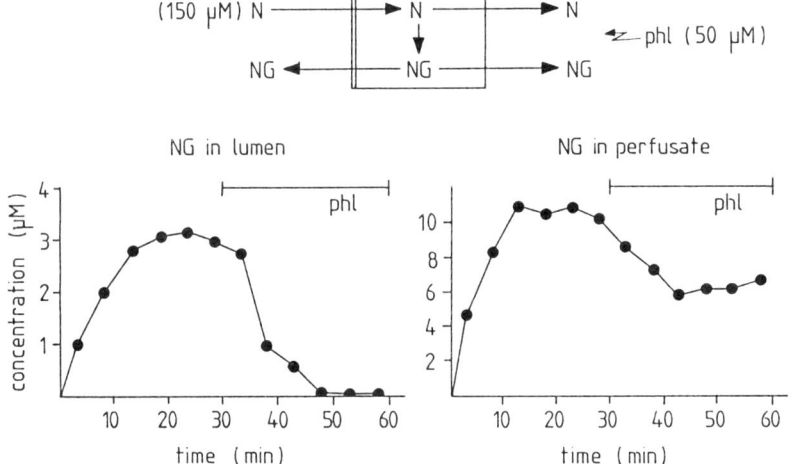

Fig. 2. Appearance of NG in the lumen (left) and perfusate (right) of the isolated intestine. Both the lumen and the vascular bed were perfused single pass (flow = 2 ml/min, lumen and 4 ml/min, vascular bed). N (150 nmol/ml) was added on the luminal side. At time = 30 min 50 nmol/ml phloridzin was added on the vascular side.

probenecid-inhibitable transport-mechanisms for NG exist in both the basolateral and the brush-border membrane. In order to investigate the possible involvement of liver-like transport systems in the renal transport of NG we also measured the renal NG-clearance in perfused kidneys of the TR$^-$ rat. Although Cl_r was lowered (1.8 ± 0.5 ml/min in the TR$^-$ rat, 2.4 ± 0.6 ml/min in the control rats), no statistically significant difference was observed. This indicates that either the renal carrier system for NG-transport was not affected by the TR$^-$ mutation or that in the kidney other carrier systems with affinity for NG do exist.

DISCUSSION AND CONCLUSIONS

In vivo metabolism of 1-naphthol

Our results indicate that conjugation of N in the rat liver, intestine and kidney was highly efficient. Metabolic Cl in these three organs was flow limited (E_h = 1.00, E_{muc} = 1.00 and E_r = 0.90). The contribution of the kidney to the systemic clearance of N *in vivo* can, therefore, be as large as 10.8 ml/min. This estimated *in vivo* Cl_r of N is larger than the value reported by Tremaine et al. (1985). However, these authors underestimate the renal metabolism of N, because only the conjugates that are directly secreted into the urine from the renal tissue are considered "nephrogenic metabolites". Our results demonstrate that these metabolites represent only a part of the conjugates that were formed in the kidney (Redegeld et al., 1988).

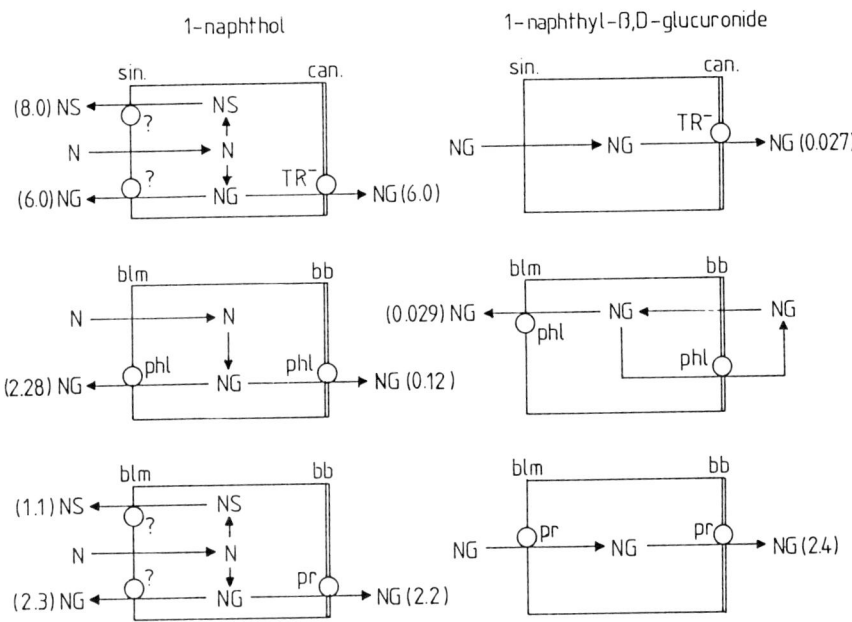

Fig. 3. Schematic representation of the Cl of 1-naphthol (N; left) and 1-naphthyl-β,D-glucuronide (NG; right) in the rat liver (top row), intestine (middle row) and kidney (bottom row). The presence of TR$^-$ mutation-, phloridzin-(phl) and probenecid-(pr) sensitive carrier-systems in the sinusoidal (sin.) and canicular (can.) membrane of the liver and the basolateral (blm) and brush border (bb) membranes of the intestine and kidney is indicated. The presence of additional carrier-systems (?) is conjectural. The numbers given in parentheses represent estimated organ clearances *in vivo* (ml/min).

The contribution of the intestinal mucosa to the systemic Cl will depend on the E of the liver. Because the mucosal blood flow (Q_{muc}) and the liver are in series the Cl_{muc} and Cl_h cannot simply be summed. The total Cl of the intestine-liver-system can be described as follows: $Cl_{tot} = E_h \cdot Q_h + E_{muc} \cdot Q_{muc} \cdot (1-E_h)$, according to Gillette (1982). It can be seen that intestinal metabolism only influences the total Cl when E_h is smaller than unity. Because $E_h = 1$ for N Cl_{tot} of the intestine-liver-system will equal Q_h (20 ml/min). Intestinal metabolism will, however, affect the appearance rate of NG in the bile. NG formed in the intestinal epithelium does not appear in the bile, while half of the NG formed in the liver enters the bile. Although Cl_{tot} remains equal when part of the N is metabolized in the intestinal epithelium (instead of in the liver), the biliary excretion of NG will decrease in the case of intestinal metabolism.

The total systemic clearance of N in the rat can be calculated to amount to 30.8 ml/min (Cl_r plus Cl_{tot} in intestine and liver). This compares favourably to the *in vivo* Cl_r of N (138 ml/min/kg) that can be calculated from the data given by Mistry and Houston (1985). This indicates that the *in vivo* Cl of N can largely be explained by metabolism in the liver, intestine and kidney. Essentially the same conclusion was reached by Tremaine et al. (1985).

Carriers for naphthyl-β,D-glucuronide

It has been suggested before that NG is most likely to leave the cell by carrier-mediated transport (Schwenk, 1985). In view of the important role of glucuronidation in drug elimination, it is rather surprising that so little direct evidence of carrier-mediated transport of glucuronides is available (reviewed by Hewitt and Hook, 1983; Klaassen and Watkins, 1984). We have now demonstrated in isolated perfused organ preparations of the rat that NG was transported in the liver canalicular membrane and in both the basolateral and the brush border membrane of the intestine and kidney by carrier-mediated mechanisms. TR⁻ rats have deficient hepatic canalicular transport of organic anions with the exception of bile salts (Jansen et al., 1987). Biliary excretion of NG was also impaired. This suggests that in the liver excretion of NG from liver into bile occurs *via* the same pathway used by bilirubin-glucuronide, S-glutathionyl-tetrabromosulfophthalein and dibromosulfophthalein. Renal tubular excretion and intestinal transport of NG was not affected in the TR⁻ rat. In an earlier study it was found that renal excretion of bilirubin glucuronides partly compensates for the defective canalicular excretion in order to keep serum bilirubin levels within reasonable limits (Jansen et al., 1985). Thus, transport mechanisms in the intestine and kidney seem to differ from the hepatic canalicular transport pathway for organic anions. Definitive proof for this has to await the purification and characterization of the carrier-proteins involved. Isolated perfused organs, on the other hand, will remain invaluable for establishing the role of carrier-mechanisms in local pharmacokinetic processes.

REFERENCES

Cassidy, M.K. and Houston, J.B. (1984): *In vivo* capacity of hepatic and extrahepatic enzymes to conjugate phenol. *Drug Metab. Dispos.* 12, 619-624.

De Vries, M.H., Groothuis, G.M.M., Mulder, G.J., Nguyen, H. and Meijer, D.K.F. (1985): Secretion of the organic anion harmol sulfate from liver into blood. Evidence for a carrier-mediated, mechanism. *Biochem. Pharmacol.* 34, 2129-2135.

De Vries, M.H., Hofman, G.A. and Koster, A.Sj. (1987): Intestinal transport of glucuronides. *Z. Gastroenterol.* 25, 623-624 (abstract).

De Vries, M.H., Hofman, G.A., Koster, A.Sj. and Noordhoek, J. (1988): Flow dependence of systemic and presystemic intestinal metabolism. *Progr. Pharmacol.* (in press).

Gillette, J.R. (1982): Sequential organ first pass effects: simple methods for constructing compartmental pharmacokinetic models form physiological models of drug disposition by several organs. *J. Pharm. Sci.* 71, 673-677.

Hartmann, F., Vieillard-Baron, D. and Heinrich, R. (1984): Isolated perfusion of the small intestine using perfluorotributylamine as artifical oxygen carrier. *Adv. Exp. Med. Biol.* 180, 711-720.

Hewitt, W.R. and Hook, J.B. (1983): The renal excretion of drugs. *Progr. Drug Metab.* 7, 11-56.

Jansen, P.L.M., Peters, W.H.M. and Lamers, W.H. (1985): Hereditary chronic conjugated hyperbilirubinemia in mutant rats caused by defective hepatic anion transport. *Hepatology* 5, 573-579.

Jansen, P.L.M., Groothuis, G.M.M., Peters, W.H.M. and Meijer, D.K.F. (1987): Selective hepatobiliary transport defect for organic anions and neutral steroids in mutant rats with hereditary-conjugated hyperbilirubinemia. *Hepatology* 7, 71-76.

Klaassen, C.D. and Watkins, J.B. (1984): Mechanisms of bile formation, hepatic uptake, and biliary excretion. *Pharmacol. Rev.* 36, 1-67.

Klippert, P.J.M. and Noordhoek, J. (1983): Influence of administration route and blood sampling site on the area under the curve. *Drug Metab. Dispos.* 11, 62-66.

Koster, A.Sj. (1985): Intestinal glucuronidation. *In vivo* and *in vitro* model systems. In *Advances in glucuronide conjugation*, ed Matern, S., Bock, K.W. and Gerok, W., pp. 177-195. Lancaster, UK: MTP-Press.

Machida, M., Morita, Y., Hayashi, M. and Awazu, S. (1982): Pharmacokinetic evidence for the occurrence of extrahepatic conjugative metabolism of p-nitrophenol in rats. *Biochem Pharmacol.* 31, 787-791.

Meijer, D.K.F., Keulemans, G.T.P. and Mulder, G.J. (1981): Isolated perfused rat liver technique. *Meth. Enzymol.* 77, 81-94.

Mistry, M. and Houston, J.B. (1985): Quantitation of extrahepatic metabolism. Pulmonary and intestinal conjugation of naphthol. *Drug Metab. Dispos.* 13, 740-745.

Mulder, G.J., Weitering, J.G., Scholtens, E., Dawson, J.R. and Pang, K.S. (1984): Extrahepatic sulfation and glucuronidation in the rat *in vivo*. Determination of the extrahepatic extraction ratio of harmol and the extrahepatic contribution to harmol conjugation. *Biochem. Pharmacol.* 33, 3081-3087.

Redegeld, F.A.M. and Noordhoek, J. (1986): Active tubular secretion of 1-naphthyl-β,D-glucuronide in the isolated perfused rat kidney. *Drug Metab. Dispos.* 14, 622-624.

Redegeld, F.A.M., De Vries, M.H., Koster, A.Sj., De Haan, J.G., Oude Elferink, R.P.J. and Jansen, P.L.M. (1987): Renal and intestinal transport of 1-naphthyl-β,D-glucuronide in the transport mutated rat. 47th. Int. Congress of Pharm. Sci. of F.I.P., p. 76 (abstract).

Redegeld, F.A.M., Hofman, G.A. and Noordhoek, J. (1988): Conjugative clearance of 1-naphthol and disposition of its glucuronide and sulfate conjugates in the isolated perfused rat kidney. *J. Pharmacol. Exp. Therap.* 244, 263-267.

Roth, R.A. and Rubin, R.J. (1976): Role of blood flow in carbon monoxide and hypoxic hypoxia-induced alterations in hexobarbital metabolism in rats. *Drug Metab. Dispos.* 4, 460-467.

Schwenk, M. (1985): Glucuronide conjugation in isolated cells from intestine, liver and kidney. In *Advances in glucuronide conjugation*, ed Matern, S., Bock, K.W. and Gerok, W., pp. 165-175. Lancaster, UK: MTP-Press.

Tremaine, L.M., Diamond, G.L. and Quebbemann, A.J. (1985): Quantitative determination of organ contribution to excretory metabolism. *J. Pharmacol. Meth.* 13, 9-35.

Wilkinson, G.R. (1987): Clearance approaches in pharmacology. *Pharmacol. Rev.* 39, 1-47.

Résumé

Le métabolisme du 1-naphtol et le transport du 1-naphtyl-β,D-glucuronide ont été étudiés sur des préparations de foie, intestin et rein perfusés et vascularisés de rat.

Dans le foie et le rein, la clearance du 1-naphtol est très efficace et approche la valeur du débit du liquide de perfusion de l'organe. Dans l'intestin, seul le perfusat à travers la muqueuse est complétement débarrassé de N. Ces résultats indiquent que la clearance du 1-naphtol, in vivo, peut être expliquée principalement par son métabolisme dans ces organes. Il a été démontré que le 1-naphtyl-β,D-glucuronide est transporté par un mécanisme mettant en jeu un transporteur au travers de la membrane canaliculaire du foie et la membrane basolatérale et bordure en brosse de l'intestin et du rein. Ces mécanismes de transport sont sensibles à l'inhibition par la phloridzine (dans l'intestin) ou le probenecid (dans le rein). Le transport au travers des membranes canaliculaires hépatiques est réduit dans les rats TR^- qui possèdent une déficience génétique pour l'excrétion biliaire d'anions organiques. Ces résultats suggèrent qu'il existe des différences considérables entre les mécanismes de transport du 1-naphtyl-β,D-glucuronide dans le foie, l'intestin et le rein.

Saturation of glucuronidation in the *in situ* intestine

Curtis D. Klaassen and Daniel Goon

University of Kansas Medical Center, Kansas City, Kansas, USA

Abstract.

Phase II biotransformation in the intestine has been demonstrated for numerous endogenous and exogenous compounds. Agents containing a phenolic moiety are particularly prone to extensive glucuronidation and sulfation in the intestine. In the present studies, an *in situ* isolated intestinal loop preparation has been used to investigate the capacity of the rat intestine to conjugate the phenolic compounds acetaminophen (AA), harmol (HA) and 1-naphthol (NA). At low doses of each compound, the respective glucuronic acid conjugate was the major intestinal metabolite formed. However, as higher doses of each compound were administered, intestinal glucuronidation became capacity-limited. Saturation of the glucuronidation pathway in the rat intestine was approached upon intraluminal administration of 14 μmol AA, 2 μmol HA and 1 μmol NA. Administration of higher doses of each agent failed to produce concomitant increases in the maximum concentration of the respective glucuronide attained in the portal circulation. The intestinal concentration of UDP-glucuronic acid (UDP-GA), the co-substrate for glucuronidation, and its immediate precursor, UDP-glucose (UDPG), were both decreased 45 percent following intraluminal exposure to 66 μmol AA. In contrast, intestinal UDPG concentrations were unchanged in rats administered HA (20 μmol) or NA (10 μmol); whereas intestinal UDP-GA concentrations were decreased 85 and 73 percent, respectively. Pretreatment of rats with *trans*-stilbene oxide (TSO), a microsomal enzyme inducer, increased the *in vitro* activity of UDP-glucuronosyltransferase (UDP-GT) directed toward AA (1.9-fold), HA (2.4-fold) and NA (1.8-fold) in isolated intestinal microsomes. Concurrently, pretreatment of rats with TSO produced no appreciable effect on either UDPG or UDP-GA concentrations in the intestine. Following TSO pretreatment, *in situ* intestinal glucuronidation of AA and HA was enhanced 2.7- and 1.5-fold, respectively. In contrast, *in situ* intestinal glucuronidation of NA was unaffected by pretreatment with TSO. Similarly, rats pretreated with 3-methylcholanthrene exhibited no increase in the *in situ* glucuronidation of NA in the intestine despite a greater than two-fold increase in UDP-GT activity in intestinal microsomes *in vitro*. Thus, capacity-limited intestinal glucuronidation of AA and HA is apparently mediated by saturation of microsomal UDP-GT; whereas glucuronidation of NA in the intestine is capacity-limited by some other mechanism, such as the availability of substrate or co-substrate.

Keywords: Glucuronidation, intestine, UDP-glucuronic acid, UDP-glucuronosyltransferase, acetaminophen, harmol, 1-naphthol

Introduction.

Historically, the ability of the rat intestine to glucuronidate xenobiotics was demonstrated initially in the mid-1950's (Hartiala, 1954; 1955; Shirai and Ohkubo, 1954). Over the ensuing years, intestinal biotransformation has gained increasing recognition as a potentially important element in the disposition of xenobiotics. Currently, it is recognized that phenolic compounds, in particular, are prone to both glucuronidation and sulfation in the intestine (Hartiala, 1973; 1975). In the studies described herein the capacity of the rat intestine to glucuronidate acetaminophen, harmol and 1-naphthol has been studied *in situ* with an isolated intestinal loop preparation with complete venous blood collection. This model system offers the distinct and powerful advantage of direct assessment of both intestinal absorption and biotransformation under conditions which closely parallel the whole animal.

Dose-Response Studies.

Initial studies were conducted to characterize intestinal glucuronidation of acetaminophen, harmol and 1-naphthol in the rat *in situ* in response to different doses of each parent compound. Under urethane-induced anesthesia, the left jugular vein was cannulated followed by isolation of the intestinal loop and cannulation of the corresponding mesenteric vein. The intestinal loop was isolated and prepared by adaptation of the methods described by Winne (1966) and Riegelman and Barr (1970). Acetaminophen (6.6-66 μmol), harmol (2-20 μmol) or 1-naphthol (0.1-10 μmol) was then injected directly into the lumen of the loop in a volume of 1.0 ml. All mesenteric venous blood exiting from the isolated intestinal segment was collected continuously for 60 min, while donor blood was infused via the jugular cannula at approximately the same rate as collected from the mesenteric cannula. At the end of 60 min, the remaining luminal fluid also was collected. Blood and luminal samples were analyzed as follows: acetaminophen and its metabolites were separated and quantitated by modification of the isocratic reverse-phase HPLC method of Howie *et al.*, (1977); harmol and its metabolites were separated by thin-layer chromatography and quantitated fluorometrically by adaptation of the method described by Mulder and Hagedoorn (1974); 1-naphthol and its biotransformation products were assayed by isocratic reverse-phase, ion-pair HPLC and UV absorbance detection at 280 nm (Rhodes and Houston, 1981) or liquid scintillation spectroscopy.

Figures 1-3 present the time-course of acetaminophen-, harmol- and naphthol-glucuronide concentrations, respectively, in the mesenteric venous (portal) blood following intraluminal administration of various doses of the respective parent compound. For all 3 compunds, the respective glucuronic acid conjugate was readily detected in the portal circulation within 3 min after intraluminal administration of the parent compound. As indicated in Fig. 1, maximal blood concentrations of acetaminophen-glucuronide were attained within 12 min after administration of all doses of acetaminophen studied. However, the maximum concentration of acetaminophen-glucuronide attained in the portal circulation upon administration of 14 μmol acetaminophen was not increased significantly when the dose was increased further to 30 and 66 μmol. In addition,

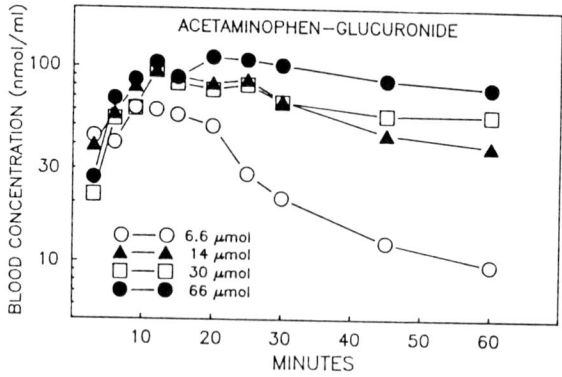

Fig. 1. Acetaminophen-glucuronide concentration in the mesenteric venous (portal) blood after intraluminal administration of various doses of acetaminophen.

no significant differences in portal blood concentration of acetaminophen-glucuronide were noted at any time between rats administered 30 or 66 μmol acetaminophen. Moreover, the cumulative formation of acetaminophen-glucuronide (*i.e.*, blood content plus luminal content) after 60 min was similar in rats administered 30 or 66 μmol acetaminophen (data not shown).

Similar to acetaminophen, harmol-glucuronide concentrations rapidly reached maximal levels within 9 min after administration of harmol and remained relatively constant throughout the remainder of the experimental period. The maximum portal blood concentration of harmol-glucuronide attained upon administration of 2 μmol harmol was not increased further by administration of 20 or 200 μmol of parent compound. Additionally, the cumulative formation of harmol-glucuronide after 60 min was similar at all doses of harmol studied (data not shown).

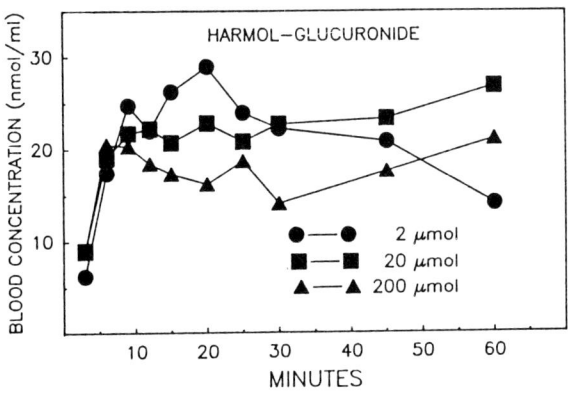

Fig. 2. Portal blood concentration of harmol-glucuronide after intraluminal administration of various doses of harmol.

The general trends noted with acetaminophen and harmol were observed also with 1-naphthol. Specifically, at all doses studied, maximal blood levels of naphthol-glucuronide were attained soon after administration of 1-naphthol (6-9 min). At all times, the concentration of naphthol-

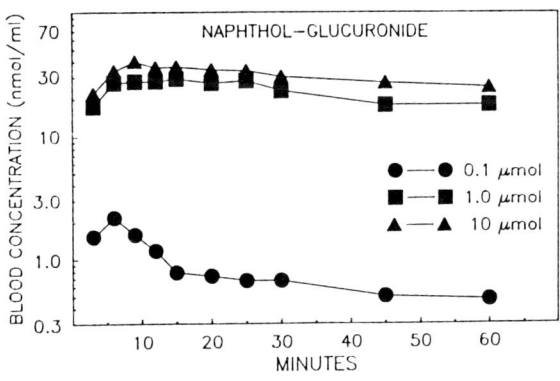

Fig. 3. Naphthol-glucuronide concentrations in the portal circulation after intraluminal administration of various doses of 1-naphthol.

161

glucuronide in the portal circulation of rats administered either 1.0 or 10 μmol 1-naphthol was at least an order of magnitude higher than in animals administered 0.1 μmol of the parent compound. However, no significant differences were noted in the blood concentration of naphthol-glucuronide upon administration of the two higher doses of 1-naphthol (1.0 and 10 μmol). Furthermore, the cumulative formation of naphthol-glucuronide after 60 min was similar after administration of 1.0 or 10 μmol 1-naphthol (data not shown).

These results demonstrate that glucuronidation of acetaminophen, harmol and 1-naphthol in the rat intestine *in situ* is capacity-limited. As the intraluminally administered dose of each compound is increased, this fact is borne out by: (1) the failure to note further increases in the maximum blood concentration attained by each glucuronic acid conjugate in the portal circulation, and (2) the similarity in cumulative formation of the respective glucuronic acid conjugate at high doses of parent compound.

Effect of Xenobiotic Exposure on Intestinal Co-substrate Levels.

In theory, in the presence of excess substrate, capacity-limited glucuronidation may result from two possible mechanisms. Specifically, glucuronidation may be limited by: the availability of the endogenous co-substrate for glucuronidation, UDP-glucuronic acid (UDP-GA); or saturation of the enzyme which catalyzes glucuronidation, UDP-glucuronosyltransferase (UDP-GT). To test the former hypothesis, intestinal concentrations of UDP-GA and its immediate precursor, UDP-glucose (UDPG), were assessed following intraluminal administration of a high dose of acetaminophen, harmol or 1-naphthol. The concentrations of UDPG and UDP-GA in intestinal loops isolated *in situ* were measured 20 min after administration of 66 μmol acetaminophen, 20 μmol harmol or 10 μmol 1-naphthol directly into the lumen of the loop. Control animals received 1.0 ml of vehicle intraluminally for 20 min. Intestinal samples were processed by modification of the procedure described by Dills and Klaassen (1985) and the concentrations of UDPG and UDP-GA determined by isocratic reverse phase, ion-pair HPLC with UV absorbance detection at 254 nm (Aw and Jones, 1982).

As shown in Fig. 4 (top panel), only acetaminophen exposure appreciably affected intestinal UDPG concentration (54 percent of control levels). In contrast, intestinal UDP-GA concentrations were decreased significantly by intraluminal exposure to all three compounds, though to varying degrees. In rats exposed to 20 μmol harmol or 10 μmol 1-naphthol, intestinal loop concentrations of UDP-GA were decreased markedly to 15 and 23 percent of control values, respectively. In comparison, intraluminal administration of acetaminophen (66 μmol) produced a more moderate decrease in intestinal co-substrate content (56 percent of control animals). The results of these studies demonstrate that intestinal UDP-GA concentrations were decreased significantly within 20 min after intraluminal administration of a relatively high dose of acetaminophen, harmol or 1-naphthol. Thus, these observations strongly imply that co-substrate depletion may be a critical factor restricting the capacity of the rat intestine to glucuronidate xenobiotics.

Role of UDP-GT Saturation in Capacity-Limited Intestinal Glucuronidation.

Although the results presented above implicate co-substrate availability as an important factor limiting the glucuronidation capacity of the rat intestine *in situ*, saturation of intestinal UDP-GT activity remains unchallenged as a potential causative mechanism. In both the liver and intestine, UDP-GT comprises a family of inducible microsomal isozymes (Dutton, 1980; Koster *et al.*, 1986). Thus, microsomal enzyme inducers can be used to assess whether the activity of UDP-GT limits the endogenous glucuronidation capacity of a particular organ or tissue. In practice, observation of enhanced glucuronide formation *in vivo* following pretreatment with an inducing agent suggests saturation of UDP-GT activity in the non-induced animal. However, many known inducers of hepatic UDP-GT activity also have the propensity to increase the concentration of UDP-GA in the liver (Watkins and Klaassen, 1982). A similar conjoined effect of microsomal enzyme inducers upon UDP-GT activity and co-substrate concentration in the intestine has not been investigated. Therefore, a series of experiments were initiated in an attempt to identify an agent(s) that would induce intestinal UDP-GT activity directed toward

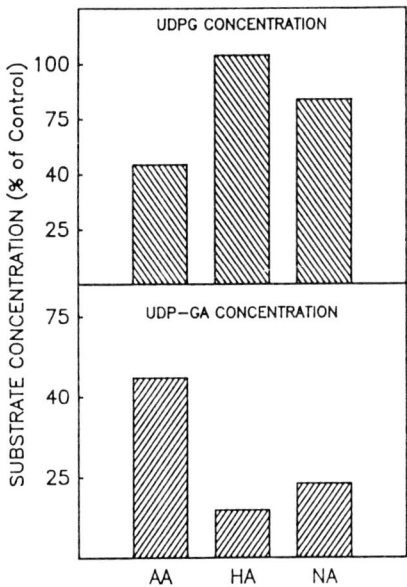

Fig. 4. Effect of acetaminophen (AA), harmol (HA) and 1-naphthol (NA) upon intestinal UDPG (upper panel) and UDP-GA concentrations (lower panel).

acetaminophen, harmol and/or 1-naphthol without concomitantly increasing intestinal UDP-GA concentration. Toward this end, rats were treated with: butylated hydroxyanisole (BHA; 1% w/w in diet for 10 days); benzo[a]pyrene (BaP; 100 mg/kg, single dose p.o.); 3-methylcholanthrene (3MC; 100 mg/kg, single dose p.o.); phenobarbital (1 mg/ml in drinking water for 4 days); pregnenolone-16α-carbonitrile (PCN; 75 mg/kg p.o. for 4 days); trans-stilbene oxide (TSO; 390 mg/kg, p.o. for 5 days); 2,3,7,8-tetrachlorodibenzo-p-dioxin (TCDD; 8 μg/kg, single dose p.o. 10 days prior); or corn oil (CON; 5 ml/kg, p.o. for 4 days). The oral route of administration was used as intestinal UDP-GT activity is enhanced more effectively when inducers are administered by this route than after intraperitoneal administration (Hietanen et al., 1980). Upon completion of inducer treatment, rats were anesthetized with urethane and two 1.0 g samples of proximal small intestinal were collected from each animal. One set of samples was processed and used for the determination of UDP-GA concentration as described above. Intestinal microsomes were prepared from the second set of samples by modification of the procedure of Lu and Levin (1972) and microsomal UDP-GT activity directed toward acetaminophen, harmol and 1-naphthol assessed in vitro. In these assays, the final incubation volume was 0.5 ml and contained Tris-HCl (200 mM, pH 7.7 at room temperature), magnesium chloride (10 mM), UDP-GA (4 mM); D-saccharic-1,4-lactone (1.25 mM), microsomal protein (0.5-4.0 mg/ml) and aglycone (5 mM acetaminophen; 0.8 mM harmol; or 1 mM [1-^{14}C]-1-naphthol, 0.2 μCi/μmol) at the final concentrations indicated. In the determination of harmol-glucuronide formation, microsomes were solubilized initially in 0.01% Triton X-100.

The results of these experiments are summarized in Fig. 5. As indicated in the upper panel, the formation of naphthol-glucuronide by intestinal microsomes in vitro was augmented substantially by treatment with BHA, BaP, 3MC or TSO in vivo. Similarly, treatment with BHA, BaP or TSO enhanced microsomal formation of acetaminophen-glucuronide and harmol-glucuronide (data not shown). However, treatment with BHA or BaP also significantly increased intestinal UDP-GA concentrations (lower panel). In contrast, neither 3MC nor TSO appreciably affected UDP-GA concentrations in the intestine. These results demonstrate that 3MC and TSO offer the advantage of selectively enhancing intestinal UDP-GT activity without concomitantly increasing intestinal UDP-GA concentration in the rat. Thus, 3MC and TSO are potentially powerful investigational tools for studying the mechanism(s) of capacity-limited glucuronidation in the rat intestine.

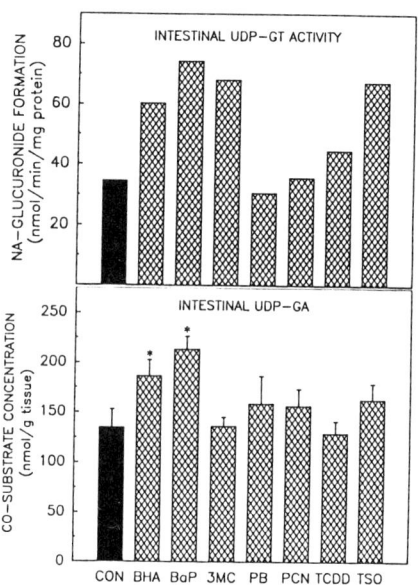

Fig. 5. Effect of various microsomal enzyme inducers upon intestinal UDP-GT activity directed toward 1-naphthol (upper panel) and intestinal UDP-GA concentration (lower panel).

Based upon the results presented, a final series of experiments were conducted to evaluate the possible role of UDP-GT activity in mediating capacity-limited intestinal glucuronidation in the rat. After pretreatment with TSO (as described above), intestinal glucuronidation of acetaminophen (66 μmol), harmol (20 μmol) and 1-naphthol (10 μmol) was assessed with the isolated intestinal loop preparation *in situ* as previously described. In addition, intestinal naphthol glucuronidation *in situ* was assessed after 3MC pretreatment. Control animals were administered corn oil p.o. for four days.

As seen in Fig. 6, neither 3MC nor TSO pretreatment augmented the portal blood concentration of naphthol-glucuronide (upper panel). Additionally, the cumulative formation of naphthol-glucuronide after 60 min was similar between control, 3MC- and TSO-pretreated rats (data not shown). In contrast, the portal blood concentrations of the glucuronic acid conjugate of both harmol and acetaminophen were altered markedly by pretreatment with TSO. Specifically, at 20 min and all later times, portal blood concentrations of harmol-glucuronide in TSO-pretreated rats

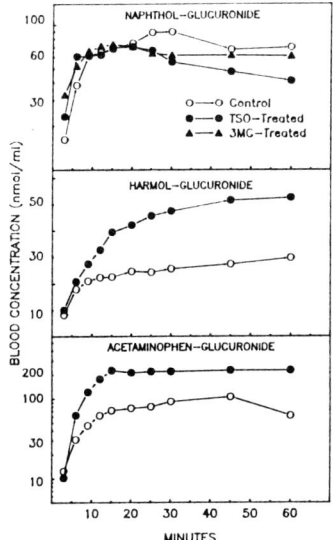

Fig. 6. Effect of UDP-GT induction upon intestinal glucuronidation of 1-naphthol (upper panel), harmol (middle panel) and acetaminophen (lower panel) *in situ.*

were approximately twice control levels (middle panel). Similarly, the concentration of acetaminophen in the portal circulation of TSO-pretreated rats was 100-200 percent greater than in control rats at 6 min and all later times (lower panel). Moreover, the cumulative formation of harmol-glucuronide and acetaminophen-glucuronide was 175 and 290 percent greater in TSO-pretreated rats, respectively, than in control animals (data not shown). These results suggest that glucuronidation of harmol and acetaminophen in the rat intestine is capacity-limited by saturation of intestinal UDP-GT activity. However, the limited capacity of the rat intestine to glucuronidate 1-naphthol appears to result from a different mechanism. Although evidence presented herein appear to imply that co-substrate availability may limit the capacity of the rat intestine to glucuronidate 1-naphthol, the observed extent of acetaminophen-glucuronide formation argues against co-substrate depletion as a primary limiting factor. Instead, the intracellular availability of 1-naphthol presents an alternative explanation. This hypothesis is supported here by the observation that less than 8 percent of the portal blood content of 1-naphthol at the end of 60 min was represented by the parent compound (data not shown). Thus, intraluminally administered 1-naphthol was nearly completely biotransformed prior to absorption into the portal circulation. In addition, Koster and Noordhoek (1983) have shown that the extent of naphthol-glucuronide formation following serosal administration of 1-naphthol was two to three times greater than after mucosal administration, suggesting that intestinal glucuronidation of 1-naphthol is limited by uptake of the substrate upon intraluminal administration.

Summary.

In conclusion, intestinal glucuronidation of acetaminophen, harmol and 1-naphthol in the rat *in situ* has been shown to be capacity-limited. Despite the observation of significantly decreased

UDP-GA concentrations in the intestine following intraluminal exposure to these compounds, the glucuronidation capacity of the rat intestine does not appear to be restricted by co-substrate availability. Instead, the results presented indicate that intestinal glucuronidation of acetaminophen and harmol is limited by the activity of UDP-GT in the intestine. However, in the case of 1-naphthol, uptake of substrate from the intestinal lumen appears to be the critical factor limiting intestinal glucuronidation in the rat.

References.

Aw, T.Y. and Jones, D.P. (1980): Direct determination of UDP-glucuronic acid in cell extracts by high-performance liquid chromatography. Anal. Biochem. 127, 32-36.

Barr, W.H. and Riegelman, S. (1970): Intestinal drug absorption and metabolism. I: Comparison of methods and models to study physiological factors of *in vitro* and *in vivo* intestinal absorption. J. Pharm. Sci. 59, 154-163.

Dills, R.L. and Klaassen, C.D. (1985): An isocratic reverse-phase high-performance liquid chromatographic assay for adenosine nucleotides in rat liver. J. Pharmacol. Methods 14, 189-197.

Dutton, G.J. (1980): Glucuronidation of Drugs and Other Compounds, pp. 137-150. Boca Raton: CRC Press.

Hartiala, K.J.W. (1954): Studies on detoxication mechanisms with special reference to the glucuronide synthesis by the mucous membranes of the intestine. Acta Physiol. Scand. Suppl. 114, 20.

Hartiala, K.J.W. (1955). Studies on detoxication mechanisms. III: Glucuronide synthesis of various organs with special reference to the detoxifying capacity of the mucous membranes of the alimentary canal. Ann. Med. Exp. Biol. Fenn. 32, 239-245.

Hartiala, K.J.W. (1973). Metabolism of hormones, drugs and other substances by the gut. Physiol. Rev. 53, 496-534.

Hartiala, K. (1977). Metabolism of foreign substances in the gastrointestinal tract. In Handbook of Physiology, Section 9: Reactions to Environmental Agents, eds. D.H.K.Lee, H.L.Falk, H.L., S.D.Murphy, and S.R.Geiger, pp. 375-388. Washington, D.C.: American Physiology Society.

Hietanen, E., Laitinen, M. and Koivusaari, U. (1980): Effect of administration route of 3-methylcholanthrene on the inducibility of intestinal drug metabolizing enzymes. Enzyme 25, 153-157.

Howie, D., Adriaenssens, P. and Prescott, L.F. (1977): Paracetamol metabolism following overdosage: Application of high-performance liquid chromatography. J. Pharm. Pharmacol. 29, 234-237.

Koster, A. Sj., and Noordhoek, J. (1983): Glucuronidation in isolated perfused rat intestinal segments after mucosal and serosal administration of 1-naphthol. J. Pharmacol. Exp. Ther. 226, 533-538.

Koster, A. Sj., Schirmer, G. and Bock, K.W. (1986): Immunochemical and functional characterization of UDP-glucuronosyltransferases from rat liver, intestine and kidney. Biochem. Pharmacol. 35, 3971-3975.

Lu, A.Y.H. and Levin, W. (1972): Partial purification of cytochrome *P*-450 and cytochrome *P*-448 from rat liver microsomes. Biochem. Biophys. Res. Commun. 46, 1334-1339.

Mulder, G.J. and Hagedoorn, A.H. (1974): UDP-glucuronyltransferase and phenolsulfotransferase *in vivo* and *in vitro*. Conjugation of harmol and harmalol. Biochem. Pharmacol. 23, 2101-2109.

Rhodes, J.C. and Houston, J.B. (1981): Quantification of naphthyl conjugates. Comparison of high-performance liquid chromatography and selected enzyme hydrolysis methods. Xenobiotica 11, 63-70.

Shirai, Y. and Ohkubo, T. (1954): Synthesis of glucuronides by tissue slices. I. J. Biochem. 41, 341-344.

Watkins, J.B. and Klaassen, C.D. (1982): Chemically-induced alteration of UDP-glucuronic acid concentration in rat liver. Drug Metab. Dispos. 11, 37-40.

Winne, D. (1966): Der Einfluss einiger Pharmaka auf die Darmdurchblutung und die Resorption tritiummarkierten Wassers aus dem Dünndarm der Ratte. Naunyn-Schmiedeberg's Arch. Pharmacol. 254, 199-224.

Résumé

Il a été démontré l'existence de biotransformation de phase II pour de nombreux xénobiotiques et composés endogènes dans l'intestin. Les substances comportant un noyau phényle sont sujettes à une glucuronoconjugaison et sulfoconjugaison extensives dans l'intestin.

Dans cette étude, une anse intestinale isolée, in situ, a été utilisée pour déterminer la capacité de l'intestin de rat à conjuguer les composés phénoliques suivants: acétaminophènes (AA), harmol (HA) et 1-naphtol (NA). A faibles doses, ces composés sont principalement glucuronoconjugués. Cependant, si la dose administrée augmente, l'intestin devient limité dans ces capacités à glucuronuconjuguer. La saturation de la voie de glucuronoconjugaison dans l'intestin de rat est obtenue par une administration intraluminale approchant 14 umoles de AA, 2 umoles de HA et 1 umole de NA. L'administration de doses supérieures, pour chaque composé, ne produit pas une augmentation simultanée du glucuronide correspondant dans la circulation portale. La concentration intestinale en acide UDP-glucuronique (UDPGA), le co-substrat de la conjugaison, et celle de son précurseur immédiat, l'UDP-glucose (UDPG), sont tous les deux diminués (45 %) après une administration luminale de AA à la dose de 66 umoles. Au contraire, la concentration instestinale en UDPG reste inchangée après administration de HA (20 umoles) et de NA (10 umoles) ; tandis que la concentration intestinale en UDPGA diminue de 85 et 73 % respectivement. Un prétraitement des rats par le trans-stilbène oxyde (TSO), un inducteur des enzymes microsomales, augmente l'activité in vitro de l'UDP-glucuronosyltransférase (UDPGT) envers AA (1,9 fois), HA (2,4 fois) et NA (1,8 fois) dans les microsomes d'intestin isolé. De même le prétraitement de rats avec TSO ne change pas de façon appréciable les concentrations intestinales en UDPG et UDPGA. Après traitement par le TSO, la glucuronoconjugaison intestinale in situ de AA et HA est augmentée de 2,7 et 1,5 fois respectivement. Au contraire, la glucuronoconjugaison dans l'intestin in situ du NA n'est pas affectée. De même, des rats prétraités par le 3-méthylcholanthrène n'ont pas de glucuronoconjugaison de NA augmentée dans l'intestin in situ, en dépit d'une augmentation supérieure à 2 fois de l'activité UDPGT dans les microsomes intestinaux in vitro. Ainsi, la glucuronoconjugaison limitée dans l'intestin de AA et HA dépend apparemment de la saturation de l'UDPGT microsomale ; tandis que la glucuronoconjugaison intestinale de NA est limitée par d'autres mécanismes telle la disponibilité en substrats et co-substrats.

Enzymatic protection of the brain : role of 1-naphthol UDP-glucuronosyltransferase from cerebral tissue and cerebral microvessels

J.-F. Ghersi-Egea*, Y. Tayarani**, J.-M. Lefauconnier** and A. Minn*

*Université de Nancy-I, Centre du Médicament, U.A. CNRS n° 597, 30 rue Lionnois, 54000 Nancy, France, and **INSERM U 26, Hôpital Fernand-Widal, 200 rue du Faubourg Saint-Denis, 75475 Paris Cedex 10, France

ABSTRACT

The brain is protected from chemical insult by the blood-brain barrier, formed by the endothelial cells of the cerebral microvasculature having tight sealed junctions and devoid of transcytosis. Some enzymes metabolizing both endogenous and exogenous substrates are present in the brain parenchyma as well as in brain microvessels, and are also involved in this protection.

Among these enzymes, we showed and characterized the isoform of UDPGT conjugating 1-naphthol in rat brain microsomes. We also showed the presence of this isoform in isolated brain microvessels, where its activity was higher than in brain homogenate. Therefore, this enzyme seems to be involved in the enzymatic blood-brain barrier.

We did not observe sex- or strain-linked variations in the rat, excepted for Gunn rats, where the genetic defect of UDPGT reported in the liver was also observed in isolated brain microvessels. The measured Km was of the same magnitude than that measured in the microsomes of both brain and liver. No activity was observed in both rabbit brain fractions.

The measurement of the uptake of 1-naphthol glucuronide by isolated microvessels showed that a weak saturable transport occurred.

KEY WORDS

UDP-Glucuronosyltransferases, Brain, Blood-brain barrier, Transport.

INTRODUCTION

The brain is a heterogenous organ protected from exogenous and endogenous chemical aggressions by the blood-brain barrier, which is constituted by the endothelial cells of cerebral capillaries. These microvessels show continuous, tightly sealed intercellular junctions and practically no transcytosis. As a consequence, polar substances present in the blood of cerebral circulation, whose liposolubility is insufficient to allow a passive diffusion across the cell phospholipid membranes, cannot reach the brain parenchyma (Oldendorf, 1977). Only nutrient substrates or precursors necessary for brain metabolism and functions can cross this barrier by the means of relatively specific transport mecanisms (Pardridge, 1984). Moreover, the endothelial cells contain enzymes which metabolize most endogenous blood-borne neuroactive substances (Lasbennes et al., 1983).

The cerebral metabolism of exogenous pharmacologically active or toxic molecules can participate to the brain protection mechanisms, as most of drug metabolizing enzymes are present, although in low quantities, in brain tissue (Mesnil et al., 1984). Glucuronides are hightly hydrophilic molecules, generally without pharmacologic or toxic properties. The study of UDPGT activities in the different cell populations of the brain is of great interest, as this enzyme is involved in both detoxification and endogenous metabolism: eventual competition, induction or inhibition of these activities may somewhat alter brain functions.

We recently characterized an isoform of UDPGT catalyzing the conjugation of 1-naphthol in the microsomal fraction isolated from the brain tissue (Ghersi-Egea et al., 1987). We showed that this 1-naphthol-UDPGT, as some other drug metabolizing enzymes, was also present in the isolated brain microvessels, where it had a higher specific activity than in the whole brain and was inducible by 3-methylcholantrene (Ghersi-Egea et al., 1988). To confirm the contribution of UDPGT to the protective functions of the blood-brain barrier, we studied the variations between species and rat strains of the UDPGT isoenzyme conjugating 1-naphthol, and we measured its kinetic parameters in isolated rat brain microvessels. We also studied the transport of 1-naphthol glucuronide through the cellular membranes of isolated microvessels.

MATERIAL AND METHODS

Sprague-Dawley rats (200 g), male Dunkin Hartley guinea pigs (450 g), (IFFA CREDO, St Germain sur l'Arbresle, France), male Wistar, Gunn heterozygous and homozygous rats (200 g, Dr. Leyten, University of Leuven, Belgium), and male Fauve de Bourgogne rabbits from local source (2.5 Kg) were used throughout.
For enzymatic determinations, the cerebral microvessel fraction was isolated according to Mrsulja et al. (1976), modified as previously described (Ghersi-Egea et al. 1988).

The activity of 1-naphthol-UDPGT was assayed at 37°C after activation with Triton X-100, using a High Performance Liquid Chromatography (HPLC) procedure for the measurement of 1-naphthol glucuronide (Ghersi-Egea et al., 1987).

The synthesis of $[^{14}C]$-1-naphthol-ß-D-glucuronide was achieved as follows: $[^{14}C]$-α-D-glucuronic acid (10 uCi, 1 umole) was incubated for 1 hour with 1-naphthol (1.75 umole) in the presence of liver activated microsomes (2 mg protein) isolated from 3-methylcholantrene pretreated rats, in a 30 mM Tris-HCl buffer, pH 7.4, containing 0.6 mM $MgCl_2$ (final volume 0.5 ml). The reaction was stopped with 0.5 ml acetonitrile, and the proteins were precipited by centrifugation. The supernatant was injected in a HPLC system using similar conditions than for the UDPGT assay. The enzymatically synthetized and purified glucuronide was collected, and the resulting fraction was evaporated to dryness under a nitrogen stream at 40°C, and dissolved in a small volume of distillated water. When this preparation was reinjected in the HPLC system, a radioactive detection, as well as an U.V. detection at 240 or 285 nm showed only one peak corresponding to the naphthol glucuronide.

The transport measurements were achieved after addition of the $[^{14}C]$-1-naphthol-ß-D-glucuronide (0.08 mM, 0.125 uCi) to a final volume of 0.250 ml of capillary suspension, according to the method of Tayarani et al. (1987).

RESULTS

1-Naphthol-UDP glucuronosyltransferase in brain microvessels.

As UDPGT is a membrane-bound enzyme, a detergent treatment of the preparation was required for removing the latency. A full activation of the enzymatic activity of cerebral microvessel fraction was obtained after Triton X-100 treatment, using a detergent to protein ratio of 0.1/1 (W/W). The measured activity was 3 times higher than in the native microvessel fraction (data not shown).

The results reported in Table I show that the 1-naphthol glucuronide formation did not change with sex or strain in rat brain microvessels, except for Gunn rats (54% decrease in

Table I. Formation of 1-naphthol glucuronide in brain microvessels from different species and strains of rat.
Specific activities are expressed in nmol/hr.mg protein as mean ± SD (n=4); ND: not detectable.

Species		Activity
Rabbit		ND
Guinea-pig		25.7 ± 1.1
Rat	(Sprague-Dawley male	15.8 ± 1.5
	(Sprague-Dawley female	15.1 ± 2.8
	(Wistar	16.7 ± 2.6
	(Gunn-heterozygous	7.7 ± 1.5
	(Gunn-homozygous	<1.5

heterozygous rat, and more than 90% decrease in homozygous rats). Thus, the genetic defect of UDPGT activity reported in the liver of Gunn rats (Weatherill and Burchell, 1978) was also observed in the endothelial cells of brain capillaries.

Some species differences were observed : for instance, no activity was detectable in rabbit brain microvessels whereas a high one was seen in those of guinea-pig.

Figure 1 shows the Hanes-Woolf representation of the affinity of UDPGT for 1-naphthol in rat brain microvessel homogenate. The apparent K_m we obtained (115 uM) was quite similar to that reported for liver or brain microsomes (Ghersi-Egea et al., 1987).

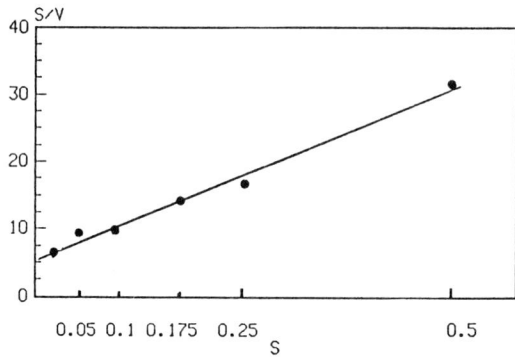

Figure 1. Hanes-Woolf representation of the affinity of UDPGT for 1-naphthol in isolated rat brain microvessels.
The concentration of UDP-glucuronic acid was 4.5 mM. Each point represents the mean of two measurements. Substrate concentrations (S) were expressed as mM, velocities (V) were expressed as nmol/hour.mg protein. The Vmax and apparent K_m were 19.3 nmol/hour.mg protein and 115 uM respectively, with a correlation coefficient r = 0.99.

[^{14}C]-1-naphthol-ß-D-glucuronide transport in isolated brain capillaries.

After incubation of the capillaries with [^{14}C]-1-naphthol-ß-D-glucuronide, a weak uptake was observed (Table II). It corresponded to 0.2 nmol/mg protein after 1 minute, and to 0.3 nmol/mg protein after 10 minutes. This uptake is low if compared to other endothelial transport systems, as those described for neutral aminoacids (total uptake 5 to 15 times higher, Tayarani et al., 1987) or for glucose (50 times higher, Betz et al., 1979). However the uptake of labelled glucuronide was reduced by 60% in the presence of 10 mM of non-labelled 1-naphthol glucuronide, indicating that the transport is saturable.

Table II : Brain capillary uptake of [^{14}C]-1-naphthol-ß-D-glucuronide.
The incubation with the labelled 1-naphthol glucuronide (0.08 mM) was carried out at various time intervals, in the absence or in the presence of a large amount of non-labelled molecule (mean of two measurements).

Total 1-naphthol glucuronide concentration		uptake (dpm/ug protein)
0.08 mM	(((	1 min : 2.6 2 min : 3.4 10 min : 4.5
10 mM	((	1 min : 1.0 10 min : 1.9

DISCUSSION

As shown in previous studies (Tayarani et al., 1987), the isolated microvessel fraction retained most of the specific properties of the intact endothelial cells. The activity of 1-naphthol-UDPGT reported in this work is that of the homogenate. It was relatively high as compared to that of brain homogenate (Vmax = 19.3 and 0.5 nmol/hour.mg protein respectively), indicating the capacity of the endothelial enzyme to efficiently protect the brain.

The other properties of the enzyme we reported here, such as optimal detergent activation, species and strains variations and Km, are similar to those we reported previously for the non capillary microsomal brain enzyme (Ghersi-Egea et al., 1987).

No detectable activity was found in both the rabbit brain microsomes and isolated brain microvessels, whereas the activity of conjugation of 1-naphthol has been reported in rabbit liver (Siest et al., 1985).

An important problem to be examined is how the brain eliminates the products of the activity of drug metabolizing enzymes. Isolated microvessels are useful for the study of transport phenomena occurring from the outside (in vivo : the brain) to the inside of endothelial cells. In these conditions, a low uptake of 1-naphthol glucuronide was observed, which seemed to be partially saturable and not only the result of a passive diffusion. This transport could be responsible at least in part for the elimination of glucuronides, both of endogenous or exogenous origin, formed by GT1 within the brain, another way of elimination being via the cerebrospinal fluid.

Although the physiological and pharmacological functions of UDPGT in the brain are poorly understood, its presence in cerebral microvessels suggests a function of this enzyme in the protection of the brain against chemical aggressions of both exogenous or endogenous origin. Some toxic or neuroactive molecules carried out by the blood of cerebral circulation may be metabolized in inactive, more water-soluble products, resulting in a role of *enzymatic blood-brain barrier* for UDPGT.

REFERENCES

Betz A.L., Csejtey J. and Goldstein G.W. (1979): Hexose transport and phosphorylation by capillaries isolated from rat brain. Amer. J. Physiol. 236, C96-C102.

Ghersi-Egea J.F., Walther B., Decolin D., Minn A. and Siest G. (1987): The activity of 1-naphthol-UDP-glucuronosyl-transferase in the rat brain. Neuropharmacology 26, 367-372.

Ghersi-Egea J.F., Minn A. and Siest G. (1988): A new aspect of the protective functions of the blood-brain barrier : activities of four drug metabolizing enzymes in isolated rat brain microvessels. Life Sci. 42, 2515-2523.

Lasbennes F., Sercombe R. and Seylaz J. (1983): Monoamine oxidase in brain microvessels determined using natural and artificial substrates : relevance to the blood-brain barrier. J. Cereb. Blood Flow Metabol. 3, 521-528.

Mesnil M., Testa B. and Jenner P. (1984): Xenobiotic metabolism by brain monooxygenases and other cerebral enzymes. In Advances in Drug Research, Academic Press, London, B. Testa Ed., vol. 13, pp 95-207.

Mrsulja B.B., Mrsulja B.J., Fujimoto T., Klatzo I. and Spatz M. (1976): Isolation of brain capillaries : a simplified technique. Brain Res. 110, 361-365.

Oldendorf W.H. (1971): Brain uptake of radiolabeled amino acids, amines and hexoses after arterial injection. Am. J. Physiol. 221, 1629-1639.

Pardridge W.M. (1984): Transport of nutrients and hormones through the blood-brain barrier. Fed. Proc. 43, 201-204.

Siest G., Boutin J.A., Magdalou J., Batt A.M., Antoine B., Fournel S. and Thomassin J. (1985): UDP-glucuronosyltransférase et glucuronoconjugaison. Thérapie 40, 139-153.

Tayarani Y., Lefauconnier J.M., Roux F. and Bourre J.M. (1987): Evidence for an alanine, serine, and cysteine system of transport in isolated brain capillaries. J. Cereb. Blood Flow Metabol. 7, 585-591.

Weatherill P.J. and Burchell B. (1978): Reactivation of a pure defective UDP-glucuronosyltransferase from homozygous Gunn rat liver. FEBS Lett. 87, 207-211.

Résumé

Le cerveau est protégé des agressions chimiques par la barrière hémoencéphalique, constituée chez les mammifères par les cellules de l'endothélium des microvaisseaux cérébraux, et caractérisée par des jonctions intercellulaires serrées et l'absence de transcytose. Certaines enzymes, capables de métaboliser des substrats exogènes, et présentes dans le tissu cérébral ou dans les capillaires cérébraux, participent également à cette protection.

Parmi celles-ci, nous avons mis en évidence et caractérisé dans les microsomes de cerveau une forme d'UDPGT conjugant le 1-naphtol. Nous avons également montré que cette isoforme est présente dans les capillaires cérébraux, où son activité est supérieure à celle de l'homogénat de cerveau total. Cette enzyme semble donc participer à la barrière hémoencéphalique enzymatique.

Il n'existe pas de variation liée au sexe ou à la souche chez le rat, excepté en ce qui concerne les rats Gunn, où la déficience génétique de l'activité UDPGT rapportée dans le foie est également observée dans les microvaisseaux cérébraux. Le K_m évalué dans les capillaires est du même ordre de grandeur que celui obtenu dans les microsomes de cerveau et de foie. L'activité mesurée est supérieure chez le cobaye, et totalement absente chez le lapin.

La mesure du prélèvement par les capillaires de cerveau du glucuronide de naphtol marqué montre qu'il existe un transport saturable de ce glucuronide à travers les membranes des cellules endothéliales cérébrales.

Difference in UDP-glucuronosyltransferases between rat and hamster

Z. Jayyosi, B. Antoine, J. Thomassin, J. Magdalou, A.-M. Batt and G. Siest

Université de Nancy, I, Centre du Médicament, U.A. CNRS n° 597, 30, rue Lionnois, Nancy, France

ABSTRACT

UDP-glucuronosyltransferase activities measured with eight aglycones have been compared in rat and hamster liver microsomes. The scale of activities, i.e. high activities towards planar aglycones (-GT1-) and lower activities for bulkier aglycones (-GT2-) observed in other mammals was also found in hamster, although glucuronidation towards testosterone, morphine and chloramphenicol was proportionally higher in this species. UDP-glucuronosyltransferase towards testosterone (17-OH steroid) was 4-fold higher in hamster than in rat liver microsomes. By contrast, no difference in glucuronidation of androsterone (3-OH steroid) could be seen. The kinetic constants for UDP-glucuronosyltransferase activity towards testosterone has been determined. No variation in the K_m values between the two species was found, only the V_{max} was markedly higher. The different profile in steroid glucuronidation potency observed between the two species could be explained by the existence of differently regulated UDP-glucuronosyltransferase isoforms active toward 3-OH or 17-OH steroids.

Partial cross immunoreactivity has been obtained between liver microsomal UDP-glucuronosyltransferase of rat and that of hamster, using an antiserum prepared against the purified rat liver enzyme. This suggests that the enzyme shares some antigenic determinants in the two species.

KEYWORDS

Hamster, Rat, UDP-glucuronosyltransferase-(testosterone), GT1, GT2.

INTRODUCTION

Conjugation reaction are of major importance in the inactivation and elimination of potentially toxic intermediates. UDP-glucuronosyltransferases (UDPGT) is involved in metabolic pathways in balance either with sulfation or with glutathion conjugation. UDPGTs catalyse conjugation of both exogenous (drugs) and endogenous (hormones, bilirubin) molecules with UDPG-glucuronic acid (UDPGa) (Siest *et al.*, 1987). The specificity of each isozyme is currently under investigation. But, untill now the more selective isoforms described so far are UDPGT(3-OH steroid) or (androsterone) by Kirkpatrick *et al.*, (1984), UDPGT(17-OH steroid) or (testosterone) by Matern *et al.*, (1982) and UDPGT(bilirubine) by Burchell (1980).

Difference in glucuronidation according to the animal used is frequently observed. For instance, when the metabolite profile of dantrolene, a unique skeletal muscle relaxant, was compared in urine of different mammals, it was observed that hamster glucuronidated this drug more efficiently than rat or mouse, since total conjugates (mercapturic acid, glucuronides) represented up to 80% of the total

metabolites in the hamster, instead of 40% only in rat (Arnold et al., 1983).
In this work, we compared the glucuronidation potency between rat and hamster, in order to understand the basis of their difference, especially in the glucuronidation of steroids.

MATERIALS AND METHODS

Chemicals: (4-^{14}C)testosterone (47mCi/m.mole) was obtained from C.E.A.(Saclay, France). All other chemicals were of analytical grade.

Animals: Male Sprague-Dawley rats (180-200g) were provided by IFFA Credo (Saint-Germain sur l'Arbresle, France). Golden Syrian hamsters (90-100g) were a gift from the Institut National de Recherche et de Sécurité (Nancy, France). Animals were allowed to food and water access *ad libitum*.
The procedure of isolation and preparation of liver microsomes has been previously described (Jayyosi et al.,1987). The protein content of the microsomal suspension was determined according to Lowry et al.(1951), with bovine serum albumin as standard.

Enzymes assays: UDPGT activities were determined according to the method described by Mulder et al.,(1975) and by Colin-Neiger et al.,(1984) using a fast analyser centrifuge (Cobas-Bio Roche). Each assay was performed at final concentrations of 0.5 mM for aglycones and 4 mM for UDPGa. Control without UDPGa was included in each run. Microsomes were previously optimally activated by Triton X-100 at a detergent/protein weight ratio of 0.4. UDPGT activity towards testosterone was also estimated by measure of the radioactive glucuronide formed according to Rao et al.,(1976) with the same substrate concentration than in the Mulder's method.

RESULTS AND DISCUSSION

Figure I summarized the results obtained for glucuronidation of 8 aglycones in rat and hamster liver microsomes. While a same decreasing scale from GT1 (umbelliferone, 1-naphthol, 4-nitrophenol) to GT2 activities occured in the two species; some GT2 activities were proportionally higher in hamster than in any other mammals tested before (Boutin et al., 1984). UDPGT activities towards morphine and

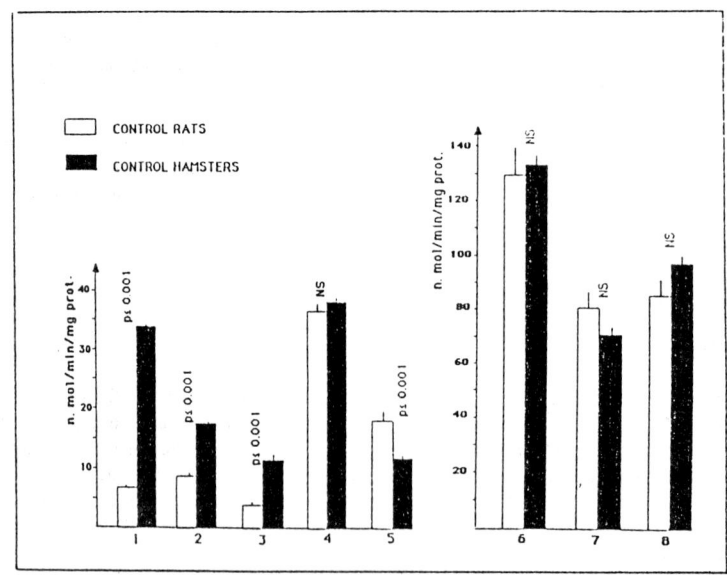

Figure 1 : UDP-GLUCURONOSYLTRANSFERASE ACTIVITIES IN CONTROL RAT AND HAMSTER LIVER MICROSOMES TOWARDS:
1) Testosterone; 2) Morphine; 3) Cloramphenicol;2) Androsterone; 5) Nopol;
6) Umbelliferone; 3) 1-Naphthol 8) 4-Nitrophenol. All substrates were at a final concentration of 0.5mM and UDPGa was 4.5mM.

chloramphenicol were 2.0 and 2.7 times higher in hamster than in rat. In contrast, we observe an opposite difference in the UDPGT activity towards androsterone (3-OH steroid) between the two species. The glucuronidation level of testosterone (17-OH steroid) was four time that commonly observed in rat. Activation of UDPGT occured for the same detergent/protein weight ratio than in rat. The reaction was performed at pH 8.8 (37°C), but did not differ at pH 7.0 (37°C). These observations were in agreement with data reported by Gabaldon et al., (1969) who found that the formation of an other steroid monoglucuronide (diethylstilbestrol) in hamster liver homogenate was 5 to 6 fold higher than in rat. This differentially "balanced" steroid conjugation capacity observed in the two species confirmed the existance of differentialy regulated UDPGT isoforms for either 3-OH or 17-OH steroids as shown by Green et al., (1985).

The determination of the kinetic constants for UDPGT-(testosterone) confirmed a higher V_{max} in hamster (Table I). Since their apprent K_m were similar in both strains, it seems that hamster possesses a higher amount of UDPGT-testosterone, than rat liver.

Kinetic constants for UDPGT activity towards testosterone in control animals.

Microsomes	K_m^{app} M^{-1}	V_{max}^{app} n.mol/min/mg prot	Vmax/Km
Rat liver microsomes	17	7.9	2.15
Hamster liver microsomes	15	32.4	0.46

The UDPGa concentration was kept at 4.5mM, whereas testosterone concentration varied from 0.01 to 0.30 mM.

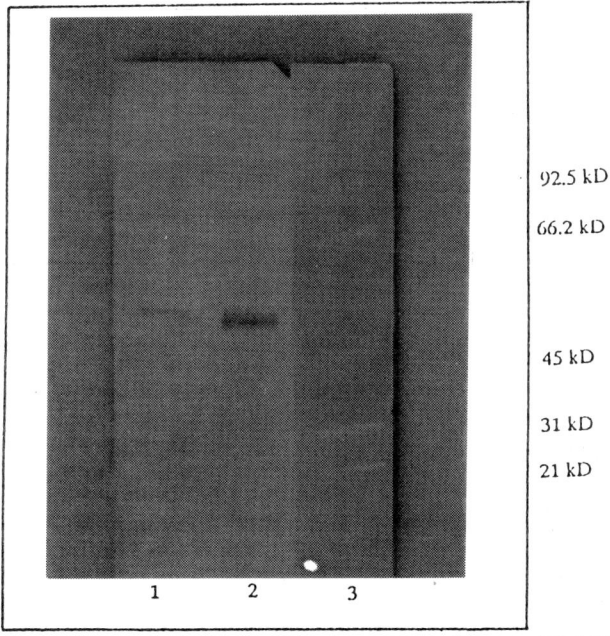

Figure 2 : Immunoblot analysis of hepatic microsomal rat and hamster UDPGT.
1-Hamster liver microsomes 2-Rat liver microsomes 3- molecular standards.

Our data suggest that the difference in the glucuronidation potency between rat and hamster could be supported by a higher amount of the UDPGT-testosterone isoenzyme in hamster. In the same way, some differences in drug metabolizing enzymes pattern between various rodents were also observed by Åstrom et al., (1987) and were interpreted at least partially, in term of difference in the metabolism of endogenous substances such as steroids.

Using an antiserum prepared against partially purified rat liver UDPGT towards phenols, we obtained a cross reactivity between liver microsomal UDP-glucuronosyltransferase of rat and that of hamster by immunoblotting ananlysis (Fig. 2). This study shows that despite discrepency between the specificity of the hamster and rat enzymes, the protein presents, however, some similar antigenic determinants.

REFERENCES

-Arnold, T.H., Miller, J., Cook, H.R., and Hamrick, M.E., (1983): Dantrolene sodium urinary metabolites and hepatotoxicity. *Res. Comm. Chem. Pathol. Pharmacol.*, 39, 381-398.

-Åstrom, A., Maner, S., and Depierre, J. W., (1987): Induction of liver microsomal epoxide hydrolase in different rodent species by 2-acetylaminofluorene or 3-methylcholanthrene, *Xenobiotica*, 17, 155-163

-Boutin, J.A., Antoine B., Batt, A.M., and Siest, G.,(1984), Heterogeneity of hepaatic microsomal UDP-glucuronosyltrans-ferase(s) activities: comparison between humaan and mammalian species activities. *Chem. Biol. Inter.*, 52, 174-184.

-Burchell, B., (1980), Isolation and purification of bilirubin UDP-glucuronosyltransferase from rat liver. *Febs Lett.* 111, 131-135.

-Colin-Neiger, A., Kauffmann, I., Boutin. J.A., Fournel, S., Siest, G., Batt, A.M., and Magdalou, J. (1984): Assessment of Mulder and Van Doorn kinetic procedure and rapid centrifugal analysis of UDP-glucuronosyltransferase activities. *J. Biochem. Biophys. Meth.*, 9, 69-79.

-Gabaldon, M., and Lacomba, T., (1969): The formation of diethylstilbestrol monoglucuronide in hamster liver homogenates. *Eur. J. Cancer*, 5, 509-513.

-Green, M.D. Falany, C.N., Kirkpatrick, R.B., and Tephly, T.R., (1985): Strain differences in purified rat hepatic 3 -hydroxysteroid UDP-glucuronosyltransferase. *Biochem. J.*, 230, 403-409.

-Jayyosi, Z., Totis, M., Souhaili, H., Goulon-Ginet, Livertoux, M.H, Batt, A.M., and Siest, G., (1987): Induction of cytochrome P-450c dependent monooxygenase activities by dantrolene in rat. *Biochem. Pharmacol.*, 36, 2481-2487.

-Kirkpatrick, R.B., Falany, C.N., and Tephly, T.R., (1984): Glucuronidation of bile acids by rat liver 3-OH androgene UDP-Glucuronosyltransferase. *J. Biol. Chem.*, 259, 6176-6180.

-Matern, H., Matern, S., and Gerok, W., (1982) Isolation and characterization of rat liver microsomal UDP-glucuronosyltransferase activity towards chenodeoxycholic acid and testosterone as a single form of enzyme. *J. Biol. Chem.*, 257, 7422-7429.

-Mulder G.D., and Van Doorn, A.B., (1975): A rapid NAD^+-linked assay for microsomal uridine diphosphate glucuronosyl- transferase of rat liver and some observation on substrate specificity of the enzyme, *Biol. J.*, 151, 131-140.

-Rao, G.S., Haueter, G., Rao, M.L., and Breuer, H., (1976): An improved assay for steroid glucuronosyltransferase in rat liver microsomes. *Anal. Biochem.*, 74, 35-40.

-Siest, G., Antoine, B., Fournel, S., Magdalou, J., and Thomassin, J., (1987) The glucuronosyltransferases : What progress can pharmacologists and toxicologists expect for from molecular biology and cellular enzymology. *Biochem.Pharmacol.*, 36, 983-989.

Résumé

Parmi les réactions de conjugaison, dont l'importance est majeure dans l'élimination potentielle des métabolites toxiques, la glucuronoconjugaison occupe une place très importante. Pour comprendre l'origine de la différence de la glucuronoconjugaison de certains médicaments entre le rat et le hamster, nous avons comparé 8 activités UDPGT hépatiques chez ces deux espèces.

La glucuronoconjugaison de la morphine et du chloramphénicol (substrat de groupe II), est deux à trois fois plus importante dans les microsomes de foie de hamsters témoins que dans ceux de foie de rats témoins. De la même façon l'activité UDPGT-(testostérone) est 4 fois plus importante dans les mêmes microsomes. Ces résultats sont confirmés en utilisant une technique de dosage par substrat radiomarqué. De plus la détermination des paramètres cinétiques (Km et Vmax) de l'UDPGT-(testostérone), a permis de conclure qu'il s'agissait de la même isoenzyme dans les deux espèces (même valeur de Km). Les UDPGT(s) conjugant les substrats plans (GT1), ont sensiblement le même taux d'activité dans les deux espèces.

Analytical and biotechnologic approaches
Approches analytiques et biotechnologiques

Structural and stereochemical aspects of acyl glucuronide formation and reactivity

J. Caldwell, N. Grubb, K.A. Sinclair, A.J. Hutt, A. Weil[1] and S. Fournel-Gigleux[2]

Department of Pharmacology and Toxicology, St. Mary's Hospital Medical School, London W2 1PG, UK
[1]*Laboratoires Fournier, Centre de Recherche, 21121 Fontaine-lès-Dijon, France*
[2]*Centre de Médicament, Université de Nancy, 54000 Nancy, France*

ABSTRACT

Studies over many years have shown the dependence of the glucuronidation of benzoic and arylacetic acid derivatives upon the structure of the acid. However, recent work with a number of aryloxyacetates has failed thus far to reveal simple predictive patterns for their conjugation. The situation is further complicated by the occurrence of substantial interspecies variability. For instance, the extensive glucuronidation of fenofibric acid, the active metabolite of the hypolipidaemic fenofibrate, was expected, but not its presence in humans and absence from rat, rabbit, guinea pig and dog.

The conjugation of chiral acids with glucuronic acid results in the formation of diastereoisomers. New methods for their separation have enabled the recognition of significant enantioselectivity with reference to the 2-aryl-propionic acids. At present, it seems most reasonable to view the glucuronidation of these pairs of stereoisomers as being carried out by the same UDPGT isoenzyme, to which the enantiomers bind differently. However, the enantioselectivity of glucuronidation in microsomal preparations does not relate clearly to the overall enantioselectivity of the reaction, which is the consequence of a number of phenomena each showing their own, different selectivities.

The acyl glucuronides produced from xenobiotic acids possess a chemical reactivity which manifests itself in various ways: case of chemical hydrolysis, intramolecular acyl migration and reaction with nucleophilic centres in proteins. Acyl glucuronides encompass a wide range of chemical reactivity e.g. the half-life for intramolecular migration varies by more than 100-fold. However, it seems that these reactivities are different, in that case of intramolecular acyl migration does not predict reactivity towards proteins.

This laboratory has for many years been interested in the metabolic behaviour of xenobiotics containing the carboxylic acid (-COOH) group. From the results of our studies and reports in the literature, it is now understood that a number of conjugation options are open to the carboxyl group, involving the formation of esters with carbohydrates (glucuronic acid, glucose, xylose, ribose), glycerol and sterols (cholesterol, bile salts and acids), amides with amino acids (glycine, glutamine, taurine, ormithine) and carnitine and thioesters with glutathione (Caldwell, Weil & Sinclair, 1987). Of these, for the great majority of compounds, two options predominate, conjugation with glucuronic acid and with various amino acids. The relative extents of these two pathways are a function of a number of chemical and biological variables, including the structure and physicochemical properties of the acid, such as log P and pKa, and the animal species (Caldwell, 1982).

For many acids, the steric environment of the -COOH group emerges as a major determinant of its glucuronic acid conjugation, and for certain classes of acids it is possible to predict the extent of glucuronidation on structural criteria (Caldwell, 1978). Thus, for benzoic acids, the covalent radius of substituents o- to the carboxyl group relates directly to glucuronidation : the larger the group, the more extensive is glucuronidation. For arylacetic acids, substitution on the methylene group α- to the carboxyl group has a similar effect. Glucuronidation of arylacetates depends upon the size of the aryl moiety, but substitution of the α carbon with a methyl group, in rodents and primates directs conjugation exclusively towards glucuronidation. An α-phenyl substituent results in glucuronidation in every species.

<u>Structure-metabolism relationships of aryloxyacetates</u>

More recently we have been examining the structure-metabolism relationships of aryloxyacetic acid congeners. These are an important group of chemicals, finding application as herbicides and hypolipidaemic drugs, but despite this there are relatively few studies of their metabolism. The information which is available indicates that their fate is similar to that of their arylacetate congeners, but that two methyl groups are required α- to the carboxyl for extensive glucuronidation (Van der Waterbeemd et al., 1986). For the p-chlorophenoxy series, the congener with a single α-methyl group is excreted unchanged, while the di-α-methyl compound (clofibric acid) is extensively glucuronidated in all species except the cat (Emudianughe et al., 1983).

We have examined the fate of fenofibrate, an aryloxyacetate hypolipidaemic, in a number of species (Weil et al., 1987, 1988). Inspection of its structure indicates three likely routes of metabolism, ester hydrolysis, carbonyl reduction and glucuronidation of the carboxylic acid. All three of these were indeed found to occur *in vivo* in animals and humans, but there occurred remarkable and unexpected species differences in their relative extents, as shown in Table 1. Fenofibrate is completely hydrolysed to fenofibric acid in all species, but this acid was only conjugated extensively with glucuronic acid in humans.

Table 1.   Metabolic fate of fenofibrate in rat, guinea pig, dog and man.

% dose as that compound in 0-24h urine of:

	Rat	Guinea pig	Dog	Man
Fenofibrate	n.d.	n.d.	n.d.	n.d.
Fenofibric acid				
free	1.5	6.5	0.3	7.8
glucuronide	0.9	5.5	n.d.	32.9
Reduced fenofibric acid				
free	5.4	28.9	4.1	3.7
glucuronide	0.3	0.9	n.d.	3.1

n.d. = not detected

(data drawn from Weil et al., 1987, 1988)

The finding that fenofibric acid undergoes very extensive glucuronic acid conjugation in man, unlike the situation encountered in laboratory animals, is not as surprising as might be thought. It is now appreciated that there are a number of types of glucuronic acid conjugates which are specific in their occurrence to primate species (Caldwell, 1985). In addition, the metabolic patterns in man of a number of xenobiotic acids, including indomethacin, indobufen, indoprofen, Myalex, isoxepac, cicloprofen and ketoprofen, are dominated by ester glucuronidation, in marked contrast to other species in which other pathways of oxidation, reduction and conjugation are prominent (Caldwell, 1978; Caldwell et al., 1988a).

Stereochemical aspects of acyl glucuronidation

There has recently been a very considerable upsurge of interest in the stereochemical aspects of drug metabolism, and this has been particularly the case with the 2-arylpropionic acids, an important group of non-steroidal anti-inflammatory drugs. These acids contain a chiral centre, and various aspects of their disposition are influenced by the absolute configuration of this chiral centre (Hutt & Caldwell, 1983; Caldwell et al., 1988b). Conjugation of these acids with glucuronic acid, which occurs naturally as a single isomer, ß-D-glucopyranosiduronic acid, produces diastereoisomers which are much more readily distinguishable than their parent enantiomers.

There is considerable evidence from the literature that there can occur considerable enantioselectivity in the glucuronidation of 2-arylpropionic acids (see Table 6 of Caldwell et al., 1988b). This has been examined in more detail with the model acid 2-phenylpropionic acid. In vivo studies have shown that there occurs stereoselective urinary excretion of the S(+)-glucuronide in the mouse but not in the rabbit (Fournel & Caldwell, 1986). In the rat, the S(+)-glucuronide predominates in the bile, but the R(-)-glucuronide is in excess in the urine (Yamaguchi & Nakamura, 1985). The glucuronidation of 2-phenylpropionic acid has been studied in rat liver microsomes and, although the two enantiomers have different V_{max} values, their K_ms are essentially identical (Fournel-Gigleux et al., 1988). Enzyme inducers had no effect on stereoselectivity. These data are consistent with the two enantiomers have the same affinity for UDPGT but adopting different orientations within the active site, so that the relative ease of transfer of glucuronic acid from UDPGA is reflected in the different K_m values.

At the present time, it is extremely difficult to relate the stereoselectivity of glucuronidation in vitro to the isomeric composition of the glucuronides found in the excreta. The composition of the excreted glucuronides will be the net product of the stereoselectivities of metabolism, protein binding and excretion, and which of these will be dominant is hard to predict.

Reactivity of acyl glucuronides

Acyl glucuronides produced from xenobiotic acids are now understood to possess an inherent chemical reactivity, which manifests itself in various ways. Like many acyl polyols, these conjugates can undergo acyl migration, in which the biosynthetic 1-O-acyl ß-D-glucopyranosiduric acids are converted to a variety of positional, geometric and stereo-isomers (Sinclair & Caldwell, 1982; Faed, 1984). This is clearly evidenced by their resistance to the hydrolytic enzyme ß-glucuronidase, unlike the biosynthetic 1-O-acyl glucuronides.

As well as intramolecular acylation of adjacent hydroxyl groups, the reactivity of acyl glucuronides can also occur towards -OH, -SH and $-NH_2$ groups in other molecules notably glutathione and proteins (Caldwell et al., 1987). In view of the possible consequences of the acylation of macromolecules, it is essential to know the magnitude of such reactions, and the relationships between the various reactivities. We have therefore initiated a comparative study of the protein binding of the glucuronides of clofibric acid and fenofibric acid, two important hypolipidaemic drugs whose chemical stability in terms of acyl migration is known. The protocol used was based very closely upon that of Benet and colleagues (Smith et al., 1986) so that the data may be compared with data for other acyl glucuronides in the literature. A detailed account of the work on fenofibryl glucuronide is presented elsewhere in this volume (Weil et al., 1988b).

The irreversible binding of 1-O-^{14}C-clofibryl-ß-D-glucopyranosiduronate (obtained biosynthetically from rabbit urine) to human plasma and human serum albumin (HSA) in vitro was determined as follows: ^{14}C-Clofibryl glucuronide (30 ug/ml) was incubated at 37°C in human plasma or HSA in 0.1M phosphate buffer, pH 7.0. 1ml aliquots were removed after 2 min and at 1, 4, 8 and 24 h. 3ml acetonitrile was added to precipitate protein and the whole centrifuged. The protein pellet was washed with 3ml aliquots of methanol/ether (3:1) 10 times to remove reversibly bound clofibric acid and conjugates. The final washed protein pellet was digested with NaOH (2ml, 1M) for 1h at 50°C, neutralized with glacial acetic acid (0.5ml) and counted for ^{14}C after the addition of scintillation fluid.

Clofibryl glucuronide is covalently bound to a small extent to plasma protein and HSA, in a time-dependent fashion, as listed in Table 3.

Table 3. Irreversible binding of clofibryl glucuronide to plasma protein and HSA

pmol clofibryl glucuronide bound/mg protein

Time	plasma	HSA
2 min	11	9
1 hr	54	45
4 hr	105	84
8 hr	111	123
24 hr	81	65

We are now in a position to compare the maximum irreversible binding of three acyl glucuronides to HSA, these studies having been performed to the same protocols, and further to compare these data with the stability of these glucuronides in pH 7.0 buffer.

Table 4 Comparative reactivity of three acyl glucuronides towards human serum albumin and acyl migration

Glucuronide of	Intramolecular rearrangement half-life (h)	Maximum irreversible binding to HSA (pmol/mg)
Zomepirac	0.98[a]	40[a]
Clofibric acid	6.7[b]	123
Fenofibric acid	34.0[b]	67[c]

a - calculated from data of Smith et al. (1986)
b - Caldwell et al. (1987)
c - Weil et al. (1988b)

Inspection of the data shown in Table 4 suggests that these two reactivities are unrelated, and that ease of intramolecular acyl migration does not predict the extent of covalent binding to plasma protein. The fuller elucidation of this discrepancy must await the comparative study of a wider range of acyl glucuronides and the systematic evaluation of the structure-activity relationships for the various reactivities involved.

References

Caldwell, J. (1978) in "Conjugation Reactions in Drug Biotransformation" (ed. A. Aitio) Elsevier, Amsterdam, p. 111-120.

Caldwell, J. (1982) in "Metabolic Basis of Detoxication" (ed. W.B. Jakoby, J.R. Bend & J. Caldwell) Academic Press, New York, p.291-306.

Caldwell, J. (1985) in "Advances in Glucuronide Conjugation" (ed. S. Matern, K.W. Bock & Gerok, W.) MTP Press, Lancaster, p. 7-20.

Caldwell, J., Weil, A. & Sinclair, K.A. (1987) in "Metabolism of Xenobiotics" (ed. J.W. Gorrod, H. Oehschlager & J. Caldwell) Taylor & Francis, London, p. 217-224.

Caldwell, J., Tanaka, Y. & Weil, A. (1988a) in "Proceedings of 2nd ISSX International Symposium", Taylor & Francis, London, in the press.

Caldwell, J., Hutt, A.J. & Fournel-Gigleux, S. (1988b) Biochem. Pharmacol. 37, 105-114.

Emudianughe, T.S., Caldwell, J., Sinclair, K.A. & Smith, R.L. (1983) Drug Metab. Dispos. 11, 97-102.

Faed, E.M. (1984) Drug Metab. Rev. 15, 1213 - 1249.

Fournel-Gigleux, S., Hamar-Hansen, C., Motassim, N., Antoine, B., Mothe, O., Decolin, D., Caldwell, J. & Siest, G. (1988) Drug Metab. Dispos. in the press.

Hutt, A.J. & Caldwell, J. (1983) J. Pharm. Pharmacol. 35, 693-704.

Sinclair, K.A. & Caldwell, J. (1982) Biochem. Pharmacol. 31, 953-957.

Smith, P.C., McDonagh, A.F. & Benet, L.Z. (1986) J. Clin. Invest. 77, 934-939.

Van der Waterbeemd, H., Testa B. & Caldwell, J. (1986) J. Pharm. Pharmacol. 38, 14-18.

Weil, A., Caldwell, J., Strolin-Benedetti, M. & Dostert P. (1987) in "Drugs Affecting Lipid Metabolism" (ed. R. Paoletti) Springer Verlag, Berlin, p. 324-327.

Weil, A., Caldwell, J. & Strolin-Benedetti, M. (1988a) Drug Metab. Dispos. 16, 302-309.

Weil, A., Guichard, J.P. & Caldwell, J. (1988b) this volume

Yamaguchi, T. & Nakamura, J. (1985) Drug Metab. Dispos. 13, 614-619.

Résumé

Les études de ces dernières années ont montré que la glucuronoconjugaison des dérivés acide benzoïque et acide aryl acétique dépendait de la structure de l'acide. Cependant un travail récent avec divers aryl oxyacétates n'a pas permis de prédire leur taux de conjugaison. Cette situation se complique davantage par l'existence de variabilité inter-espèce appréciable. Par exemple, on peut s'attendre à une glucuronoconjugaison extensive de l'acide fénofibrique, le métabolite actif de l'hypolipémiant fénofibrate ; cependant on ne peut prédire qu'il est glucuronoconjugué chez l'homme de façon intensive et pas chez le rat, le lapin, le cobaye et le chien.

La conjugaison des acides chiraux à l'acide glucuronique provoque la formation de diastéréoisomères. De nouvelles méthodes de séparation ont permis de mettre en évidence une énantio sélectivité significative dans le cas des acides 2-aryl propioniques. A présent, il semble plus raisonnable de penser que la glucuronoconjugaison de ces paires de stéréoisomères est catalysée par la même isoenzyme d'UDPGT à laquelle se fixent de façon différente les énantiomères. Toutefois l'énantio sélectivité de la glucuronoconjugaison dans les préparations microsomales ne reflète pas clairement l'énantio sélectivité d'ensemble de la réaction qui est la conséquence d'un nombre de phénomènes, chacun montrant ses propres et différentes sélectivités.

Les acyl glucuronides formés à partir de xénobiotiques acides possèdent une réactivité chimique qui se manifeste de plusieurs façons : facilité d'hydrolyse chimique, migration intramoléculaire du groupement acyle et réaction avec les structures nucléophiles des protéines. Les acyl glucuronides présentent des réactivités chimiques à des degrés divers, ainsi la demi vie de la migration intramoléculaire peut varier plus de 100 fois. Cependant il semble que ces réactivités soient différentes car la facilité avec laquelle s'effectue la migration intramoléculaire du groupement acyle n'est pas un gage de réactivité envers les protéines.

Immunochemical characterization of UDP-glucuronyl transferase by monoclonal antibody techniques

Helmuth H.G. van Es, Wilbert H.M. Peters*, Bart G. Goldhoorn, Marianne Paul-Abrahamse, Ronald P.J. Oude Elferink and Peter L.M. Jansen

*Divisions of Gastrointestinal and Liver Diseases, Academic Medical Center, Meibergdreef 9, 1105 AZ Amsterdam and *St. Radboud Hospital, University of Nijmegen, Nijmegen, The Netherlands*

ABSTRACT

In order to study the heterogeneity of the UDP-glucuronyltransferase (UDPGT) system, we have used different approaches for the production of monoclonal and polyclonal antibodies. Firstly, mice were immunized with crude human liver microsomes and the resulting hybridoma media were tested for their ability to inhibit the glucuronidation of para-nitrophenol. This resulted in a hybridoma clone, WP1, secreting a UDPGT specific antibody. Besides the inhibition of bilirubin- and phenol-conjugating UDPGT activities, three immunoreactive polypeptides are visualized by immunoblot analysis of human liver microsomes. Using immobilized WP1, UDPGT was immunopurified from human liver microsomes. This resulted in a catalytically inactive UDPGT preparation which was used as antigen to produce other monoclonal and polyclonal antibodies. One MAb, HEB7 and a polyclonal antiserum were obtained. HEB7 reacts with both human and rat UDPGT in contrast to WP1 which is human specific. With immunoblot analysis a 53 kDa and a clofibrate inducible 54 kDa polypeptide are recognized by MAb HEB7 and the polyclonal antiserum in Wistar rat liver microsomes. Both polypeptides are absent from Gunn rat liver microsomes.

KEYWORDS

Monoclonal antibodies, immunopurification, Gunn rat

ABBREVIATIONS

MAb, monoclonal antibody; ELISA, enzyme linked immunosorbent assay; PNP, para-nitrophenol; 4-MU, 4-methylumbelliferone; UDPGA, uridine 5' diphosphate glucuronic acid; UDPGT, uridine 5' diphosphate glucuronyltransferase.

INTRODUCTION

The introduction of the hybridoma technology as developed by Kohler and Milstein (1975) has given an impulse to many areas of biology, biochemistry and medicine. Because of the specificity and versatility of monoclonal antibodies (MABs) many different applications have arisen. Purification of proteins using immobilized MAbs, cloning of cDNA's using cDNA expression libraries, studies of hereditary diseases at the level of proteins and epitope mapping are only a few of the numerous applications. The use of monoclonal antibodies has also proven to be fruitful for the characterization of heterogeneous enzyme systems like for example cytochrome P450 (Friedman et al., 1983). UDP-glucuronyltransferase (UDPGT, EC 2.4.1.17) is a membrane-bound enzyme system concentrated in the lipid bilayer of the endoplasmatic reticulum of cells of liver, intestine, kidney and other tissues (Dutton, 1980). It consists of several isoenzymes with distinct substrate specificities (Roy Chowdhury et al., 1986). Comparison of cDNA deduced amino acid sequences reveals that different isoenzymes have a high homology (Burchell et al., 1987). We report on the development of two MABs and a polyclonal antiserum specific for UDPGT. These antibodies have been used to study the heterogeneity of UDPGT and its hereditary defects in man and in the rat.

METHODS

Immunization with microsomes isolated from human liver
The monoclonal antibody WP1 was obtained by immunizing mice with microsomal proteins isolated from human liver. The splenocytes of these mice were fused with myeloma cells. Screening for UDPGT specific antibodies was performed by testing the hybridoma media for their capability of inhibiting the glucuronidation of para-nitrophenol (PNP) (Peters et al., 1987a).

Inhibition of glucuronidation by WP1
Sodium dodecyl sulphate (SDS) activated human liver microsomes were incubated with different amounts of WP1 ascites protein for 1 h at 20°C. Subsequently, UDPGT activities for various substrates were assayed (Peters et al., 1987a).

Immunoprecipitation experiments
Immunoprecipitation of UDPGT activities from solubilized microsomal membranes was performed by using monoclonal antibodies from ascites covalently coupled to Sepharose 4B beads (van Es et al., submitted).

Immunopurification of human hepatic UDPGT
Triton X-100 solubilized microsomal proteins isolated from human liver were centrifuged for 30 min at 100,000 g and the supernatant was applied to a column of Sepharose 4B immobilized WP1 at 20°C. After immunoabsorption of UDPGT, the column was washed sequentially with 5 bed volumes of 50 mM Tris-HCl pH 7.8, 250 mM sucrose, 2 mM EDTA, 1% Triton X-100 and 5 bed volumes of the same buffer but containing 0.1% Triton X-100. Immunobound human UDPGT was eluted with 2 M $MgCl_2$, 50 mM Tris-HCl pH 7.0 and 0.1% Triton X-100. Detection of eluted UDPGT was performed by means of an Enzyme Linked Immunosorbent Assay (ELISA).

Immunization with immunopurified UDPGT
Immunopurified human liver UDPGT obtained as described above was injected into mice and splenocytes were fused with myeloma cells. The resulting hybridomas were screened for UDPGT specific antibodies by testing the hybridoma media for recognition of the immunopurified UDPGT in an ELISA. The same immunopurified UDPGT preparation was used to immunize rabbits (van Es et al., submitted).

Immunoblot analysis
SDS-polyacrylamide gel electrophoresis followed by Coomassie brilliant blue protein staining or immunoblotting of the resolved proteins on nitrocellulose was carried out according to Laemmli (1970) and Towbin et al. (1979). Immunostaining was performed using the alkaline phosphatase method as supplied by Promega, Madison, USA.

RESULTS

Table 1 shows the maximum percentage of inhibition of UDPGT activities by MAb WP1 which can be achieved in SDS solubilized human liver microsomes. These data suggest that WP1 recognizes the human UDPGT isoenzymes which glucuronidate phenolic compounds and bilirubin. In rat liver microsomes no inhibition was observed. The possibility was investigated that WP1 and UDPGA have a common binding site. These experiments showed that the maximal inhibition was clearly dependent on the UDPGA concentration and varied from 67% at 2 mM UDPGA to less than 40% at 32 mM UDPGA. With PNP as the varying substrate (0.25-4.0 mM) and a fixed UDPGA concentration (4 mM), the inhibition pattern was not variable (data not shown). These experiments indicate that binding of WP1 may occur at or near the UDPGA binding site.

Table 1. Inhibition and immunoprecipitation of UDPGT activities by the MAb WP1. PB = phenobarbital; 3-MC = 3-methylcholantrene; ND = not done.

Tissue	Substrate	Maximal inhibition %	Maximal precipitation %
Human liver	PNP	75	75
	Bilirubin	67	ND
	4-MU	55	75
	Testosterone	0	ND
	Estrone	0	ND
	Phenolphtalein	0	ND
Rat liver			
Untreated	PNP	0	0
PB treated	PNP	0	ND
3MC treated	PNP	0	ND

Using WP1, in an immunoblot analysis three immunoreactive polypeptides of 57, 54 and 53 kDa and one polypeptide of 54 kDa were detected in human liver and kidney microsomes respectively (Fig. 1). No reaction was seen with microsomes isolated from human testis. Microsomes from testis are capable of glucuronidating testosterone, estriol, androsterone and estrone (data not shown).

To investigate whether WP1 can be used as a tool for the preparative purification of UDPGT from human liver, immunoprecipitation experiments were performed with WP1 immobilized to Sepharose 4B beads. With solubilized microsomes, WP1 beads were able to precipitate 75% of the UDPGT-activity towards PNP, a representative substrate for the phenol UDPGT as present in rat tissue (Roy Chowdhury et al., 1986; Coughtrie et al., 1987a). A similar fraction of UDPGT activity towards 4-MU was precipitated (Table 1). The non-precipitable UDPGT activity towards PNP and 4-MU may represent other isoenzyme(s) which are not recognized by WP1. Using immobilized WP1, an immunopurification procedure for human UDPGT was developed. Human liver microsomes solubilized with Triton X-100 were applied to a column of immobilized WP1. The column was washed and the immunobound UDPGT was eluted with 2 M $MgCl_2$. A typical example of such an immunopurification of UDPGT is depicted in Fig. 2. Some immunoreactive material is eluted before applying 2 M $MgCl_2$. However, this is not seen when less microsomal protein is applied, suggesting that it is caused by overloading the column (data not shown).

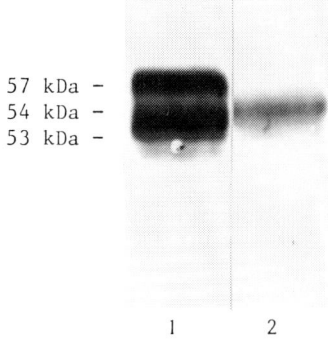

Fig. 1. Immunoblot analysis of human liver and human kidney microsomes using WP1. Lane 1: human liver microsomes (10 µg); lane 2: human kidney microsomes (20 µg).

SDS-polyacrylamide gel electrophoresis of the immunopurified human UDPGT and subsequent staining of the resolved proteins revealed that within the limits of resolution three polypeptides with a distinct molecular weight are purified (Fig. 2). These proteins have an apparent molecular weight of 57, 54 and 53 kDa.

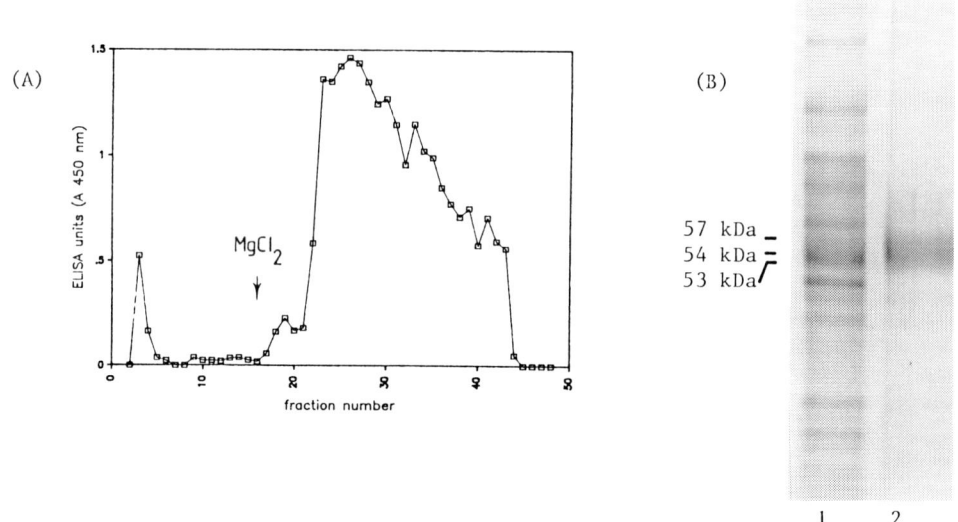

Fig. 2. (A) Immunopurification of UDPGT from Triton X-100 solubilized human hepatic microsomes on immobilized WP1. Solubilized microsomes were applied to the column and unbound material was removed by washing. The immunobound UDPGT was eluted with 2 M $MgCl_2$ (arrow). UDPGT in the fractions was detected in an ELISA as described in Methods. Data are from a single representative experiment.
(B) SDS-PAGE of microsomes and immunopurified UDPGT from human liver. UDPGT was immunopurified from microsomes as shown in Fig. 2A. Lane 1: human liver microsomes (20 µg); lane 2: immuno-purified UDPGT 5 µg).

Immunopurified human UDPGT was injected into mice in order to obtain new monoclonal antibodies. Screening of the hybridoma media for anti-UDPGT-antibodies was carried out using an ELISA with the immunopurified human liver UDPGT as antigen. Subsequent cloning of the hybrid cells resulted in a stable, positive hybridoma-clone, HEB7. This antibody reacts with UDPGT from both human and rat liver microsomes. Using immobilized HEB7, 90 and 60% of the UDPGT-activity towards PNP and 4-MU respectively can be precipitated from solubilized rat liver microsomes. Immunoblot analysis reveals the heavy staining of a 53 kDa polypeptide and several less stained polypeptides in liver microsomes from Wistar rats (Fig. 3, lane 1). A 54 kDa polypeptide is visualized when liver microsomes from clofibrate treated Wistar rats were used (Fig. 3, lane 2). These immunoreactive polypeptides are not visualized with hepatic microsomes from untreated Gunn rats (Fig. 3, lane 3). Treatment of Gunn rats with clofibrate did not have any effect. The differential effect of clofibrate treatment on different immunoreactive polypeptides is accompanied by a 1.5 to 2.5 fold induction of the UDPGT activity towards bilirubin (not shown; Coughtrie et al., 1987b).

A polyclonal antiserum was obtained by injecting rabbits with the immunopurified human UDPGT. Immunoblotting with these polyclonal antibodies reveals five polypeptides with Wistar rat liver microsomes (Fig. 3, lane 4). Again, clofibrate induces a 54 kDa polypeptide (Fig. 3, lane 5) and this polypeptide is not detected in Gunn rat liver microsomes (lane 6) as was observed with the monoclonal antibody HEB7. Treatment of Gunn rats with clofibrate had no effect (data not shown).

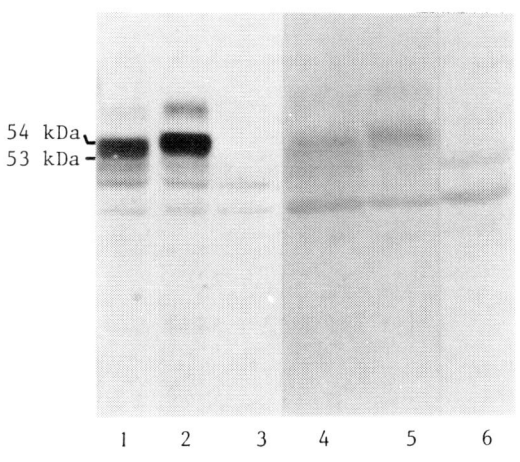

Fig. 3. Immunoblot analysis of microsomes isolated from Wistar and Gunn rat liver. Lanes 1 and 4: hepatic microsomes from Wistar rat (20 µg); lanes 2 and 5: hepatic microsomes from clofibrate treated Wistar rat (20 µg); lanes 3 and 6: Gunn rat liver microsomes (20 µg). Lanes 1, 2 and 3 were incubated with the monoclonal antibody HEB7 and lanes 4, 5 and 6 were incubated with the polyclonal antibodies.

DISCUSSION

The monoclonal antibody WP1 is specific for UDPGT from human origin as shown by the inhibition of PNP, 4-MU and bilirubin glucuronidation by human liver microsomes. This specificity is also reflected by the ability of immobilized WP1 to precipitate UDPGT activity. This antibody does not react with UDPGT's from rat.

Immunoblot analysis of human microsomes with this antibody reveals 57, 54 and 53 kDa polypeptides in hepatic microsomes and a 54 kDa polypeptide in renal microsomes (Fig. 2b). The absence of the 57 and 53 kDa polypeptide in renal microsomes is in accordance with the absence of at least one known UDPGT activity: bilirubin (Peters et al., 1987b).

The UDPGT-specificity of WP1 was used to develop an immunopurification procedure. Immunopurification as reported in this paper is a powerful method for preparative purification of certain UDPGT's from human tissues. With this method the 54 kDa polypeptide from human kidney could also be purified (data not shown). The method described here does not allow the purification of biologically active UDPGT's. This is probably caused by extensive delipidation due to the high concentrations of Triton X-100 used during chromatography. Inactivation by delipidation is a well known feature of UDPGT's (Wood et al., 1985; Jansen and Arias, 1975). Using the immunopurified human hepatic UDPGT as antigen a new MAb (HEB7) was obtained with the following characteristics: (a) ELISA-experiments showed that this antibody recognizes immunopurified UDPGT; (b) immunoprecipitation experiments using immobilized HEB7: 90 and 60% of the UDPGT activity towards PNP and 4-MU can be precipitated from solubilized rat liver microsomes; (c) immunoblot analysis of rat liver microsomes show that HEB7 reacts with at least two polypeptides: a 54 kDa clofibrate inducible polypeptide and a 53 kDa polypeptide. These two polypeptides are absent when microsomes isolated from Gunn rat liver are analysed with either HEB7 or the polyclonal antiserum as the primary antibody. This correlates well with the absence and strongly lowered UDPGT activities towards bilirubin and phenolic compounds respectively, which was found by us (data not shown) and others (Coughtrie et al., 1987b; Roy Chowdhury et al., 1987).

Recently it has been postulated that these two polypeptides (54 and 53 kDa) correspond with the bilirubin- and the phenol-UDPGT isoenzyme, respectively (Coughtrie et al., 1987b).

It is interesting to note that using different preparations for immunization (non purified human microsomal proteins versus immunopurified human liver UDPGT's) and different methods of screening for anti-UDPGT antibodies (UDPGT inhibition assay versus ELISA) resulted in two monoclonal antibodies with different characteristics. Furthermore, we have produced a panel of specific monoclonal and polyclonal antibodies without purifying UDPGT by conventional means.

Confusion exists concerning the nature of the UDPGT defect in the Gunn rat. Roy Chowdhury et al. performed chromatofocusing experiments with Gunn rat microsomal proteins (Roy Chowdhury et al., 1987). Immunoblot analysis of the purified chromatofocusing fractions using a polyclonal antiserum suggests the presence of a mutated inactive bilirubin and phenol UDPGT. These results contradict ours and those of Coughtrie et al. which suggest the complete absence of both isoenzymes (Fig. 3) (Coughtrie et al., 1987b). These contradictory results could be explained by the existence of different Gunn rat strains (Roy Chowdhury et al., 1987). This would however mean that two different mutations have led to two identical phenotypes. Another possibility is that the antibodies we used cannot recognize the mutated UDPGT's in contrast to those of Roy Chowdhury et al. Indeed the antiserum of Roy Chowdhury et al. was raised against a UDPGT preparation purified from rat liver with activity for 1-naphtol, testosterone, beta-oestradiol, androsterone and aniline (Roy Chowdhury et al., 1983). The antisera from the group of Burchell (1984; Coughtrie et al., 1987b) were raised against other rat UDPGT preparations, namely: a liver preparation glucuronidating testosterone and PNP and a preparation isolated from rat kidney, glucuronidating 1-naphtol and bilirubin. Furthermore, our antiserum was raised against UDPGT's from human origin.

Therefore it cannot be excluded that in the antiserum of Roy Chowdhury et al. antibodies are present, which do not react with a determinant involved in the mutation. These antibodies could be absent in the other antisera. Exchange of antisera would probably solve this problem. Thus if the isoenzymes for glucuronidation of bilirubin and phenolic compounds are present at all in Gunn rat liver microsomes they must at least have undergone considerable changes.

REFERENCES

Burchell, B., Kennedy, S., Jackson, M. and McCarthy, L. (1984): The biosynthesis and induction of microsomal UDP-glucuronyltransferase in avian liver. Biochem. Soc. Transactions 12, 50-53.

Burchell, B., Coughtrie, M.H.W., Jackson, M.R., Shepherd, S.R.P., Harding, D. and Hume, R. (1987): Genetic deficiency of bilirubin glucuronidation in rats and humans. Molec. Aspects Med. 9, 429-455.

Coughtrie, M.W.H., Burchell, B. and Bend, J.R. (1987a): Purification and properties of rat kidney UDP-glucuronosyltransferase. Biochem. Pharmacol. 36, 245-251.

Coughtrie, M.W.H., Burchell, B., Shepherd, I.M. and Bend, J.R. (1987b): Defective induction of phenol glucuronidation by 3-methylcholantrene in Gunn rats is due to the absence of a specific UDP-glucuronyltransferase isoenzyme. Mol. Pharmacol. 31, 585-591.

Dutton, G.J. (1980): The glucuronidation of drugs and other compounds, Boca Raton, FL: CRC Press.

Friedman, F.K., Robinson, R.C., Park, S.S. and Gelboin, H.V. (1983): Monoclonal antibody-directed immunopurification and identification of cytochromes P-450. Biochem. Biophys. Res. Commun. 116, 859-865.

Jansen, P.L.M. and Arias, I.M. (1975): Delipidation and reactivation of UDP-glucuronyltransferase from rat liver. Biochem. Biophys. Acta 391, 28-38.

Kohler, G. and Milstein, C. (1975): Continuous cultures of fused cells secreting antibody of predefined specificity. Nature 256, 495.

Laemmli, U.K. (1970): Cleavage of structural proteins during the assembly of the head of bacteriophage T4. Nature 227, 680-685.

Peters, W.H.M., Allebes, W.A., Jansen, P.L.M., Poels, L.G. and Capel, P.J.A. (1987a): Characterization and tissue specificity of a monoclonal antibody against human uridine 5'-diphosphate-glucuronyltransferase. Gastroenterol. 93, 162-169.

Peters, W.H.M. and Jansen, P.L.M. (1987b): Immunocharacterization of UDP-glucuronyltransferase isoenzymes in human liver, intestine and kidney. Biochem. Pharmacol. 37, 564-567.

Roy Chowdhury, J., Roy Chowdhury, N., Moscioni, A.D., Tukey, R., Tephly, T.R. and Arias, I.M. (1983): Differential regulation by triiodothyronine of substrate specific uridine diphosphoglucuronate glucuronyltransferase in rat liver. Biochim. Biophys. Acta 761, 58-65.

Roy Chowdhury, J., Roy Chowdhury, N., Falany, C.N., Tephly, T.R. and Arias, I.M. (1986): Isolation and characterization of multiple forms of rat liver UDP-glucuronate glucuronosyltransferase. Biochem. J. 233, 827-837.

Roy Chowdhury, N., Gross, F., Moscioni, A.D., Kram, M., Arias, I.M. and Roy Chowdhury, J. (1987): Isolation of multiple normal and functionally defective forms of uridine diphosphate-glucuronyltransferase from inbred Gunn rats. Clin. Invest. 79, 327-334.

Towbin, H., Staehlin, T. and Gordon, J. (1979): Electrophoretic transfer of proteins for polyacrylamide gels to nitrocellulose sheets: Procedure and some applications. Proc. Natl. Acad. Sci. USA 76, 4350-4354.

Wood, G.C., Scott, G. and Graham, A.B. (1985): Phospholipid regulation of UDP-glucuronyltransferase. In <u>Advances in glucuronide conjugation</u>, Falk symposium 40, ed S. Matern, K.W. Bock and W. Gerok, pp 83-91. Lancaster: MTP Press.

Résumé

Dans le but d'étudier l'hétérogénéité des UDP-glucuronosyltransférases (UDPGT), nous avons utilisé différentes approches pour la production d'anticorps mono- et polyclonaux. D'abord, les souris ont été immunisées par des microsomes hépatiques humains et les hybridomes correspondants ont été testés pour leur pouvoir d'inhiber la conjugaison du para-nitrophénol. Un clone WP1 secrétant un anticorps spécifique anti UDPGT a été développé. L'inhibition des formes d'UDPGT conjuguant la bilirubine et les phénols est accompagnée de la présence après immunoblot de trois polypeptides immuno-réactifs. L'UDPGT a été purifiée à partir de microsomes hépatiques humains en utilisant WP1 immobilisé. Ceci nous conduisit en une préparation d'UDPGT biologiquement inactive qui fut utilisée comme antigène pour produire d'autres anticorps poly- et monoclonaux. Un MAb, HEB7 et un antisérum polyclonal ont été obtenus. HEB7 réagit avec l'UDPGT d'homme ou de rat, alors que WP1 est spécifique de la protéine humaine. Par immunoblot, ce polypeptide de 53 kDa et un de 54 kDa induit par le clofibrate sont reconnus par MAb, HEB7 et le sérum polyclonal dans les microsomes hépatiques de rats Wistar. Les deux polypeptides sont absents dans les microsomes hépatiques de rat Gunn.

New chromatographic methods for *in vitro* glucuronidation studies

Alain Nicolas and Pierre Leroy

Laboratoire de Chimie Analytique, UA CNRS 597, Faculté des Sciences Pharmaceutiques et Biologiques, BP 403, 54001 Nancy Cedex, France

ABSTRACT

Two versatile high-performance liquid chromatography (HPLC) techniques have been respectively elaborated to reduce glucuronide analysis time and to enhance their detection sensitivity. An ion-pair reversed-phase (RP) HPLC system using an hydrophobic counter-ion (cethexonium bromide) and a high content of methanol in mobile phase was found to provide short elution time. Pre-column labelling of the carboxylic group with 4-bromomethyl-7-methoxycoumarin (BrMmc) affords a sensitivity of 10 pmol for each conjugate injected. These methods have been applied to follow glucuronidation of aromatic steroid and terpene aglycones in Wistar rat and human hepatic microsomal preparations.

KEY WORDS

HPLC - steroid and terpene glucuronides - ion pairing - pre-column labelling - human liver microsomes.

INTRODUCTION

UDP glucuronosyltransferase exhibits a very broad specificity, thus suggesting the existence of multiple forms. Its heterogeneity is investigated by numerous in vitro assays using a great variety of structurally different aglycones. The measurement of activities requires fast, general, selective and sensitive analytical methods. Those based upon the analysis of the intact glucuronides are more advisable and many direct HPLC assays have been reported. However, they present some disadvantages :
- they have been generally elaborated on an individual basis and require quite different elution or detection conditions for each conjugate measured ;
- the reversed-phase systems require long analysis time for the elution of apolar aglycones such as naphthol, testosterone (often more than one hour (Baker, 1981)).
- the detection generally relies upon the spectral properties of the aglycone since the sugar moiety of these conjugates exhibits only a weak UV absorbance at about 200 nm due to the carbonyl group. So, there is a loss of selectivity when low UV wavelength is used to increase sensitivity.

Moreover, conjugates of aglycones without chromophores need radiolabelling with ^{14}C-UDPGA (Hamar-Hansen et al., 1986, Coughtrie et al., 1986) for their detection, but these techniques are costly and time-consuming.

To overcome these difficulties two HPLC systems have been developed :
- an ion-pairing reversed-phase technique providing short analysis time ;
- a pre-column chemical derivatization of glucuronic acid moiety which affords sensitive detection.

MATERIAL AND METHODS

Chemicals and reagents

All chemicals and solvents were of analytical reagent grade and were used without further treatment, except for acetone, which was dried over molecular sieves 3 Å. (±) Menthol glucuronide ammonium salt, phenol, phenolphtaleine, androsterone, estrone and testosterone glucuronide sodium salts, Tris-HCl, Triton X-100 were supplied by Sigma (St Louis, MO, USA). 4-Bromomethyl-7-methoxycoumarin (BrMmc) and 18-crown-6 were purchased from Fluka (Buchs, Switzerland). Cethexonium bromide (hexadecyl (2-hydroxycyclohexyl) dimethylammonium bromide) was obtained from Cooper (Melun, France). Uridine disphosphoglucuronic acid (UDPGA) sodium salt and 3-((3-cholamidopropyl)dimethylammonio)-1-propansulfonate (CHAPS) were obtained from Boehringer (Mannheim, FRG). 2-naphthol, cyclohexanol and (-) borneol glucuronides were synthetized as previously described (Leroy, 1982).

Animals and treatment

Mature male Wistar rats (180-200 g) from Iffa Credo (St Germain l'Arbresle, France) were fed with a commercial diet (U.A.R. Villemoisson, France) and had free access to tap water. For induction purpose, they received a daily i.p. injection of phenobarbital (80 mg/kg) in aqueous sodium chloride solution (0.9 %, w/v) for four days. They were decapited and hepatectomized on the fifth day.

Preparation of microsomal fractions

Hepatic microsomes were prepared by conventional ultracentrifugation technique as previously described (Hogelboom, 1955) and their protein content was measured by the technique of Lowry et al. with bovine serum albumin as the standard. They were frozen (-20°C) and used within four weeks.

Biochemical assays

Microsomal fractions were diluted with 75 mM Tris-HCl buffer pH 7.4 containing 5 mM magnesium chloride, to a final protein concentration of 5 mg.ml^{-1}. Triton X-100 was added to the microsomal suspension in a detergent : protein ratio of 0.4 (w/w) when the glucuronidation of terpenes was studied. In the case of steroids, CHAPS amount varied to obtain different detergent : protein ratios (0 to 2.0, w/w). The mixture was allowed to stand for 20 min at 0°C to complete maximal activation.

The activated microsomal preparations were diluted with Tris-HCl, $MgCl_2$ buffer to obtain various protein concentrations in the range 0.125 to 1 mg per tube, and added with 0.035 ml of 100 mM aqueous solution of UDPGA. The mixture was pre-incubated in a shaking water-bath at 37°C for 5 min before addition of variable amounts of the aglycone solution dissolved in ethanol-water (40:60, V/V). The final reaction volume was adjusted to 1.0 ml with Tris-HCl, $MgCl_2$ buffer and the incubation was run at 37°C for 5 to 30 min. The reaction was stopped by addition of 0.15 ml of 0.15 M hydrochloric acid and placing the flask on ice. Control reaction tubes without aglycone, spiked with known amounts of standard glucuronides were prepared and treated in a similar way to the biochemical assays in order to obtain calibration curves. Stock solutions of standard glucuronides were prepared at a concentration of 0.1 mg.ml^{-1} in ethanol-acetonitrile (1:1, V/V) and diluted with the same solvents.

In all cases, an internal standard was used, chosen according to the glucuronide measured : borneol glucuronide for menthol glucuronide, testosterone glucuronide for estrone and androsterone glucuronides and vice versa. Microsomal mixtures resulting from the incubation step were mixed with 0.2 ml of the internal standard stock solution before the analytical procedure was run.

Extraction of glucuronides from incubation medium
Glucuronides were extracted with octadecylsilica cartridges (Sep-Pak C_{18}, Waters-Millipore, Milford, MA, USA). They were pre-wetted before use with 5 ml of methanol-water (4:1, V/V). The acidified incubation medium was transferred to a cartridge which was washed after 15 min with 3 ml of HPLC-grade water ; residual water was removed by flushing with air by means of a syringe. The conjugates were eluted with 3 ml of methanol containing 0.1 % (V/V) triethylamine. The eluate was evaporated to dryness under nitrogen.

Pre-column labelling procedure
The reaction was performed in a 5 ml flask fitted with a screw-cap and protected from light by aluminium foil. The dried residue obtained from the extraction step was dissolved in 0.02 ml of N,N-dimethylformamide and 0.05 ml of acetone. Then, 0.02 ml of 1.5 mg.ml^{-1} BrMmc, 0.01 ml of 1.0 mg.ml^{-1} 18-crown-6 solutions in acetone and 5 mg of potassium carbonate were added. The reaction vial was heated at 70°C for 30 min, then cooled in ice and an aliquot was injected into the HPLC system.

High-performance liquid chromatography (HPLC) analysis
The HPLC system consisted of a ternary solvent delivery pump (Model SP 8700 ; Spectra-Physics, Santa Clara, CA, USA), an injection valve with a 10-µl sample loop (Model 7125 ; Rheodyne, Cotati, CA, USA), a UV-VIS detector (Model LC 313, Merck-Clevenot, Nogent-sur-Marne, France), a conductimetric detector (Model Tridet, Perkin Elmer, CT, USA) or a fluorimetric detector (Model Spectraflow 980, Kratos, NJ, USA). The reversed-phase and normal-phase columns, respectively packed with LiChrospher 100 CH-18 (Hibar RT 250x4 mm I.D., 5 µm) and LiChrospher 100 DIOL (LiChrocart 250x4 mm I.D., 5 µm), were purchased from E. Merck (Darmstadt, FRG). Guard columns (4x4 mm I.D.) prefilled with LiChrospher 100 RP-18 or DIOL, were used in all chromatographic analyses.

Mobile phases were filtered through a 0.45 µm microfilter (Type SM, Sartorius, Palaiseau, France). Mobile phases in ion-pairing system were methanol-0.01 M phosphate buffer pH 6.0 (70:30 or 75:25, V/V) mixtures containing cethexonium bromide (2.5 mM) and used at a flow rate of 1 ml.min^{-1}. Various chromatographic conditions after pre-column labelling are detailed in Table 2.

The spectrophotometric detector was set at 328 nm and the fluorimetric one at 328 nm for excitation and 370 nm (long pass filter) for emission. The chromatograms were recorded at 20 ± 2°C ; all calculations were made with an integrator (Model 5020, Spectra-Physics).

Statistical analysis
Apparent kinetic constants were calculated by linear least-squares regression analysis from values of double reciprocal plots corresponding to at least six different aglycone concentrations.

Method reproducibility for calculation of UDP-glucuronosyltransferase activities (expressed as nmol glucuronide.min^{-1}. mg protein $^{-1}$) was checked with four parallel assays realized with the same microsomal fraction. Values represent the mean ± standard deviation (SD).
Differences between groups of values or between a value and the control level were considered significant when $P \leq 0.05$ (Student's t-test).

RESULTS AND DISCUSSION

Chromatographic conditions
The development of HPLC systems has been aimed for two main purposes : reducing analysis time and enhancing detection sensitivity.

RP-HPLC using cethexonium bromide as ion-pairing reagent
Usual ion-pairing reagents for RP-HPLC of glucuronides are tetrabutylammonium bromide and sodium dodecylsulphate for conjugates whose aglycone has an amino group (e.g. morphine : Liu et al., 1984). A long elution time of apolar aglycones results from their use. This disadvantage was resolved by choosing an hydrophobic counter-ion, cethexonium bromide :

$$\left[(CH_3)_2\overset{C_{16}H_{33}}{\underset{}{N^+}}\underset{OH}{\bigcirc} \right] Br^-$$

A high content of methanol (65 to 75 %) in the mobile phase consequently decreases the retention time of aglycones. Phenolic and steroid compounds are even eluted faster than their respective conjugate. Capacity factors of a variety of aglycones and their conjugate are given in Table 1.

Table 1. Capacity factors (K') of various aglycones and their glucuronic acid congujates in the ion-pair HPLC system.

compound	class	capacity factor (K')		detection mode
		aglycone	conjugate	
menthol		ND*	6.9 (1)	
borneol	alcoholic	ND	4.9 (1)	conductimetric
cyclohexanol		ND	3.4 (1)	
phenol		0.4	1.9 (1)	
acetaminophen		0.05	1.5 (1)	
thymol		1.9	4.9 (1)	
4-hydroxy phenobarbital	aromatic	0.3	2.5 (2)	UV
4-hydroxy phenytoin		0.3	2.1 (2)	
phenolphthalein		0.3	1.9 (1)	
2-naphtol		1.0	3.8 (1)	
morphine		0.6	1.0 (1)	
estrone		1.5	3.7 (1)	
testosterone	steroid	1.5	4.1 (1)	UV
androsterone		1.6	4.3 (1)	
clofibric acid	carboxylic acid	5.8	4.5 (2)	UV

(1) : methanol content of mobile phase = 75 %
(2) : methanol content of mobile phase = 70 %
(*) : not detected

No loss of selectivity for the glucuronide versus other components of microsomal suspensions is observed as shown in Fig. 1.

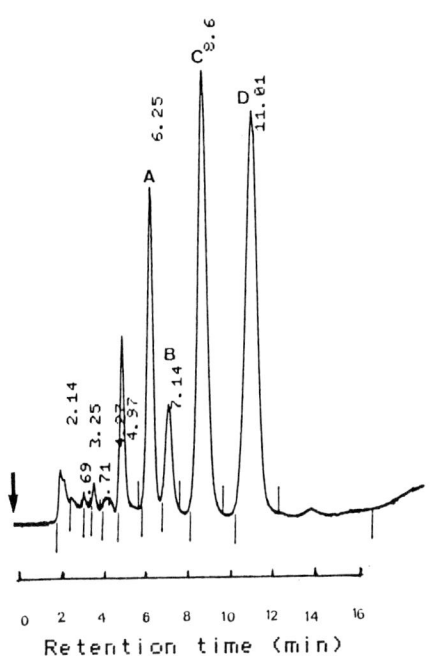

Fig. 1. Typical chromatograms obtained by injection of extracts from incubation of microsomal preparations.
A : testosterone
B : UDPGA
C : 2-naphthol glucuronide (internal standard)
D : testosterone glucuronide

Pre-column labelling with 4-bromomethyl-7-hydroxycoumarin (BrMmc)
The carboxylic group of glucuronic acid conjugate was esterified as indicated in the following scheme :

Optimum reaction conditions, structural data of resulting esters and extraction procedures from microsomal preparations have been already described (Leroy et al., 1986, Chakir et al., 1987).

Capacity factors (k') obtained for the various glucuronides tested in the two chromatographic modes are indicated in Table 2.

205

Table 2. Capacity factors (k') of Mmc-glucuronide esters.

Derivative : Mmc- glucuronide ester of	Chromatographic mode			
	Normal-phase(*)		Reversed-phase(**)	
	Mobile phase : hexane-ethanol (V/V)	k'	Mobile phase : methanol-water (V/V)	k'
menthol	80 : 20	6.0	75 : 25	7.3
borneol	80 : 20	7.0	75 : 25	5.2
androsterone	70 : 30	6.2	75 : 25	5.1
testosterone	70 : 30	6.6	75 : 25	4.8
estrone	70 : 30	7.6	70 : 30	8.0
phenol	70 : 30	4.7	65 : 35	2.6

* NP column : LiChrospher DIOL (5 μm) 250 x 4 mm I.D.
** RP column : LiChrospher 100 CH-18 (5 μm) 250 x 4 mm I.D.
Flow rate of mobile phases : 1.2 ml.min^{-1}

Spectrophotometric detection of esters provides high selectivity and sensitivity for biochemical assays due to the wavelength (λ = 328 nm) and the molar extinction coefficient (about 10^4 M^{-1} cm^{-1}). 10 pmol of each derivatized conjugate were detected in a signal-to-noise ratio of 10. Fluorimetric detection does not increase sensitivity and needs use of reversed-phase columns and a high water content in mobile phases to reach a maximum level.

Typical elution profiles of glucuronides extracted from microsomal preparations and derivatized with BrMmc are shown in Fig. 2.

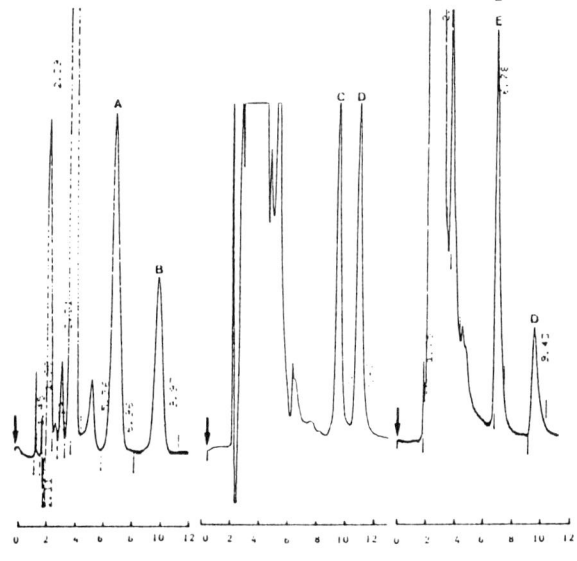

Retention time (min)

Fig. 2. Typical chromatograms obtained by injection of derivatized extracts from incubation of microsomal preparations
  I : borneol (A) and menthol (B) glucuronides in the RP-HPLC system
  II : testosterone (C), estrone (D) and androsterone (E) glucuronides in the NP-HPLC system

Biochemical results

Activation of UDP glucuronosyltransferase was achieved with two detergents : the non ionic detergent Triton X-100 as previously described (Boutin et al., 1984) for terpenes and the zwitterionic detergent CHAPS for steroids. This latter appears more advisable since it has a wider optimum activation range (detergent : protein ratios from 0.5 to 1.0 (w/w)) than Triton X-100. A value of 0.8 was retained for further experiments. The apparent kinetic parameters calculated for the studied substrates (Table 3) afford some information on UDP-glucuronosyltransferase mechanism.

Table 3. Apparent kinetic parameters of UDP-glucuronosyltransferase toward terpenes and steroids in hepatic microsomal fractions of adult Wistar rats.

Aglycones	concentration range ($\mu mol.ml^{-1}$)	Km (mM)		Vmax (nmol min^{-1} (mg protein)$^{-1}$)	
		C*	PB**	C*	PB**
menthol	0.05 to 0.80	0.07	0.12	11.00	16.20
borneol	0.06 to 0.60	0.16	0.27	20.20	28.50
testosterone	0.022 to 0.200	0.04	0.08	4.65	11.70
estrone	0.01 to 0.10	0.08	0.11	0.83	1.50
androsterone	0.007 to 0.056	0.02	–	6.06	–

* C : control rats
** PB : phenobarbital treated rats
Protein and UDPGA concentrations were 0.5 $mg.ml^{-1}$ and 3.5 mM respectively. Incubation time was 15 min.

The analysis of Km values revealed that the affinity of all the substrates considered in this study was quite similar. Only the Vmax values were different and terpenes were conjugated much faster than steroids. Glucuronidation of estrone proceeded at a very low rate. PB treatment did not change the Km value ; only the Vmax was substantially increased, thus suggesting an induction of the enzyme forms responsible for glucuronidation of terpenes and endogenous steroids.

Some remarkable feature characterize the metabolism of androsterone in Wistar rats as previously demonstrated (Matsui et al., 1986). In this study, activities measured on ten hepatic microsomal fraction batches exhibit two classes (Table 4).

Table 4. Classification of hepatic UDP-glucuronosyltransferase activities (nmol min^{-1} (mg protein)$^{-1}$) toward androsterone, measured for ten adult Wistar rats, into high-activity and low-activity groups.

High-activity*	Low-activity*	
4.90 ± 0.30	0.53 ± 0.02	0.45 ± 0.02
6.50 ± 0.20	0.55 ± 0.02	0.46 ± 0.02
4.51 ± 0.21	0.43 ± 0.01	0.32 ± 0.01
	1.02 ± 0.05	

(*) : mean + SD, calculated for four parallel assays.

Activities of UDP-glucuronosyltransferase were measured in microsomal fractions of human liver. Values as low as 0.02 nmol min^{-1}(mg protein)$^{-1}$ of testosterone glucuronide were measured by using pre-column labelling (Table 5).

Table 5. Activities of UDP-glucuronosyltransferase (nmol min^{-1}(mg protein)$^{-1}$) toward terpenes and steroids in microsomal fractions of human liver.

Sex	tumoral disease	Aglycone			
		menthol	borneol	testosterone	estrone
female	−	0.80 ± 0.03	1.01 ± 0.04	0.02 ± 0.01	ND
female	+	4.43 ± 0.32	4.71 ± 0.04	0.12 ± 0.02	0.10 ± 0.01
male	+	1.10 ± 0.02	1.27 ± 0.03	1.08 ± 0.04	0.15 ± 0.01

CONCLUSION

The two HPLC systems are versatile : they have been successfully applied to the analysis of a great variety of glucuronic acid conjugates. They present some advantages versus previously reported techniques. First, the use of cethexonium bromide as ion-pairing compound instead of usual reagents shortens elution time of apolar aglycones. Then, pre-column labelling of glucuronides is a simple and efficient approach for the enhancement of sensitivity. Limits of detection are in the pmol range per injection compared with 0.2 nmol in the case of testosterone glucuronide by direct UV spectrophotometric detection. Post-column reactions are under investigation to combine the selectivity of ion-pairing system with a highly sensitive detection. They rely upon the periodic oxidation of vicinal hydroxyl groups of the glucuronic acid moiety followed by either a condensation of the resulting aldehydic compounds with dimedone and fluorimetric detection, or the reaction of α-hydroxycarbonyl compounds with lucigenin and a chemiluminescence measurement.

REFERENCES

Baker J.K. (1981) : Estimation of high-performance liquid chromatographic retention indices of glucuronide metabolites. J. Liq. Chromatogr. 4, 271-278.

Boutin J.A., Antoine B., Batt A.M., Siest G. (1984) : Heterogeneity of hepatic microsomal UDP-glucuronosyltransferase(s) activities : comparison between human and mammalian species activities. Chem. Biol. Interact 52, 173-184.

Chakir S., Leroy P., Nicolas A., Ziegler J.M., Labory Ph. (1987) : High-performance liquid chromatographic analysis of glucuronic acid conjugates after derivatization with 4-bromomethyl-7-methoxycoumarin. J. Chromatogr. 395, 553-561.

Coughtrie M.W.H., Burchell B., Bend J.R. (1986) : A general assay for UDP-glucuronosyltransferase activity using polar amino-cyano stationary phase HPLC and UDP(U-^{14}C)glucuronic acid. Anal. Biochem. 159, 198-205.

Hamar-Hansen C., Fournel S., Magdalou J., Boutin J.A., Siest G. (1986) : Liquid chromatographic assay for the measurement of glucuronidation of arylcarboxylic acids using uridine diphospho-(U-^{14}C)glucuronic acid. J. Chromatogr. 383, 51-60.

Hogeboom G.H. (1955) : Fractionation of cell components of animal tissues. Methods Enzymol. 1, 16-19.

Leroy P. (1982) : Apport de l'oxydation periodique à la régénération de composés hydroxylés à partir de leur glucuronoconjugué obtenu par synthèse. 3rd cycle thesis, NANCY.

Leroy P., Chakir S., Nicolas A. (1986) : Measurement of the formation of menthol glucuronide in vitro, by reversed-phase high-performance liquid chromatography after pre-column labelling with 4-bromomethyl-7-methoxy-coumarin. J. Chromatogr. 351, 267-274.

Liu Z., Franklin M.R. (1984) : Separation of four glucuronides in a single sample by high-pressure liquid chromatography and its use in the determination of UDP-glucuronosyltransferase activity toward four aglycones. Anal. Biochem. 142, 340-346.

Matsui M., Nagai F. (1986) : Genetic deficiency of androsterone UDP-glucuronosyltransferase activity in Wistar rats is due to the loss of enzyme protein. Biochem. J. 234, 139-144.

Résumé

Deux systèmes de chromatographie liquide haute performance (CLHP) ont été développés afin de s'appliquer à une grande variété de glucuronides et de résoudre les difficultés rencontrées avec les techniques précédemment décrites (à savoir principalement des temps d'élution élevés pour les aglycones apolaires et une sensibilité de détection réduite pour les conjugués ayant une faible absorbance UV). Un système à polarité de phases inversée avec appariement d'ions utilisant un contre-ion apolaire (bromure de céthexonium) et un pourcentage élevé de méthanol dans la phase mobile permet de réduire considérablement la durée d'analyse. Une réaction d'estérification du groupe carboxyle au moyen de bromométhyl-4 méthoxy-7 coumarine réalisée en mode pré-colonne permet d'atteindre une limite de détection de 10 pmol de chaque glucuronide injecté. Ces méthodes ont été utilisées pour la mesure de la glucuronoconjugaison d'aglycones à structure stéroïdique, aromatique et terpénique dans des préparations microsomales provenant de foies de rat Wistar et d'Homme.

Fast atom bombardment mass spectrometry with B/E linked scanning of ether — and thiophenol — linked glucuronides

R.B. Van Breemen

Department of Chemistry, North Carolina State University, Raleigh, North Carolina 27695-8204, USA

ABSTRACT

Glucuronide molecular ions, formed by fast atom bombardment mass spectrometry, fragment at or near the glycosidic bond to produce daughter ions confirming the molecular weights of the glucuronic acid and aglycone moieties. Because matrix ions, chemical noise, or ions from contaminants sometimes hinder the identification of sample fragment ions, the MS/MS technique of B/E linked scanning with collisional activation was used to obtain daughter ion spectra of both positive and negative molecular ions of three ether-linked glucuronides and one thiophenol glucuronide. These daughter ion mass spectra were free from matrix or other contaminating ions. The B/E linked scans of the natriated molecular ion, $[M+Na]^+$, provided fragment ions confirming the molecular weights of both the aglycon and glucuronic acid groups, whereas the linked scans of molecular ions $[M+H]^+$ and $[M+NH_4]^+$ formed a less complete set of fragment ions for some glucuronides. In the negative ion B/E linked scans of $[M-H]^-$, fragmentation formed daughter ions corresponding to the glucuronic acid group and the aglycon.

KEYWORDS

glucuronide, mass spectrometry, MS/MS, fast atom bombardment

INTRODUCTION

Glucuronides are enzymatically-formed conjugates of a variety of endogenous and xenobiotic compounds with glucuronic acid. Because the polarity of glucuronides has historically hindered their characterization, chemical or enzymatic hydrolysis is often carried out prior to analysis of the released aglycone. As one alternative, the polar groups on the intact glucuronide are sometimes derivatized to increase thermal stability and volatility prior to purification by gas chromatography (Imanari and Tamura, 1967) and then analysis by electron impact or chemical ionization mass spectrometry (Fenselau and Johnson, 1980). Mass spectrometry is a highly sensitive physicochemical technique typically requiring microgram or smaller quantities of sample. In recent years, desorption ionization techniques have been developed for mass spectrometry so that underivatized, polar, and thermally labile compounds like glucuronides can be analyzed directly. Examples of these soft ionization methods applied to glucuronide analysis include laser desorption (van Breemen, et al., 1984), thermospray (Liberato, et al., 1983), and fast atom bombardment (Fenselau, et al., 1983).

Fast atom bombardment (FAB) has become the most widely used desorption ionization method for the analysis of biological molecules (Fenselau and Cotter, 1987). In FAB, sample ionization occurs as a result of bombardment by a beam of high energy atoms (usually argon or xenon at 3-10 KV). Both positive and negative ions can be formed. To facilitate ionization, organic compounds like glucuronides are bombarded while dissolved in a liquid matrix. Matrix ions are formed along with sample ions, and considerable chemical noise results from the ionization process. Because the intensity of matrix ions rapidly decreases with increasing molecular weight, glucuronide molecular ions are usually easy to distinguish. However, fragment ions derived from glucuronide molecular ions are often obscured by the matrix ions. These fragment ions, which contain structurally significant information, may be easily distinguished and the chemical background noise reduced by the use of mass spectrometry/mass spectrometry (MS/MS) techniques. MS/MS is facilitated by the sustained sample ionization provided by FAB (Carr, et.al., 1985).

Tandem and hybrid mass spectrometers have been developed for MS/MS studies, but ordinary double-focussing instruments can also be used for MS/MS measurements such as B/E linked scans in which the magnetic field (B) and the electric field (E) are scanned at a constant ratio. In this investigation, a double-focussing mass spectrometer was used to detect daughter (or fragment) ions of glucuronide molecular ion precursors. Both positive and negative ion B/E linked scans were recorded and compared to ordinary FAB mass spectra.

MATERIALS AND METHODS

Positive and negative ion fast atom bombardment mass spectra including B/E linked scans were acquired using a JEOL (Tokyo, Japan) JMS-HX110 double-focussing mass spectrometer equipped with a high field magnet, collision chamber in the first field-free region, and JMA-DA5000 data system. A mixture of cesium iodide and potassium iodide was used for calibration of positive ion FAB spectra, and negative ion FAB spectra were calibrated using sodium iodide in glycerol. The accelerating voltage was 10 KeV, and the resolving power was 1000.

Xenon gas at 3 KV was used for FAB ionization. Approximately 3 µg of glucuronide was introduced into the mass spectrometer for each positive ion FAB analysis and 1 µg for each negative ion analysis. Thioglycerol (1 µl) was used as the matrix.

For B/E linked scans, precursor ions were formed by FAB in the ionization source, and fragmentation in the first field-free region was enhanced by collisional activation. The helium gas pressure in the collision cell was increased until the precursor ion abundance was attenuated 70%. Mass spectra were recorded at constant B/E at unit resolution by the data system.

Chloramphenicol glucuronide, 11-ketoandrosterone glucuronide, menthol glucuronide, p-aminophenyl-1-thioglucuronide, glycerol, and thioglycerol were purchased from Sigma Chemical Company (St. Louis, MO, USA). Cesium iodide, potassium iodide, and sodium iodide were obtained from Fluka Chemical Corporation (Ronkonkoma, NY, USA).

RESULTS AND DISCUSSION

The molecular ion species in the FAB mass specta of four underivatized glucuronides of chloramphenicol, 11-ketoandrosterone, menthol and p-aminophenyl-1-thiol were abundant and easily discernable. Characteristic of FAB (Barber, et al., 1982), multiple molecular cations were observed in positive ion spectra, which were formed by addition of protons, NH_4^+, Na^+, or K^+, to the glucuronide molecule (Fig. 1). Molecular ion radicals, which have been observed for some glucuronides (van Breemen, et al., 1988) were not detected for these glucuronides. Although addition of ammonium or alkali metal salts to the sample or matrix would enhance the formation of $[M+NH_4]^+$, $[M+Na]^+$, etc., in these spectra, NH_4^+, Na^+, and K^+ arose from impurities in the sample, matrix, and/or the mass spectrometer. The multiplicity of molecular ions in positive ion FAB helped to confirm the molecular weight of the sample, but reduced the intensity of any one molecular ion, and lowered the sensitivity of the analysis. In negative ion FAB, molecular ion species, $[M-H]^-$, predominated, which were formed by loss of the acidic proton from the glucuronic acid moiety (Fig. 4). Because of the greater abundance of these anions compared to the corresponding molecular cations in positive ion FAB, approximately one-third as much sample (1 µg) was used for each negative ion FAB analysis compared to positive ion FAB.

Ordinary FAB spectra of glucuronides typically contain considerable chemical noise and matrix ions as shown in Figs. 1 and 4. The MS/MS technique of B/E linked scanning with collisional activation was used to reduce the background noise and eliminate interfering ions such as those derived from the thioglycerol matrix. Figures 2, 3 and 5 show B/E linked scans of different molecular ions of 11-ketoandrosterone glucuronide. The precursor ion, which was the molecular ion in each of these spectra, appears off-scale so that the daughter ions may be easily observed.

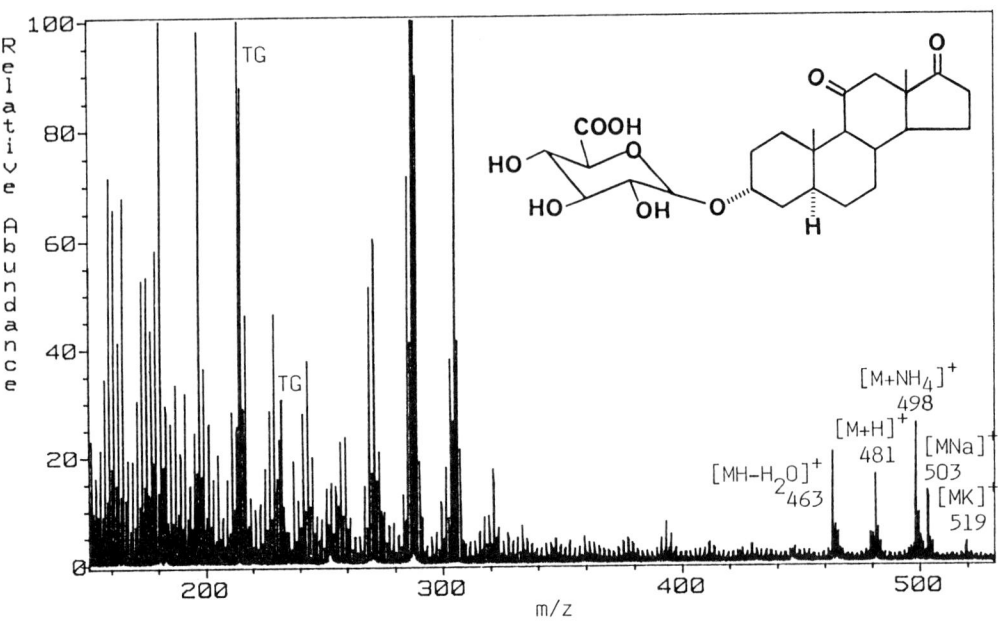

Fig. 1 Positive ion fast atom bombardment mass spectrum of 11-ketoandrosterone glucuronide. (TG=thioglycerol matrix ion)

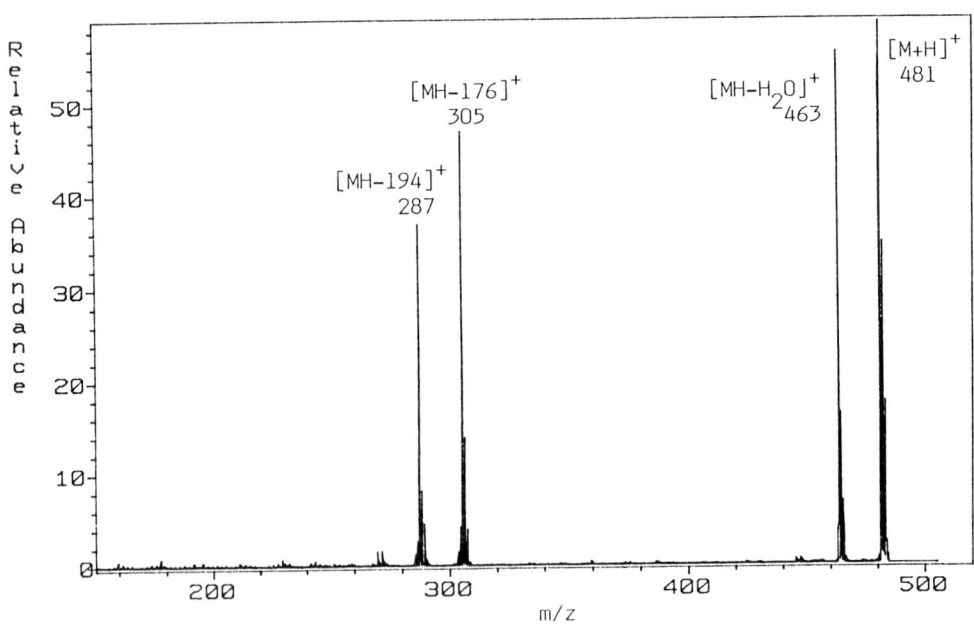

Fig. 2 B/E linked scan of [M+H]$^+$ following collisional activation. Positive ion fast atom bombardment mass spectrum of 11-ketoandrosterone glucuronide.

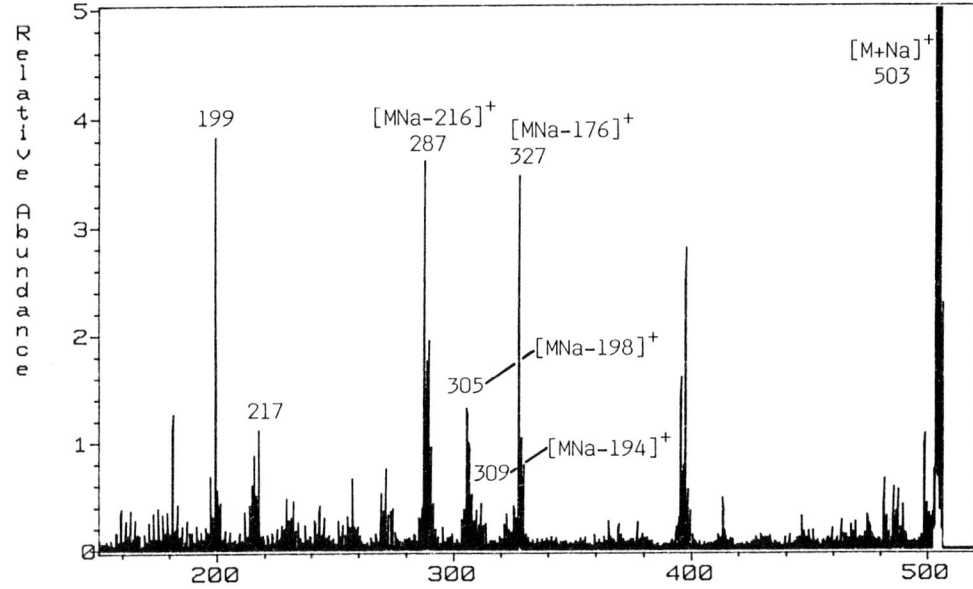

Fig. 3 B/E linked scan of [M+Na]$^+$ following collisional activation. Positive ion fast atom bombardment mass spectrum of 11-ketoandrosterone glucuronide.

Table 1. Daughter ions formed by cleavage at or near the glycosidic bond of the glucuronides of chloramphenicol, 11-ketoandrosterone, menthol, or p-aminothiophenol are summarized according to their precursor (parent) ions. B/E linked scanning following FAB ionization and collisional activation was used to measure daughter ions of particular molecular ion precursors.

Precursor Ion	Aglycon Fragment Ions	Glucuronic Acid Fragment Ions
[M+H]$^+$	[MH-176]$^+$ [MH-194]$^+$	m/z 195 177
[M+Na]$^+$	[MNa-176]$^+$ [MNa-194]$^+$ [MNa-198]$^+$ [MNa-216]$^+$	m/z 217 199
[M+NH$_4$]$^+$	[MNH$_4$-193]$^+$ [MNH$_4$-211]$^+$	m/z 195 177
[M-H]$^-$	[M-177]$^-$ [M-195]$^-$	m/z 193 or 191 159

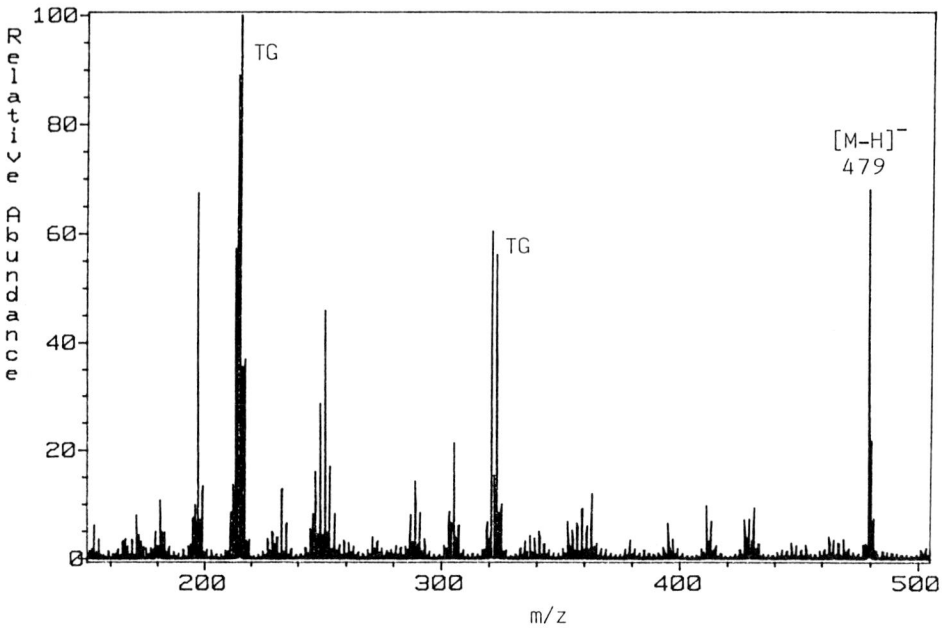

Fig. 4 Negative ion fast atom bombardment mass spectrum of 11-ketoandrosterone glucuronide. (TG=thioglycerol matrix ion)

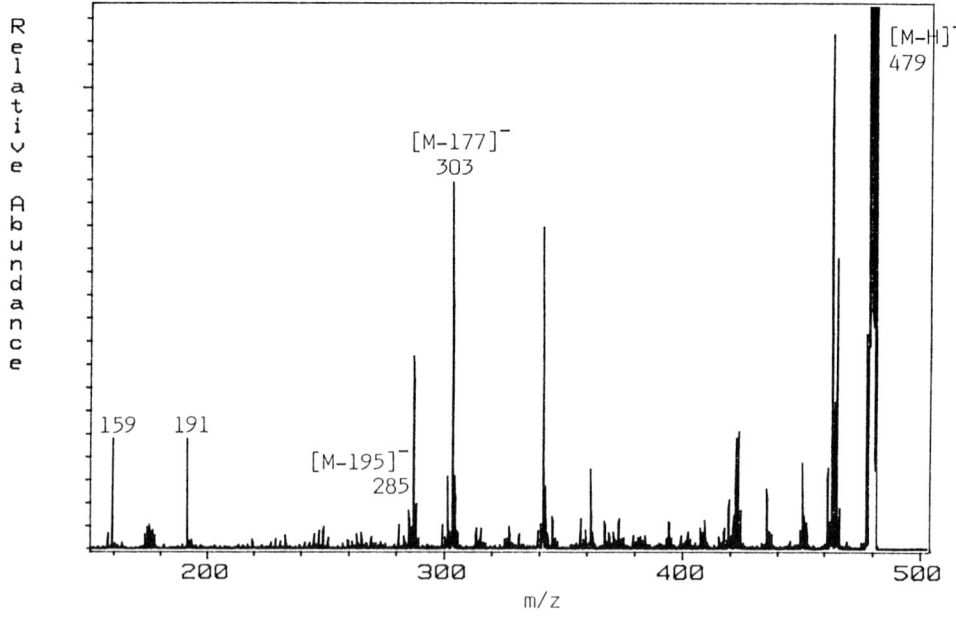

Fig. 5 B/E linked scan of [M-H]$^-$ following collisional activation. Negative ion fast atom bombardment mass spectrum of 11-ketoandrosterone glucuronide.

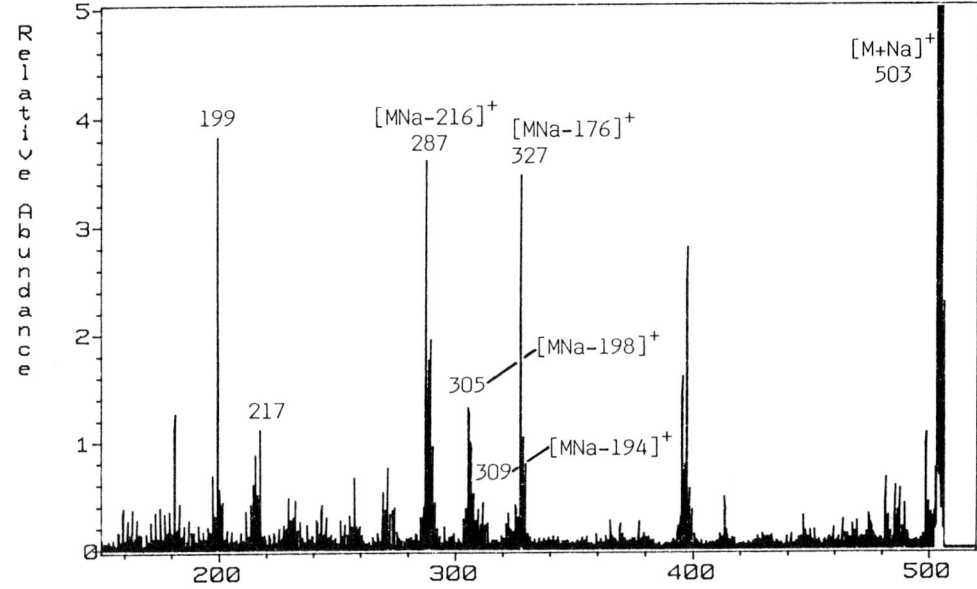

Fig. 3 B/E linked scan of [M+Na]$^+$ following collisional activation. Positive ion fast atom bombardment mass spectrum of 11-ketoandrosterone glucuronide.

Table 1. Daughter ions formed by cleavage at or near the glycosidic bond of the glucuronides of chloramphenicol, 11-ketoandrosterone, menthol, or p-aminothiophenol are summarized according to their precursor (parent) ions. B/E linked scanning following FAB ionization and collisional activation was used to measure daughter ions of particular molecular ion precursors.

Precursor Ion	Aglycon Fragment Ions	Glucuronic Acid Fragment Ions
[M+H]$^+$	[MH−176]$^+$ [MH−194]$^+$	m/z 195 177
[M+Na]$^+$	[MNa−176]$^+$ [MNa−194]$^+$ [MNa−198]$^+$ [MNa−216]$^+$	m/z 217 199
[M+NH$_4$]$^+$	[MNH$_4$−193]$^+$ [MNH$_4$−211]$^+$	m/z 195 177
[M−H]$^-$	[M−177]$^-$ [M−195]$^-$	m/z 193 or 191 159

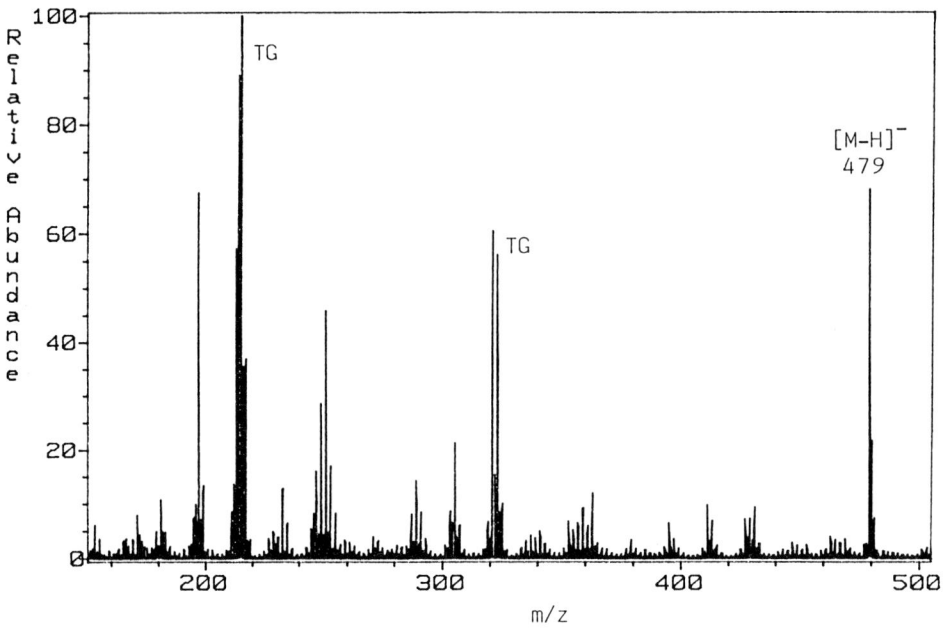

Fig. 4 Negative ion fast atom bombardment mass spectrum of 11-ketoandrosterone glucuronide. (TG=thioglycerol matrix ion)

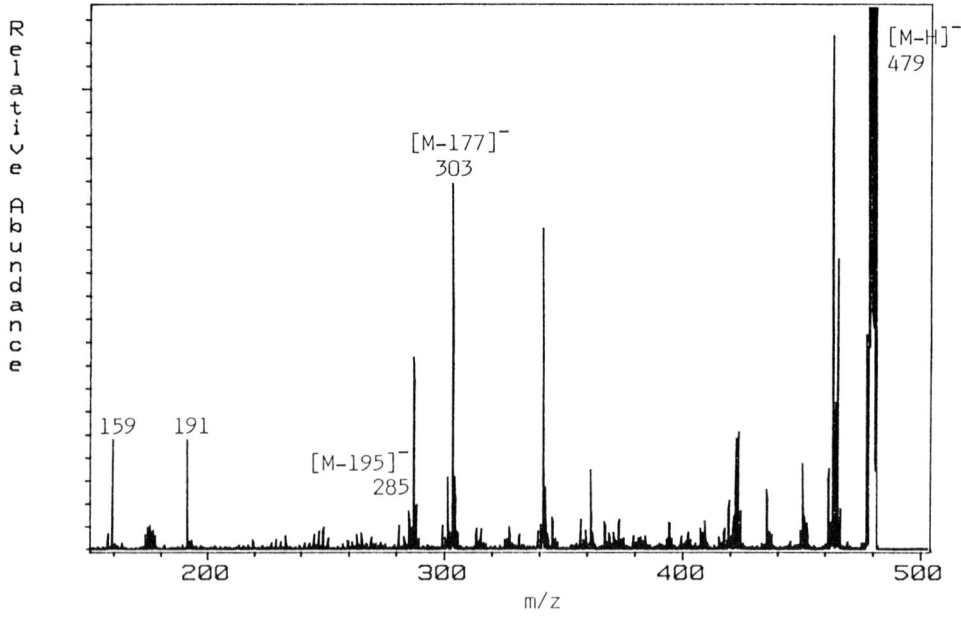

Fig. 5 B/E linked scan of $[M-H]^-$ following collisional activation. Negative ion fast atom bombardment mass spectrum of 11-ketoandrosterone glucuronide.

Fragmentation pathways involving cleavage at or near the glycosidic bond have been reported to be characteristic of FAB spectra of glucuronides (Fenselau, et al., 1983; van Breemen, et al., 1988). For the glucuronides of chloramphenicol, 11-ketoandrosterone, menthol, and p-aminothiophenol, Table 1 summarizes these characteristic daughter ions of particular molecular ion precursors, which were detected by using B/E linked scanning following FAB ionization. Aglycone fragment ions, $[MH-176]^+$ and/or $[MH-194]^+$, were observed for all samples except menthol glucuronide. Daughter ions corresponding to the glucuronic acid moiety weighing 195 and 177 mass units were detected in the linked scans of protonated molecular ions of menthol glucuronide and p-nitrophenylthioglucuronide but not the other two samples.

The multiplicity of molecular cation species was used to advantage by comparing the B/E linked scans of the precursor ions $[M+H]^+$, $[M+NH_4]^+$, and $[M+Na]^+$. Molecular ions $[M+H]^+$ and $[M+Na]^+$ have been shown to form different fragment ions for some compounds (Harada, et al., 1985). Daughter ion spectra of $[M+NH_4]^+$ ions were similar to the protonated molecular ion linked scans although they tended to contain more abundant glucuronic acid fragment ions (data not shown). However, the B/E linked scans of $[M+Na]^+$ ions contained daughter ions corresponding to both the aglycone and the glucuronic acid moieties for all four glucuronides (Table 1). Daughter ions in these spectra included $[MNa-176]^+$, $[MNa-194]^+$, $[MNa-198]^+$, and/or $[MNa-216]^+$ for the aglycone species and glucuronic acid ions weighing 217 and 199 mass units. $[M+H]^+$ and $[M+NH_4]^+$ ions readily eliminated a molecule of water whereas $[M+Na]^+$ ions did not.

B/E linked scans of negative molecular ions, $[M-H]^-$, also contained daughter ions corresponding to both the aglycone and glucuronic acid moieties following cleavage at or near the glycosidic bond (Table 1) Aglycone ions $[M-177]^-$ and $[M-195]^-$ were detected as well as the glucuronic acid species weighing 159 mass units. Other glucuronic acid fragment ions weighing either 191 or 193 mass units were observed in these spectra.

CONCLUSIONS

Although ordinary FAB mass spectra of glucuronides contain abundant molecular ions, fragment ions containing important structural information that can help confirm the presence of glucuronic acid and the molecular weight of the aglycone can be obscured by contaminant ions and ions derived from the matrix. MS/MS techniques such as B/E linked scanning with collisional activation can provide daughter ion spectra of selected molecular ion precursors that are free from matrix ions or other contaminating ions. $[M+Na]^+$ and $[M-H]^-$ ions form daughter ions confirming the molecular weights of both aglycone and glucuronic acid moieties. The set of fragment ions from $[M+H]^+$ or $[M+NH_4]^+$ precursors appears to be less informative for certain oxygen and sulfur-linked glucuronides than daughter ion spectra of $[M+Na]^+$ and $[M-H]^-$ ions.

ACKNOWLEDGMENT

Mass spectra were obtained at the Mass Spectrometry Laboratory for Biotechnology Research supported by the North Carolina Biotechnology Center.

REFERENCES

Barber, M.; Bordoli, R.S.; Elliot, G.J.; Sedgwick, R.D., and Tyler, A.N. (1982): Fast atom bombardment mass spectrometry. Anal. Chem. 54, 645A-657A.

Carr, S.A.; Reinhold, V.N.; Green, B.N., and Hass, J.R. (1985): Enhancement of structural information in FAB ionized carbohydrate samples by neutral gas collision. Biomed. Mass Spectrom. 12, 288-295.

Fenselau, C., and Johnson, L.P. (1980): Analysis of intact glucuronides by mass spectrometry and gas chromatography mass spectrometry. Drug Metab. Dispos. 8, 274-283.

Fenselau, C.; Yelle, L.; Stogniew, M.; Liberato, D.; Lehman, J.; Feng, P., and Colvin, M. Jr. (1983): Analysis of glucuronides by fast atom bombardment. Int. J. Mass Spectrom. Ion Phys. 46, 411-414.

Fenselau, C., and Cotter, R.J. (1987): Chemical aspects of fast atom bombardment. Chem. Rev. 87, 501-512.

Harada, K.; Kimura, I.; Matsuda, K., and Suzuki, M. (1985): Structural investigation of the antibiotic sporaviridin: 11-molecular secondary ion mass spectral studies on the constituent pentasaccharides viridopentaoses. Org. Mass Spectrom. 20, 582-588.

Imanari, T., and Tamura, Z. (1967): Gas chromatography of glucuronides. Chem. Pharm. Bull. 15, 1677-1681.

Liberato, D.J.; Fenselau, C.C.; Vestal, M.L., and Yergey, A.L. (1983): Characterization of glucuronides with a thermospray liquid chromatography/mass spectrometry interface. Anal. Chem. 55, 1741-1744.

van Breemen, R.B.; Tabet, J.-C., and Cotter, R.J. (1984): Characterization of oxygen-linked glucuronides by laser desorption mass spectrometry. Biomed. Mass Spectrom. 11, 278-283.

van Breemen, R.B.; Stogniew, M., and Fenselau, C. (1988): Characterization of acyl-linked glucuronides by electron impact and fast atom bombardment mass spectrometry. Biomed. Environ. Mass Spectrom. in press.

Résumé

Les ions moléculaires de glucuronides formés par ionisation FAB en spectrométrie de masse se fragmentent au niveau ou à proximité de la liaison glucosidique pour produire des ions fils qui confirment les masses moléculaires des parties acide glucuronique et aglycone. L'identification des ions fragments est parfois impossible en raison des ions provenant de la matrice, du bruit chimique ou de contaminants. Le balayage avec couplage des champs B/E en MS-MS et l'activation par collision sont utilisés pour obtenir des spectres d'ions fils à partir des ions moléculaires, en mode positif et négatif, de trois éthers de glucuronide et d'un S-glucuronide de thiophénol. Les spectres d'ions fils obtenus sont exempts d'ions de matrice ou de contaminants. Les spectres en mode B/E de l'ion moléculaire lié au sodium $[M+Na]^+$ présentent des ions qui confirment les masses moléculaires des groupements aglycone et acide glucuronique, alors que les spectres des ions $[M+H]^+$ et $[M+NH_4]^+$ montrent des ensembles moins complets d'ions fragments pour quelques glucuronides. Les spectres en technique B/E en mode négatif obtenus à partir de l'ion $[M-H]^-$ montrent une fragmentation en ions fils qui correspond aux groupements acide glucuronique et aglycone.

Modulation of UDP-glucuronosyltransferase kinetic by the lipid composition of the microsomal membranes in rat liver

J. Magdalou, B. Faye, B. Antoine and G. Siest

Centre du Médicament, U.A. CNRS n° 597, Faculté des Sciences Pharmaceutiques et Biologiques, 30 rue Lionnois, 54000 Nancy, France

ABSTRACT

This study was carried out to investigate the *in vitro* effect of cholesterol concentration of microsomal membranes on the kinetic properties of UDP-glucuronosyltransferase (4-nitrophenol). For this purpose, rat liver microsomes were incubated with liposomes different in their relative content in phosphatidylcholine and cholesterol. Upon incubation, the microsomes were enriched or depleted in cholesterol. Cholesterol/phospholipid molar ratio was 0.22 in control microsomes and varied from 0.15 to 0.31 after interaction with liposomes. A depletion in cholesterol of about 32% did not change the kinetic parameters. By contrast, cholesterol incorporation significantly stimulated by 34% the V_{max} of 4-nitrophenol glucuronidation for the latent enzyme. The Hill coefficient, which reflects the organization state of the membrane, was subsequently increased. Cholesterol incorporation also increased the V_{max} (46%) in maximally activated microsomes by Triton X-100, and decreased the dissociation constants $K_{UDP-glucuronic\ acid}$ and $K_{4-nitrophenol}$. The results indicate that changes in membrane cholesterol content modified the kinetic properties of UDP-glucuronosyltransferase.

KEYWORDS

Cholesterol incorporation in membranes -lipid exchange-enzyme kinetic-liposomes

INTRODUCTION

UDP-glucuronosyltransferase (UDPGT) is associated to the subcellular membranes of the hepatocytes, mainly the endoplasmic reticulum (Antoine et al., 1983). Because of this membrane situation, the enzyme is strictly lipidodependent. In microsomes the enzyme is latent; but any modification of the lipid environment by detergents or phospholipases dramatically activates the enzyme (Magdalou et al., 1979). The latency/activation of UDPGT has been explained either by changes in the protein conformation, or by facilitation of the accessibility of UDP-glucuronic acid to the active site (Vessey and Zakim, 1978; Berry and Hallinan, 1976). Nevertheless, whatever the hypothesis postulated, it appears that lipid-protein interactions play a major role in glucuronidation reaction. Untill now the effects of membrane phospholipids on UDPGT kinetic has been considered in microsomes (Zakim and Vessey, 1975a) or after purification (Magdalou et al., 1982a). The physicochemical properties of the membranes itself, and especially the tansition state gel-liquid of the lipid phase were also suspected to alter the catalytic behavior of UDPGT (Zakim and Vessey, 1987b). Recently, Castuma and Brenner (1986) pointed out the role of cholesterol, as a membrane condensing agent of the lipid bilayer, on the modulation of glucuronidation reaction in guinea pigs. This work was carried out to precise the *in vitro* effect of incorporation of cholesterol or phosphatidylcholine in microsomes on the V_{max} and dissociation constants for glucuronidation of 4-nitrophenol. The results were related to the organisation state of the lipid phase estimated from the determination of the Hill coefficient.

MATERIAL AND METHODS

Preparation of the enzyme fraction

Male wistar rats, 180-200 g (Domaine des Oncins, St. Germain l'Abresle, France) were housed in cages with kiln-pine shavings as bedding in an environmentally controled room (12 hr light cycle, 22°C). They were killed by decapitation and their liver was quickly removed and homogenized in 0.250 M sucrose with a Potter-Elvejhem apparatus (1500 rpm, 3 strokes), in ice. The microsomal fraction was prepared by differential ultracentrifugations. The pellets were homogenized in 0.250 M sucrose, 1mM Tris-HCl buffer, pH 7.4.

Determination of enzyme activity

Glucuronidation of 4-nitrophenol (Merck, Darmstadt, FRG) was followed according to the method of Frei (1966) on an Aminco DW2 spectrophotometer. The co-substrat UDP-glucuronic acid was provided by Boehringer (Mannheim, FRG). Latent activity of UDPGT was measured without any detergent. Glucuronidation of the fully activated enzyme was followed after addition of Triton X-100 (Sigma, St. Louis MO), at the optimal detergent/weight ratio of 0.4. The value of activity at V_{max} and that of the dissociation constants were determined for an enzyme with a rapid equilibrium, random order kinetic mechanism.

Determination of membrane lipid composition and incorporation of cholesterol to microsomes

Extraction separation and quantification of phospholipids from microsomes were carried out as previously described (Thomassin *et al.*, 1986). Total cholesterol was evaluated by the technique of Klose *et al.* (1975). Enrichment of microsomes in phosphatidylcholine and cholesterol was achieved by incubation of microsomes with liposomes whose cholesterol/phospholipids composition varied. For liposome preparation, 43 moles of a chloroform solution of pure egg-phosphatidylcholine (Sigma, St.Louis, MO) was evaporated to dryness under reduced pressure. Cholesterol (0 to 200 moles, Merck, Darmstadt, FRG) was added at this stage and suspended in 10 mM Tris-HCl, pH 7.4 containing 100 mM KCl, 1mM ascorbate. The mixture was vigorously agitated with a vortex and sonicated for 20 min under nitrogen with a titanium-probe sonicator (MSE, UK) . The suspension was centrifuged at 20°C for 30 min at 100,000 x g in an ultracentrifuge Beckman L5-75 B equipped with a 50 Ti rotor. The clear supernatant was taken as the liposome fraction. Incorporation of cholesterol and phosphatidylcholine into microsomes was performed by lipid exchange according to Archakov *et al.* (1983). Briefly, the liposomes were incubated with microsomes at 30°C for 120 min in 180 mM Tris-HCl buffer, pH 7.4 containing 1mM EDTA, 1mM dithiothreitol (Sigma, St. Louis, MO, USA). Non incorporated liposomes were removed by centrifugation for 180 min at 115,000 x g in the same buffer containing 0.5 M sucrose. The lipid composition of this final preparation was measured as previously described.

RESULTS AND DISCUSSION

Upon incubation of liver microsomes with liposomes containing egg phosphatidylcholine or cholesterol, the amounts in phospholipids and cholesterol were markedly increased by 93% and 108%, respectively in the membrane bilayers (Table 1). The corresponding cholesterol/phospholipids varied from 0.22 in control microsomes to 0.15 in phospholipid-enriched microsomes and 0.31 in cholesterol-enriched microsomes. In these conditions the value of V_{max} for glucuronidation of 4-nitrophenol by the latent enzyme as well as the Hill coefficient were not affected by addition of phosphatidylcholine in the microsomal membranes (Table 2).

Table 1. Lipid composition of liver microsomes upon incubation with liposomes

Microsomal Fractions	[a]Total Cholesterol	[a]Total Phospholipids	Cholesterol/Phospholipid (Molar ratio)
Controls	83 ± 19	375 ± 56	0.22
Phospholipid enriched	106 ± 9	723 ± 98[b]	0.15
Phospholipid and cholesterol enriched	173 ± 7[b]	564 ± 78[b]	0.31

[a] The results were expressed in nmol/mg protein. Values are the mean ± SD for three independent experiments. [b] $p<0.05$, significantly different from controls.

Table 2. Détermination of the kinetic constants for glucuronidation of 4-nitrophenol in microsomes different in lipid composition.

Microsomal Fractions	[a]Latent enzyme		[a]Triton X-100 activated enzyme				
	V_{max}	Hill coefficient	V_{max}	K_{UDPGA}	K'_{UDPGA}	K_{4-NP}	K'_{4-NP}
Controls	2.67 ± 0.29	0.43 ± 0.03	28	0.28	0.24	0.10	0.08
Phospholipid enriched	3.03 ± 0.68	0.39 ± 0.02	32	0.58	0.11	0.26	0.05
Phospholipid and cholesterol enriched	4.07 ± 0.45[b]	0.54 ± 0.06[b]	41	0.19	0.37	0.04	0.08

[a] The activity at V_{max} were expressed as nmol 4-nitrophenol (4-NP) conjugated/min/mg protein ; the dissociation constants K, for an enzyme with a rapid equilibrium, random order kinetic mechanism, were in mM. Values are the mean ± SD for three independent experiments.
[b] $p<0.05$, significantly different from controls. UDPGA, UDP-Glucuronic acid.

This suggests that, despite phospholipid incorporation to the microsomal membranes, the organisation of the lipid phase, as indicated from the Hill coefficient, and the velocity of the reaction were not apparently changed. By contrast, V_{max} was significantly enhanced by 52% after cholesterol addition. At the same time, the Hill coefficient was increased by 25% when cholesterol-enriched microsomes were used. After fully activation of UDPGT by Triton X-100, changes in phosphatidylcholine and cholesterol concentrations modified both the dissociation constants of the different enzyme-substrates complexes and the V_{max}. The affinity of the free enzyme towards UDP-glucuronic acid and 4-nitrophenol was increased by cholesterol addition, whereas the affinity of UDPGT already saturated by one substrate for the second substrate was decreased after addition of phosphatidylcholine and increased after cholesterol addition. Cholesterol is known for changing the physicochemical properties of the membranes (Cullis et al., 1978). This was supported in this study, by an increase in the value of the Hill coefficient, thus suggesting an increase in the membrane viscosity. Cholesterol incorporation has been associated to shift the glucuronidation reaction from non-Michaelian to Michaelian kinetic in guinea pig liver microsomes (Castuma and Brenner, 1986). The 25% increase in the Hill coefficient found in this work also suggested this evolution. This could be of relevant importance for UDPGT present in membranes rich in cholesterol, such as the plasma membranes (Magdalou et al., 1982b; Antoine et al., 1984).

REFERENCES

Antoine, B., Magdalou, J. and Siest G.(1983): Functional heterogeneity of UDP-glucuronosyltransferases in different membranes of rat liver. Biochem. Pharmacol. 32, 2629-2632.

Antoine, B., Magdalou, J. and Siest, G. (1984): Kinetic properties of UDP-glucuronosyltransferase(s) in different membranes of rat liver cells. Xenobiotica 14, 575-579.

Archakov, A. I., Borodin, E. A., Dobretsov, G. E., Karasevich E. I. and Karyakin, A. V.(1983): The influence of cholesterol incorporation and removal on lipid-bilayer viscosity and electron transfer in rat-liver microsomes. Eur. J. Biochem. 134, 89-95.

Berry, C. and Hallinan, T.(1976): Summary of a novel, three-component regulatory model for uridine diphosphate glucuronyltransferase. Biochem. Soc. Trans. 4, 650-652.

Castuma, C. E. and Brenner, R. R.(1986): Cholesterol-dependent modification of microsomal dynamics and UDP-glucuronyltransferase. Biochemistry 25, 4733-4738.

Cullis, P. R., Van Dijck, P. W. M., De Kruijff, B. and De Gier, J.(1978): Effects of cholesterol on the properties of equimolar mixtures of synthetic phosphatidylethanolamine and phosphatidylcholine. A ^{31}P NMR and differential scanning calorimetry study. Biochim. Biophys. Acta 513, 21-30.

Frei, J. and Falcao, L.(1966): Leucocyte et glucuronoconjugaison. Helv. Physiol. Pharmacol. Acta 24, 84-85.

Klose, S., Hagen, A. and Greif, H.(1975): Méthode de dosage colorimétrique du cholestérol par voie entiè rement enzymatique adaptée à tous les types d'auto-analyseurs. In Organisation des Laboratoires et Interprétation des Résultats, ed G. Siest, pp 505-507. Paris: L'Expansion Scientifique Française.

Magdalou, J., Balland, M., Thirion, C. and Siest, G.(1979): Effects of membrane perturbants on UDP-glucuronyltransferase activity in rat-liver microsomes. Chem. Biol. Interac. 27, 255-268.

Magdalou, J., Hochman, Y. and Zakim, D.(1982a): Factors modulating the catalytic activity of a pure form of UDP-glucuronyltransferase. J. Biol. Chem. 257, 13624-13629.

Magdalou, J., Antoine, B., Ratanasavanh, D. and Siest, G. (1982b): Phenobarbital induction of cytochrome P-450 and UDP-glucuronyltransferase in rabbit liver plasma membranes. Enzyme 28, 41-47.

Thomassin, J., Dragacci, S., Faye, B., Magdalou, J. and Siest G.(1986): Kinetic constant determination of liver microsomal and purified UDP-glucuronyltransferase after phenobarbital and 3-methylcho lanthrene treatments in rats. Comp. Biochem. Physiol. 83, 127-131.

Vessey, D. A. and Zakim, D. (1978): Are glucuronidation reactions compartimented? In Conjugation Reactions in Drug Biotransformation., ed A. Aitio, pp 247-255. Elsevier/North Holland Biomedical Press.

Zakim, D. and Vessey D. A.(1975a): Regulation of microsomal enzymes by phospholipids. IX. Production of uniquely modified forms of microsomal UDP-glucuronyltransferase by treatment with phospholipase A and detergents. Biochim. Biophys. Acta 410, 61-73.

Zakim, D. and Vessey, D. A.(1975b): The effect of a temperature-induced phase change within the membrane lipids on the regulatory properties of microsomal uridine diphosphate glucuronyltransferase. J. Biol. Chem. 250, 342-343.

Résumé

Cette étude a pour but de mettre en évidence l'effet de la composition lipidique, en particulier de la teneur en cholesterol des microsomes hépatiques, sur les propriétés cinétiques de l'UDP-glucuronosyltransférase. A cette fin les microsomes sont incubés en présence de liposomes différant par leur composition relative en phosphatidylcholine et cholestérol. Après échange de lipides entre les deux types de membranes, le rapport molaire cholestérol:phospholipides varie de 0,15 à 0,31; ce rapport étant égal à 0.22 dans les microsomes natifs. Une déplétion (32%) en cholestérol ne modifie pas les paramètres cinétiques de la conjugaison du 4-nitrophénol. Au contraire, l'incorporation de cholestérol stimule de façon significative (34%) la V_{max} de l'enzyme latente. Le coefficient de Hill, qui reflète l'état d'organisation de la membrane des microsomes, est augmenté. L'addition de cholestérol augmente également la V_{max} (46%) de l'enzyme activée par un détergent Triton X-100, et diminue les constantes de dissociation $K_{acide\ UDP-glucuronique}$ et $K_{4-nitrophénol}$ mesurées pour un système enzymatique en équilibre rapide dont les deux substrats se fixent au hasard. Les résultats montrent que la variation en cholestérol membranaire modifie les propriétés cinétiques de l'UDP-glucuronosyltransferase.

Reconstitution of UDP-glucose-sterol-β-D-glucosyltransferase into lipid vesicles and regulation by phospholipids

A. Ury, P. Ullmann, P. Bouvier-Nave and P. Benveniste

Laboratoire de Biochimie Végétale, U.A. 1182 du CNRS, Institut de Botanique, 28, rue Goethe, 67083, Strasbourg, France

ABSTRACT

The UDP-glucose-sterol-glucosyltransferase (UDPG-SGTase) of maize coleoptiles microsomes was partially purified in the detergent Triton X-100 ; the resulting enzyme preparation was strongly delipidated and inactivated (Ullmann, P., Bouvier-Navé, P. and Benveniste, P. (1987) - Plant Physiol., 85, 51-55). This enzyme preparation was then incorporated into unilamellar phospholipid vesicles by removing detergents from Octylglucoside / Triton X-100 / Phospholipid / Sterol / Enzyme mixed micelles by chromatography over Sephadex G-50. This treatment leads to almost complete removal of detergents. Activity coelutes with liposomes of 260 Å average diameter on Sephacryl S-1000 column. Furthermore, in flotation experiments on metrizamide density gradients, active enzyme is recovered with the lipid fraction, thus confirming the incorporation of UDPG-SGTase into the vesicles bilayer. The integrity of these liposomes is established by trapping 5,5'-Dithiobis (2-nitrobenzoic acid) (DTNB) into their internal volume. p-Chloro-mercuriphenyl-sulfonic acid (pCMBS) treatment of intact vesicles strongly suggests the asymmetrical orientation of the enzyme with its active site facing outward. Our results indicate that the reconstituted UDPG-SGTase activity can be activated in a large extent by negatively charged phospholipids, as shown by measurement of kinetic parameters of the reaction.

INTRODUCTION

Steryl glucosides and acylated steryl glucosides are present with free and esterified sterols in all plant tissues investigated so far, but not in animals. The physiological role of these glucosylated compounds is still to be defined. The glucosylation of sterols is catalyzed by UDPG-SGTase, a plasma membrane-bound enzyme of plant cells :

$$Sterol \ + \ UDP\text{-}glucose \longrightarrow Steryl \ glucoside \ + \ UDP \ .$$

This enzyme, solubilized in Triton X-100 and partially purified by chromatography on DEAE-cellulose, exhibits a lipid-dependence in micellar conditions. A preferential affinity for negatively charged phospholipids has been shown (Ullmann et al., 1987). The kind of reaction catalyzed by UDPG-SGTase and its requirement for phospholipids present some analogy with those of UDP-glucuronyltransferase (Erickson et al., 1978). To investigate its regulation by lipids in more physiological conditions (bilayers instead of micelles), incorporation of the enzyme into liposomes was performed.

MATERIALS AND METHODS

The UDPG-SGTase preparation used for the reconstitution corresponds to the enriched fractions after a DEAE cellulose DE 52 purification step (Ullmann et al., 1987). The reconstitution procedure was performed as described by Green and Bell (1984) with some modifications. Lipids used for proteoliposomes formation are soybean phosphatidylcholine (PC), phosphatidylglycerol (PG) and phosphatidic acid (PA) from egg yolk lecithin. Sterols consist in 92% β-sitosterol and 8% campesterol. Vesicles size was determined by gel filtration using Sephacryl S-1000 chromatography (Reynolds et al., 1983) and their integrity was established according to Ganong and Bell (1984) using DTNB. For UDPG-SGTase assay, UDP$[^{14}C]$glucose (40 µl) at different concentrations is added to proteoliposomes (160 µl) corresponding to the void volume peak of the Sephadex G-50 column. The reaction is run at 30°C for 15 min and stopped by boiling the mixture for 1 min. Reaction products are extracted as previously described (Ullmann et al., 1987).

RESULTS AND DISCUSSION

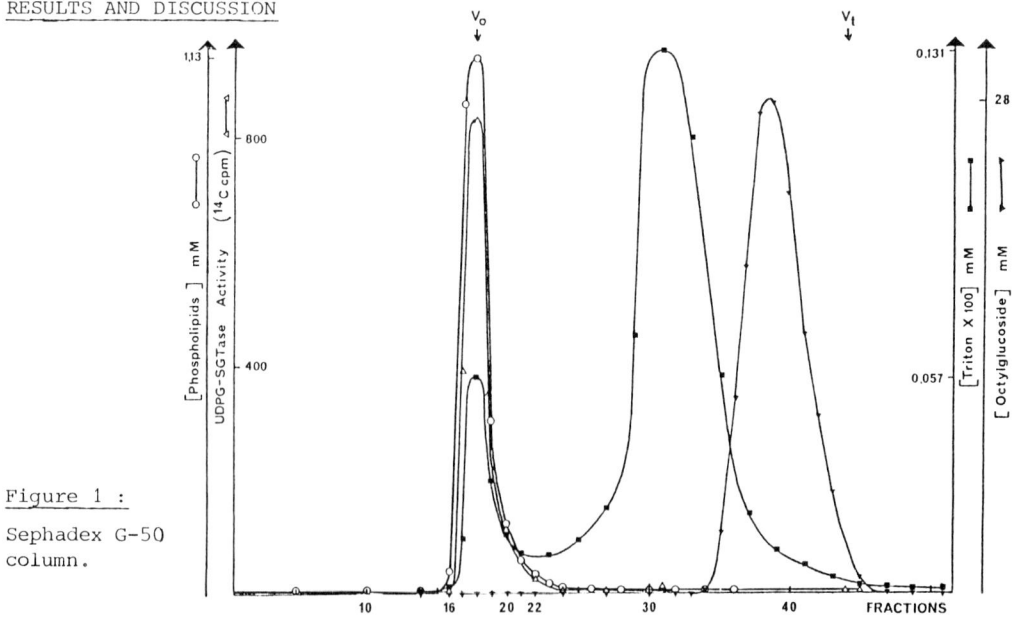

Figure 1 :

Sephadex G-50 column.

Reconstitution into single-walled vesicles - Successful reconstitution of UDPG-SGTase into single-walled vesicles is achieved by passing an Octylglucoside / Triton X-100 / Phospholipid / Sterol / Enzyme mixture through a Sephadex G-50 (Green and Bell, 1984). Enzyme activity coelutes with lipids in the void volume of the column and is well separated from Triton X-100 and Octylglucoside peaks (Fig.1). The resulting vesicles containing active UDPG-SGTase have less than 1 Triton X-100 and 1,5 Octylglucoside molecules / 20 lipid molecules.

Two results demonstrate that the UDPG-SGTase is incorporated into the vesicles bilayer : activity (i) coelutes with the vesicles in the included volume of Sephacryl S-1000 column (Fig.2) and (ii) is recovered with the lipid fraction, in flotation experiments on metrizamide density gradients (data not shown).

Characterization of UDPG-SGTase containing liposomes - Sephacryl S-1000 gel exclusion chromatography was also used to determine proteoliposomes size (Reynolds et al., 1983). The peak of activity elutes with a maximum at Kd = 0,61 correlating to an average vesicles diameter of 260 Å (Fig.2).

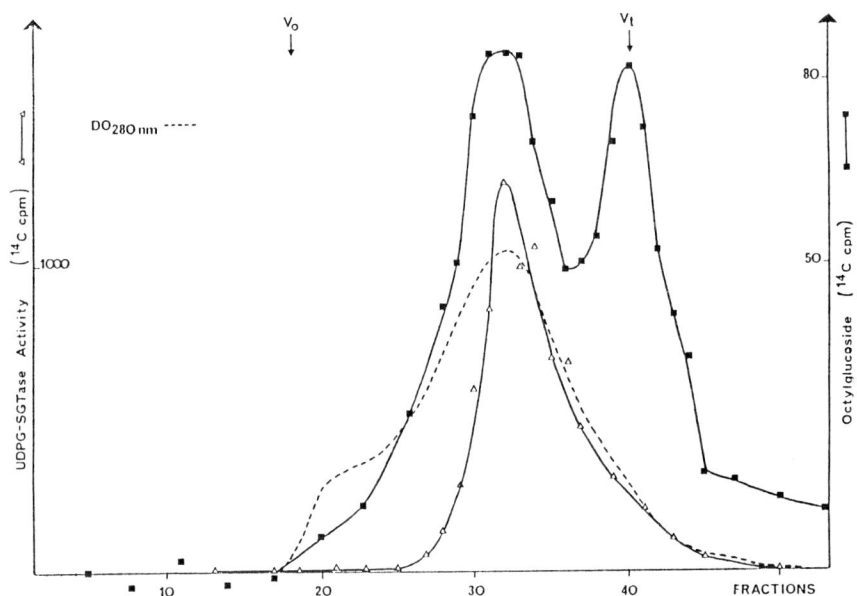

Figure 2 : Sephacryl S-1000 column

Vesicle integrity was investigated by monitoring the leakage of DTNB that is incorporated into the vesicles during the reconstitution procedure (Ganong and Bell, 1984). When vesicles are stored at 4°C, the half-life for release of DTNB is 25 days (data not shown), thus indicating that the liposomes are tightly sealed. The orientation of the active site of UDPG-SGTase within the vesicles bilayer was determined by measuring the activity remaining after treating vesicles with pCMBS. Under the conditions of treatment (10 min at 4°C), pCMBS is unable to penetrate the tightly sealed vesicles (Giaquinta, 1976). For all of them, differing in phospholipid composition, more than 95% of the UDPG-SGTase activity is lost ; this result strongly suggests that the enzyme is reconstituted asymmetrically with its active site facing outward.

Effect of Phospholipids on Reconstituted UDPG-SGTase activity - To examine the modulation of UDPG-SGTase kinetic parameters by negatively charged phospholipids, the enzyme was reconstituted into a variety of phospholipid vesicles (Table I). Results clearly show a large increase of Vmax and Km_{UDPG} induced by either PG or PA, with a maximum increase at a PC/PG (PA) molar ratio of 3/1.

Vesicle composition	Molar ratio	Apparent Vmax (pmol/mg prot./s)	Km-UDPG (µM)
PC		13	36
PC/PG	9/1	60	75
	3/1	167	143
	1/1	133	125
PC/PA	9/1	54	60
	3/1	56	87
	1/1	6	38

Table I : Effect of vesicle phospholipid composition on UDPG-SGTase kinetic parameters. For all the vesicles, lipids analysis showed that : (i) the final molar ratio PL/sterol is 3,5:1, (ii) the final PL concentrations are similar and (iii) the different molar ratios PC/negatively charged PL are conserved through the reconstitution step.

CONCLUSION

In order to gain insight into the regulation of UDPG-SGTase activity by phospholipids we have reconstituted the purified enzyme into well characterized liposomes. Our results clearly indicate a strong stimulation of the enzyme by negatively charged phospholipids, thus confirming previous results obtained in micellar conditions. The decrease of affinity for UDPG and the increase of Vmax induced by negatively charged phospholipids are reminiscent of the results reported for UDP-Glucuronyltransferase (Hochman et al., 1981).

REFERENCES

ERICKSON, R.H., ZAKIM, D. and VESSEY, D.A. (1978) : Biochem., 17, 3706-3711.
GANONG, B.R. and BELL, R.M. (1984) : Biochemistry, 23, 4977-4983.
GIAQUINTA, R. (1976) : Plant Physiol., 57, 872-875.
GREEN, P.R. and BELL, R.M. (1984) : J. Biol. Chem., 259, 14688-14694.
HOCHMAN, Y., ZAKIM, D. and VESSEY, D.A. (1981) : J. Biol. Chem., 256, 4783-4788.
REYNOLDS, J.A., NOZAKI, Y. and TANFORD, C. (1983) : Anal. Biochem., 130, 471-474.
ULLMANN, P., BOUVIER-NAVE, P. and BENVENISTE, P. (1987) : Plant Physiol., 85, 51-55.

Résumé

L'UDPG-SGTase de microsomes de coléoptiles de maïs a été délipidée et partiellement purifiée dans du Triton X-100, puis incorporée dans des vésicules phospholipidiques par élimination des détergents à partir d'un mélange Octylglucoside / Triton X-100 / Phospholipides / Stérols / Enzyme par chromatographie sur gel de Sephadex G-50. Ce traitement conduit à l'élimination quasi totale des détergents. Sur colonne de Sephacryl S-1000, l'activité coélue avec les liposomes de 260 Å de diamètre moyen. Par ailleurs, dans des expériences de flottation sur gradients de densité en metrizamide, l'activité enzymatique est récupérée avec la fraction lipidique, confirmant ainsi l'incorporation de l'UDPG-SGTase dans la bicouche des vésicules. L'intégrité de ces liposomes est établie en encapsulant du DTNB dans leur volume interne. Le traitement de ces vésicules au pCMBS suggère fortement une orientation asymétrique de l'enzyme avec son site actif situé vers l'extérieur. La détermination des paramètres cinétiques de la réaction montre une forte activation de l'UDPG-SGTase par les phospholipides chargés négativement.

Monoclonal antibodies to rat liver 4-nitrophenol UDP-glucuronosyltransferase

L. von Meyerinck, C. Augustin[2], M. Schulz[2], F. Donn[3], H.F. Benthe, and A. Schmoldt[2]

Departments of Pharmacology and Legal Medicine[2], University of Hamburg, D-2000 Hamburg 20, Martinistrasse 52, FRG and Marienhospital[3], Alfredstr. 6, D-2000 Hamburg 76, FRG

SUMMARY

Two monoclonal antibodies were developed for purified rat liver 4-nitrophenol UDP-glucuronyltransferase. The antibodies anti-rat-pnpgt-67-mab and anti-rat-pnpgt-96 mab were specific for 4-nitrophenol UDP-glucuronyltransferase in Western-blot experiments. Whereas anti-rat-pnpgt-96-mab recognized two bands, anti-rat-pnpgt-67-mab recognized only one band. Both antibodies verified their characteristics when microsomes from differentially induced animals were investigated and staining was maximal in 5,6-benzoflavone treated animals.

MOTS CLEFS

monoclonal antibodies - UDP-glucuronyltransferase - UDP-glucuronosyltransferase glucuronidation - western blotting

INTRODUCTION

Monoclonal antibodies to UDP-glucuronosyltransferases are still rare: According to our knowledge only Peters et al. (1987) published results about a monoclonal antibody, which enabled the tissue immunostaining of an enzyme form. The antibody further inhibited 4-nitrophenol-, 4-methylumbeliferron-, and bilirubin-glucuronidation. This paper did not show any Western-blot results.
Monoclonal antibodies proved to be a useful tool in the research of the cytochrome P-450 isoenzyme forms as described by Gelboin and Friedman (1985).
We were interested, whether it is possible to improve the immunological detection of 4-nitrophenol UDP-glucuronosyltransferase with monoclonal antibodies in comparison to heterosera raised against this enzyme form so far.

MATERIAL AND METHODS

IMMUNISATION
Immunisation of 4 female Balb/c mice was carried out with 20 µg of purified 4-nitrophenol UDP-glucuronosyltransferase according to Falany and Tephly (1983) with Freund complete adjuvant on day one and further ip injections on day 8, 15 and 23 with the same antigen in incomplete Freund adjuvant. On day 30 the mice received final boostering injections with pure antigen and were sacrificed three days later.

FUSION OF HYBRIDOMAS
The fusion of the hybridoma cell lines was performed according to the technique of Köhler and Milstein (1975) with X63-AG.8.653 myeloma cells. The fused cells were placed in high dilution into ten 24-well plates and grown for ten days with hypoxanthine-aminopterine-thymidine addition in RPMI-1254 medium with 20 % fetal calf serum for ten days and further grown in the same medium without aminopterine. All wells were screened for antibody secretion with the dot-blot-technique. All cell culture media were from GIBCO, Karlsruhe, F.R.G..

Screening of the clones was performed with dot-blot-technique with custom-made 96-well dot-blot-apparatus' similar to the models available for nick-translation.

SDS-POLYACRYLAMIDE GELELECTROPHORESIS
8 µg samples of microsomes induced with phenobarbital (80 mg/kg day for four days ip in 0.9 % NaCl) or 5,6-benzoflavone (40 mg/kg day for four days ip in peanut oil) were run on each well of a conventional vertical slab gel electrophoresis chamber (Mini-Protean II, BIORAD, Munich, F.R.G.) on 6 x 8 cm gels of 0.75 mm gauge, 10 % separation gels and 3 % stacking gels according to the guidelines of the manufacturer with 100 V for 5 min and 200 V for 45 min as outlined by Laemmli (1970). Samples were pretreated by the addition of ß-mercaptoethanol and SDS to final concentrations of 5 % and 1 %, respectively, and placed in a boiling water bath for 10 min. Prestained gelelectrophoresis standards were from GIBCO-BRL (Karlsruhe, F.R.G.) and were pretreated equally. Gels were removed from the apparatus when the bromphenolblue stained front migrated close to the bottom. If not otherwise quoted, all electrophoresis chemicals were from BIORAD, Munich, F.R.G..

WESTERN BLOT ANALYSIS
The removed gels were placed onto layers of filter paper on a semi-dry blotter (SARTORIUS, Göttingen F.R.G.), soaked in the appropriated buffers recommended by the manufacturer. Transfer was performed to nitrocellulose BA 85 for 1 hour at room temperature with 0.8 mA/cm^2 current, typically about 40 mA. Gels were removed and stained: 3 times 10 min washings in TBS to remove traces of transfer buffer, one hour blocking of excess binding sites of the nitrocellulose with 2 % BSA in TTBS, overnight incubation in the appropriate antibody solution, 3 times 10 min washings in TTBS, secondary antibody reaction with a goat-anti-mouse alkaline phosphatase-conjugate in a 20,000-fold dilution in TTBS. Staining was obtained following three last washings for 10 min in TBS pH 9.4 with 0.4 M nitrobluetetrazolium and 0.38 M of the toluedene salt of 5-bromo-4-chloro-indolylphosphate according to Leary et al. (1983).

RESULTS

The experimental design as outlined above enabled us to resolve two monoclonal hybridoma cell lines anti-rat-pnpgt-67-mab and anti-rat-pnpgt-96-mab. Both these cell lines secreted antibodies which recognized 4-nitrophenol-UDP-glucuronosyltransferase. Anti-rat-pnpgt-96-mab stained two bands of this enzyme in differentially induced rat liver microsomes (figure 1, upper panel): whereas the signal was faint in control- and phenobarbital-microsomes the signal was increased heavily in 5,6-benzoflavone treated microsomes and further proved the induction process of the 3-methylcholanthrene-type. Anti-rat-pnpgt-67-mab (figure 1, lower panel) differentiated these two bands: whereas the upper band was stained only faint in all microsomes tested, the lower band was stained according to the type of induction and was heavily increased in microsomes of 5,6-benzoflavone-treated rats.

Subisotyping of the antibodies showed them to be of different IgG-subtypes: Whereas anti-rat-pnpgt-67-mab is an IgG2B subtype, the anti-rat-pnpgt-96-mab is of IgG3 subtype.

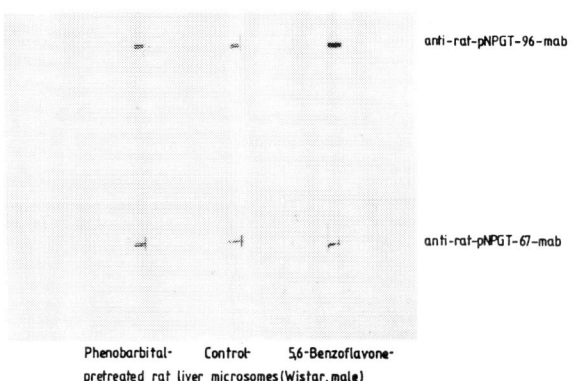

Fig. 1: Western-blots with anti-rat-pnpgt-96-mab (upper lane) and anti-rat-pnpgt-67-mab (lower lane) of male Wistar rat liver microsomes of animals pretreated with either 5,6-benzoflavone or phenobarbital or untreated. The detection system consists of the appropriate monoclonal antibody and an alkaline phosphatase conjugated goat-anti-mouse heteroserum. For all other methodological details see the Materials and Methods section.

REFERENCES

C.N.Falany and T.R.Tephly (1983): Separation, purification and characterization of three different isoenzymes of UDP-GT from rat liver microsomes. Arch. Biochem. Biophys. 227, 248-258.
H.V.Gelboin and F.K.Friedman (1985): Monoclonal antibodies for studies on xenobiotics and endobiotic metabolism. Biochem. Pharmacol. 13, 2225-2234.
G.Köhler and C.Milstein (1975): Continuous cultures of fused cells secreting antibody of predifined specificity. Nature 256, 495-497.
U.K.Laemmli (1970): Cleavage of structural proteins during the assembly of the head of bacteriophage T4. Nature 227, 680-685.
J.J. Leary (1983): Histochemical detection of antibodies by alkaline phospatase staining. Proc. Natl. Acad. Sci. 80, 4045-4049.
W.H.M.Peters, W.A.Allebes, P.L.M.Jansen, L.G.Poles and P.J.A.Capel (1987): Characterization and tissue specificity of a monoclonal antibody against human UDPGT. Gastroenterology 93, 162-169.

Résumé

Deux anticorps monoclonaux ont été développés contre l'UDP-glucuronosyl-transférase (4-nitrophénol) purifiée de foie de rat. Par Western Blot, nous avons montré que l'anticorps anti-rat-pnpgt-67 mab et anti-rat-pnpgt-96 mab sont spécifiques de la forme d'UDP glucuronosyltransférase conjugant le 4-nitrophénol.
Si l'anti-rat-pnpgt-96 mab reconnaît deux bandes, l'anti-rat-pnpgt-67 mab n'en reconnaît qu'une seule.
Ces caractéristiques ont été vérifiées sur des microsomes d'animaux traités par différents inducteurs ; la reconnaissance était maximale pour des animaux traités à la 5,6-benzoflavone.

Interactions between fenofibryl glucuronide and human serum albumin or human plasma

A. Weil, J.P. Guichard and J. Caldwell*

Laboratoires Fournier, Centre de Recherches, Daix, 21121 Fontaine-lès-Dijon, France
*Department of Pharmacology & Toxicology, St. Mary's Hospital Medical School, London W2 1PG, England, UK

ABSTRACT

Interactions between fenofibryl glucuronide and human serum albumin (HSA) or human plasma lead to the following reactions (i) acyl migration of the aglycone from position 1 to positions 2, 3 and 4 of the glucuronic acid moiety, (ii) hydrolysis of the glycosidic bond, and (iii) covalent binding of fenofibric acid to the HSA molecule or plasma proteins. Comparison of the rate of these reactions with those for other acyl glucuronides to be found in the literature indicates that fenofibryl glucuronide is a stable example of an acyl glucuronide.

KEYWORDS

Fenofibrate, reactivity of acyl glucuronide, HSA, plasma

INTRODUCTION

Fenofibrate is a hypolipidaemic drug structurally related to clofibrate. Fenofibrate exerts its activity through its hydrolysis product fenofibric acid. Early studies revealed that the major metabolite of fenofibrate in human urine is the glucuronide of fenofibric acid (Weil et al., 1988). There has been considerable speculation in the literature in recent years about the possible role of ester glucuronides. These conjugates possess a chemical reactivity which may manifest itself in three ways (i) spontaneous chemical hydrolysis to liberate the aglycone from the glucuronide molecule (Upton et al., 1980), (ii) intramolecular rearrangement of the conjugate where the acyl moiety migrates from hydroxyl to adjacent hydroxyl (Compernolle et al., 1978 ; Sinclair & Caldwell, 1982), (iii) acyl group donation to nucleophilic centres in macromolecules such as proteins (Stogniew & Fenselau, 1982). Recently, it was demonstrated that spontaneous hydrolysis and rearrangement were catalysed by human plasma, and more specifically, human serum albumin (HSA). It was further noted in the reactions of some acyl glucuronides with HSA, that some of the substrate became irreversibly bound to the albumin (van Breemen & Fenselau, 1985 ; Ruelius et al., 1986 ; Smith et al., 1986 ; Wells et al., 1987). In the present study, we have examined the reactivity of fenofibryl glucuronide in human plasma and HSA solution at 37 °C to estimate the fraction covalently bound to proteins and the products of degradation of fenofibryl glucuronide.

MATERIALS AND METHODS

Materials
Labelled 1-0-fenofibryl-β-D-glucuronide (FAG, MW = 494) was purified from human urine by preparative HPLC, identified by FAB-MS, ^{1}H-NMR and ^{13}C-NMR, chemical and enzymatic treatments and kept at -20°C in acetate buffer, pH 5. [^{14}C]-Fenofibric acid (FA, MW = 318) was dissolved in isopropyl alcohol. Human plasma was collected from volunteers into heparinized tubes (10 U/ml). Human serum albumin (HSA) (fraction V essentially fatty acid free) and β-glucuronidase (from Helix Pomatia, type H_1) were purchased from Sigma (La Verpillière, France). Solvents used for analysis were HPLC grade, and all other chemicals were reagent grade.

Buffer incubation
FAG was incubated in 0.1 M Tris/Maleate buffer pH 7.4 and pH 8.3 at 37°C (30 µg/ml, FAG equivalents, 16 000 dpm/ml). After 1, 2, 4, 8, 24, 48 h, 1 ml aliquots were passed on C18 Sep-pak cartridges (Waters, St Quentin-en-Yvelines, France), eluted with 1 ml methanol, evaporated under a stream of nitrogen, and the residues taken up in 200 µl HPLC mobile phase for analysis.

Plasma incubation
The protein concentration (91.7 mg/ml) was determined by the method of Lowry (Lowry et al., 1951). Incubation of radiolabelled FA and FAG were conducted at a concentration of 31 µg/ml (FAG equivalents, 16 000 dpm/ml), and 30 µg/ml (FA equivalents 35 000 dpm/ml), in human plasma at 37°C. 1 ml FAG aliquots taken after 1, 4, 8 and 24 h of incubation and 1 ml FA aliquot taken after 24 h were added to 3 ml acetonitrile to precipitate proteins and centrifuged. The protein pellet was washed 5 times with 3 ml acetone/water/acetic acid (89 : 10 : 1, by vol.) and twice with 3 ml methanol/ether (3 : 1, by vol.) to remove reversibly bound FA and conjugates. The washed protein pellet was digested with 2 ml of 1M NaOH for 1 h at 50°C, neutralized with 1 ml glacial acetic acid, and suspended in 15 ml scintillation fluid (Instagel, Packard-Chrompack, Les Ulis, France) for counting. Irreversible binding is expressed as the fraction of the total radioactivity added to 1 ml of the incubation which became irreversibly bound.
The acetonitrile supernatant was concentrated under a stream of nitrogen. The residues were taken up in 200 µl HPLC mobile phase. After counting, a fraction of this solution was analyzed by HPLC.

HSA incubation
Duplicate incubations of radiolabelled FAG were conducted at a concentration of 31.8 µg/ml (FAG equivalents, 16 000 dpm/ml) with 0.5 mM (3 g/100 ml) HSA in 0.10 M Phosphate buffer, pH 7 at 37°C and with buffer only. 1 ml FAG aliquots were taken after 1, 4, 8 and 24 h of incubation. Control incubation of radiolabelled FA were conducted at a concentration of 30 µg/ml (FA equivalents, 35 000 dpm/ml) with 0.5 mM (3 g/100 ml) HSA in 0.10 M phosphate buffer, pH 7 at 37°C for 24 h. The same procedure as for plasma incubations was followed for extraction, counting and analysis. Drug not removed from plasma protein or HSA by the washing procedure but liberated only on treatment with strong base was defined as "irreversibly bound".

HPLC
HPLC employed a Spectra Physics 8000B Liquid chromatograph (Les Ulis, France) and a model 770 spectrophotometric detector set on 290 nm. The column was a C8 Nucleosil 5 µ, 250 x 4.6 mm (SFCC, Gagny, France) cooled at 4°C during analysis. The mobile phase was acetonitrile : 10 mM phosphate buffer pH 7.5 (45 : 55, by vol.) containing 0.005 M tetrabutylammonium bromide for ion pair chromatography (Fluka-Labex, Riedisheim

France), flow rate 1 ml/min. Fractions were collected every 0.5 min with a Gilson model 201 collector (Villiers-le-Bel, France) and quantitated by liquid scintillation counting. Peaks were identified after β-glucuronidase and mild alkaline treatments. Peaks assigments for isomers were based on their time of appearance after incubation in buffer.

RESULTS

Incubation of fenofibryl glucuronide with human plasma showed a rapid decline of the concentration of the parent 1-0-fenofibryl glucuronide with simultaneous appearance of β-glucuronidase resistant products over the first 4 hours. Subsequently, there was a slow decline in the concentration of resistant products while the fenofibric acid concentration continued to increase. By 24 hours under these conditions, most of the fenofibryl glucuronide was converted to the aglycone. The concentration of covalently bound drug remained low after 24 h incubation (Fig. 1).

When fenofibryl glucuronide was incubated with human serum albumin there was a slow decline of the concentration of the parent 1-0-fenofibryl glucuronide with simultaneous appearance of β-glucuronidase resistant products (isomeric esters), the aglycone and covalently bound drug over 24 hours (Fig. 2). Control incubation in phosphate buffer pH 7 showed a similar decline of the fenofibryl glucuronide concentration with concomitant appearance of products of degradation.

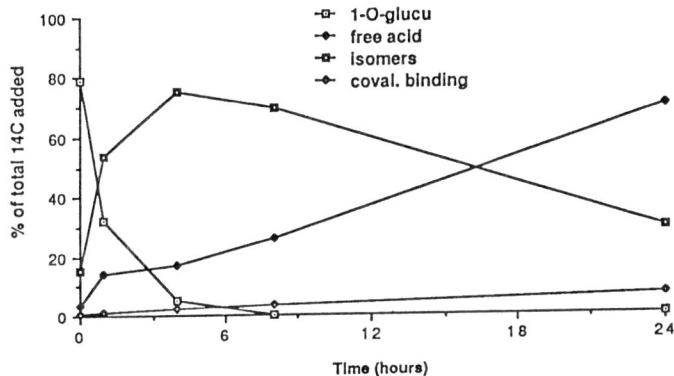

Figure 1 : 24 hr time course of the reactions of fenofibryl glucuronide in the presence of human plasma, 37°C

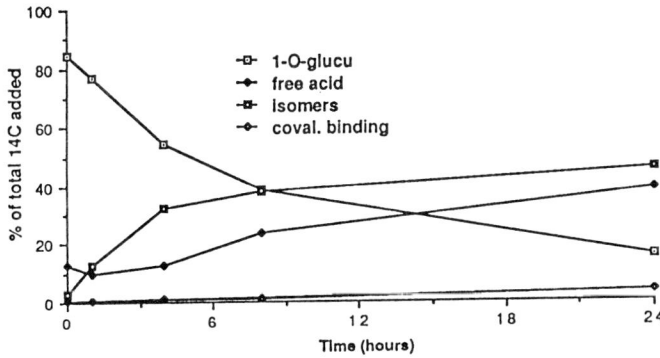

Figure 2 : 24 hr time course of the reactions of fenofibryl glucuronide in the presence of HSA (0,5 mM) in 0.1 M phosphate buffer, pH 7, 37°C

DISCUSSION

Fenofibryl glucuronide undergoes intramolecular rearrangement, hydrolytic cleavage and covalent binding to HSA and plasma proteins (Table I). Comparison of the rate of these reactions with those for other acyl glucuronides to be found in the literature indicates that fenofibryl glucuronide is a stable example of an acyl glucuronide (Caldwell et al., 1988). Furthermore, fenofibryl glucuronide is not detected in plasma of man and occurrence in man "in vivo" of the reactions described above is, therefore, highly unlikely.

		Time	% 14C bound	pmol FAG or FA bound/ mg protein
HSA		1 hr	0.4	8.5
		4 hr	1.0	21.4
		8 hr	1.4	30.1
		24 hr	3.3	70.8
	"Blank" FA	24 hr	2.0	62.9
Human plasma proteins		1 hr	1.3	8.9
		4 hr	2.3	15.8
		8 hr	3.6	24.7
		24 hr	6.7	45.7
	"Blank" FA	24 hr	1.3	13.4

Table I : Irreversible binding of fenofibric acid to human serum albumin (HSA) or plasma proteins. [^{14}C] fenofibryl glucuronide was incubated with HSA or human plasma at 37°C. [^{14}C] fenofibric acid was incubated with HSA or human plasma for 24 hr as a "blank" control of incubation.

REFERENCES

van Breemen, R.B. & Fenselau, C. (1985) : Drug Metab. Dispos. 13, 318.
Caldwell, J., Sinclair, K.A. & Weil, A. (1988) In : Metabolism of Xenobiotics, ed Gorroa, J.W., Oelschläger, H. & Caldwell, J. Taylor & Francis, London.
Compernolle, F., Van Hees, G.P., Blanckaert, N. & Heirwegh, K.P.M. (1978) : Biochem. J. 171, 185.
Lowry, O.H., Rosebrough, N.J., Farr, A.L. & Randall, R.J. (1951) : J. Biol. Chem. 193, 265.
Ruelius, H.W., Kirkman, S.K., Young, E.M. & Janssen, F.W. (1986) In Biological Reactive Intermediates III, ed Kocsis J.J., Jollow D.J., Witmer C.M., Nelson J.O. & Snyder R., Plenum Press, New York, p 431.
Sinclair, K.A. & Caldwell, J. (1982) : Biochem. Pharmacol. 31, 953.
Smith, P.C., McDonaugh, A.F. & Benet, L.Z. (1986) : J. Clin. Invest. 77: 934.
Stogniew, M. & Fenselau, C. (1982) : Drug Metab. Dispos. 10, 609.
Upton, R.A., Buskin, J.N., Williams, R.L., Holford, N.H.G. & Riegelman S. (1980) : J. Pharm. Sci. 69, 1254.
Weil, A., Caldwell, J. & Strolin Benedetti, M. (1988) : Drug Metab. Dispos., in press.
Wells, D.S., Janssen, F.W. & Ruelius, H.W. (1987) : Xenobiotica 17, 1437.

AKNOWLEDGEMENTS

This work was supported in part by a grant from the Groupement d' Intérêt Scientifique en Toxicologie Cellulaire de Dijon (GIS).

RESUME

Le fénofibryl glucuronide incubé en présence d'albumine de sérum humain ou de plasma humain subit les réactions suivantes (i) migration de l'aglycone de la position 1 aux positions 2, 3 et 4 de l'acide glucuronique, (ii) hydrolyse de la liaison glycosidique, et (iii) liaison covalente de l'acide fenofibrique à l'albumine et aux protéines plasmatiques. La comparaison de la vitesse de ces réactions avec celles d'autres acyl glucuronides trouvées dans la littérature indique que le fénofibryl glucuronide est un exemple d'acyl glucuronide stable.

Toxicological, pharmacological and physiopathological applications

Applications en toxicologie, pharmacologie et en physiopathologie

Rat and human liver UDP-glucuronosyltransferases inducible by 3-methylcholanthrene-type inducers

Karl Walter Bock*, Sabine Krull, Ursula Jongepier and Gerhard Schirmer

Departments of Toxicology, University of Tübingen Wilhelmstraße 56, D-7400 Tübingen, FRG and of Pharmacology and Toxicology, University of Göttingen, Robert-Koch-Straße 40, D-3400 Göttingen, FRG*

ABSTRACT

Advances have been made recently in the purification of rat UDP-glucuronosyltransferase (GT) isozymes. In the case of the 3-methylcholanthrene(MC)-inducible isozyme of GT (GT_{MC}) evidence accumulates that it is coinduced with P450 isozymes. GT_{MC} may be part of an adaptive program which evolved to efficiently eliminate and detoxify planar aromatic compounds. However, several observations are difficult to reconcile with one single GT_{MC} enzyme form. (a) Benzo(a)pyrene-3,6-quinol monoglucuronide (QMG) and diglucuronide (QDG) formation are markedly induced by MC-treatment of rats. However, the ratio of QDG/QMG is increased upon induction although both reactions appear to be catalyzed by highly purified GT_{MC} (monomeric Mr 55000). (b) QDG/QMG ratios vary in different organs such as kidney and liver and in different species. For example, QDG formation is negligible in the mouse and in man. (c) GT_{MC} appears to be permanently increased after initiation of hepatocarcinogenesis. In rat liver nodules and in differentiated hepatocellular carcinomas QDG/QMG ratios are increased. However, immunoblot analysis suggests that an immunochemically related GT_{MC} with smaller molecular weight (Mr 53000) is preferentially increased in liver nodules.

Paracetamol glucuronidation is increased in heavy smokers indicating that the responsible GT isozyme is inducible by MC-type inducers. Separation of human GT isozymes by chromatofocusing suggests that paracetamol glucuronidation is mostly catalyzed by the unspecific enzyme 2 (Mr 54000) which preferentially conjugates 4-aminobiphenyl.

KEYWORDS

UDP-glucuronosyltransferase, 3-methylcholanthrene-inducible isozyme, rat liver and kidney, human liver, benzo(a)pyrene-3,6-quinol, paracetamol, isozyme alterations in hepatocarcinogenesis.

INTRODUCTION

Glucuronide formation represents a major pathway in phase II of drug metabolism and an important detoxication reaction (Dutton, 1980). It is catalyzed by microsomal UDP-glucuronosyltransferase (GT, EC 2.4.1.17) which consists of a family of isozymes with different substrate specificities and differential inducibility by xenobiotics, such as phenobarbital and 3-methylcholanthrene (MC; Bock et al., 1973, 1979; Wishart 1978; Falany and Tephly, 1983; Iyanagi et al., 1986). MC is used as a prototype inducer for a large group of planar aromatic compounds including plant constituents such as β-naphthoflavone and halogenated hydrocarbons such as 3,4,7,8-tetrachloro-p-dibenzodioxin. MC-inducible GT isozymes (GT_{MC}, which have also been termed p-nitrophenol-GT, Falany and Tephly 1983 or GT1, Bock et al., 1979) appear to be almost ubiquitously present in tissues (Bock et al., 1980; Dutton, 1980). Recently, the complete amino acid sequence of GT_{MC} has been elucidated from the corresponding cDNA clones (Iyanagi et al., 1986). Evidence accumulates that GT_{MC} is coinduced with MC-inducible isozymes of cytochrome P450 (Owens, 1977; Nebert and Gonzalez, 1987). These coinduced isozymes may be part of an adaptive program which has evolved to efficiently detoxify planar aromatic compounds present in the diet and combustion products (Legraverend, 1983, Lilienblum et al., 1985, 1987). Interestingly GT_{MC} appears to be permanently increased after initiation of rat hepatocarcinogenesis (Bock et al., 1982, Yin et al., 1982, Fischer et al. 1985). However, several observations are difficult to reconcile with one single GT_{MC} enzyme form. The present investigation summarizes these observations and suggests possible explanations. In addition, it was investigated whether MC-inducible isozymes exist in man. Glucuronidation of the widely used analgesic paracetamol has been found to be increased in people eating brussels sprouts and cabbage (Pantuck et al., 1984) and in heavy smokers (Bock et al., 1987) who are presumably exposed to MC-type inducers. Recently two isozymes have been characterized from human liver (Irshaid and Tephly, 1987). It was therefore of interest to identify the isozyme(s) responsible for increased paracetamol glucuronidation in smokers.

METHODS

GT_{MC} was purified from Emulgen 911-solubilized male Wistar rat liver microsomes by chromatofocusing and subsequently purified by affinity chromatography (Bock et al., 1988a). Similarly human liver GT activities were separated by chromatofocusing (Irshaid and Tephly, 1987).
GT activities were assayed by previously described methods (for references see Bock and Bock-Hennig, 1987; Irshaid and Tephly, 1987). At low enzyme concentrations paracetamol was assayed by HPLC using ^{14}C-paracetamol. Benzpyrene-3,6-quinol was assayed according to Lilienblum et al. (1985) and testosterone-GT according to Rao et al.(1976).
Immunoblot analysis was carried out as described, using anti-GT_{MC} antibodies (Bock et al., 1988a).

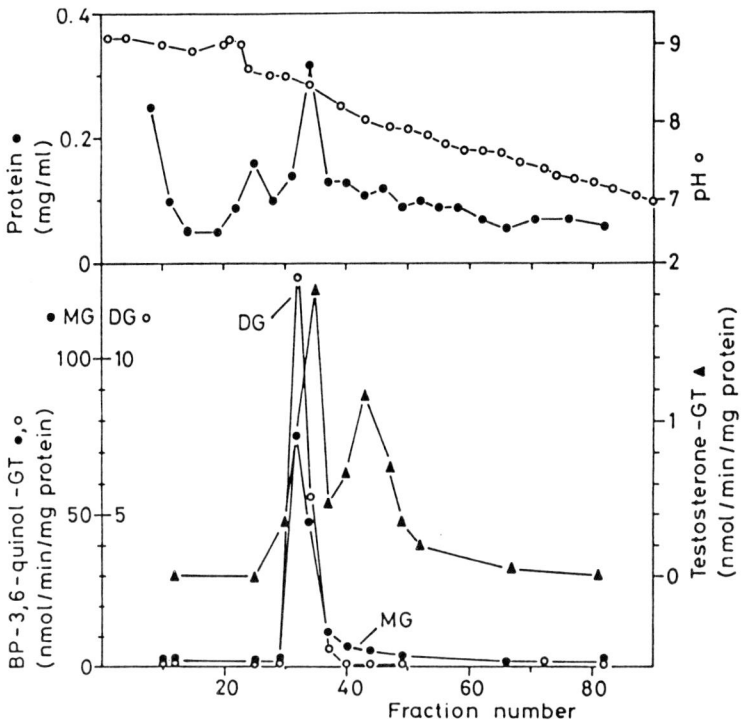

Fig. 1. <u>Separation by chromatofocusing of rat liver GT activities from MC-treated rats.</u>
Emulgen 911-solubilized microsomes (110 mg protein) were applied to a chromatofocusing column PBE 94 and eluted with Polybuffer 96-HAc, pH 7.0, to generate a pH 9-7 gradient. GT activities were determined using the substrates listed.

RESULTS AND DISCUSSION

Rat GT_{MC}
When GT activities are separated by chromatofocusing, benzo(a)-pyrene-3,6-quinol monoglucuronide (QMG) and diglucuronide (QDG) formation was catalyzed by enzyme fractions eluting at about pI 8.5 (Fig. 1) which also conjugate 4-methylumbelliferone (not shown). These fractions were distinct from those conjugating testosterone. The large induction factors by MC-treatment (about 10-fold for QMG formation and 40-fold for QDG formation, which are due to increased V_{max} and not to apparent Km) suggested that benzo(a)pyrene-3,6-quinol may be a selective substrate for GT_{MC} (Lilienblum et al., 1985). Induction factors of 5- to 8-fold have also been found for a number of phenolic metabolites of polycyclic aromatic hydrocarbons (Lilienblum et al., 1987). However, the exceptionally high increase of QDG formation and the selective inhibition of this reaction by dicoumarol

Table 1. GT activity towards benzo(a)pyrene-3,6-quinol (Q) and its response to inducing agents in rat and human tissues
Means ± SD (n=4) are listed. Induction factors are given in parenthesis. QMG, monoglucuronide; QDG, diglucuronide.

Tissue	Inducer	GT activity (QMG formation)		QDG/QMG
		(nmol/min/mg protein)		(%)
Rat liver	Controls	5.6 ± 0.9		4
	Phenobarbital	10.9 ± 3.3	(2)	4
	MC	51.8 ± 15.4	(9)	20
Rat liver	Controls	6.6 ± 0.9		4
	A1254	59.7 ± 11.3	(9)	23
Rat kidney	Controls	1.0 ± 0.1		5
	A1254	1.8 ± 0.3	(2)	8
Rat liver nodules	-	17.7 ± 1.6		8
Carcinoma 1	-	47		14
Carcinoma 2	-	30		42
Human liver	Controls (n=7)	1.3 ± 0.5		0.5
	Phenytoin or Pentobarbital	2.9 ± 0.7	(2)	0.9
	Smoker (20 cigarettes/day)	2.4	(2)	0.8

has been interpreted as evidence for at least two different forms of GT_{MC} (Segura-Aquilar et al.,1987).

Mono- and diglucuronide formation is also known with endogenous substrates such as bilirubin and steroids (Dutton 1980). In the case of bilirubin higher induction factors are found for bilirubin DG formation than for bilirubin MG formation in liver microsomes from phenobarbital-treated rats (Blanckaert et al., 1979). Bilirubin mono- and diglucuronide formation may be catalyzed by a single GT isozyme (Burchell and Blanckaert, 1984). A similar situation may exist in the case of benzo(a)pyrene-3,6-quinol glucuronidation. However, the different induction factors cannot be readily explained. One explanation may be the following: GT isozymes are possibly incorporated as oligomeric complexes into the microsomal membrane (Peters et al., 1984). Perhaps induction leads to the formation of oligomeric complexes favouring diconjugate formation.

QDG/QMG ratios have been calculated from initial rates of QMG and QDG formation and compared in various tissues and species (Table 1). Using QDG/QMG as a functional probe the question was asked: Are GT_{MC} isozymes identical in different tissues? Coughtrie et al. (1986) purified GT_{MC} from rat kidney and found properties similar to the liver enzyme, although some differences were also

Table 2: <u>Separation of human liver GT activities by chromatofocusing.</u> Representative determinations of 6 chromatographic separations are listed.

	Substrate	GT activities			
		Microsomes	Enzyme 1	Enzyme 2	Enzyme 2 / Enzyme 1
		(nmol/min/mg protein)			
a)	Aminobiphenyl	3.6	0.7	1.1	1.6
	Paracetamol	0.21	0.1	0.15	1.5
	Benzo(a)pyrene-3,6-quinol	1.3	1.0	1.1	1.1
b)	Estriol	2.2	0.6	0.3	0.5
	Methylumbelliferone	14	30	11	0.4

noted. When Aroclor 1254 (500 mg/kg) was used as a MC-type inducer it markedly increased QDG/QMG in liver but the increase in kidney was much smaller (Koster et al., 1986). Conversion of QMG to QDG was almost negligible in mouse (not shown) and man.

GT_{MC} is permanently increased after initiation of hepatocarcinogenesis in rat liver foci (Fischer et al., 1985), liver nodules and some hepatomas (Bock et al., 1982) and in differentiated hepatocellular carcinomas (Bock et al. 1988b). QMG and QDG was also markedly increased in liver nodules and differentiated hepatocellular carcinomas (Table 1), supporting the notion of increased GT_{MC} in these tissues. Furthermore, in differentiated hepatocellular carcinomas increased GT_{MC} (Mr 55000) was supported by immunoblot analysis of GT polypeptides. However, in rat liver nodules a new GT_{MC} polypeptide (Mr 53000) was preferentially stained by anti-GT_{MC} antibodies. This MC-inducible polypeptide could also be recognized in normal liver in overstained immunoblots (Bock et al., 1988b). However, GT_{MC} is a glycoprotein (Iyanagi et al., 1986). It is therefore conceivable that the new GT_{MC} polypeptide (Mr 53000), which is immunochemically related to the 55 kDa polypeptide (Bock et al., 1988b) may be a posttranscriptional modification of GT_{MC}.

Comparative investigations of GT_{MC} at the gene and protein levels may be useful to answer the question whether the above discrepancies are due to different GT_{MC} isozymes or to posttranscriptional modifications of a common GT_{MC} isozyme. Search for regulatory elements in the 5'-flanking region of GT_{MC}, similar to those found in the case of a MC-inducible isozyme of P450 (P450IA1; Sogawa et al., 1986; Nebert and Gonzalez, 1987), may lead to the elucidation of the mechanism of coinduction of P450I and GT_{MC}. Furthermore, studies with cloned cDNA to GT_{MC} may be essential to explore the permanent increase of GT_{MC} in liver foci and nodules. In addition to posttranscriptional modification of the gene product the permanent increase of GT activation in liver foci and nodules may be related to alterations of regulatory systems. For example, in the case of MC-inducible quinone reductase or DT diaphorase the gene has been found to be hypomethylated in liver nodules (Williams et al., 1986). Permanent alterations in regulatory systems of drug metabolizing enzymes and of growth controlling components may be important preneoplastic phenomena (Farber, 1984).

Human GT_{MC}
Based on differential inducibility by phenobarbital-type inducers indirect evidence was obtained for 3 groups of human liver GT activities towards (a) bilirubin, (b) morphine and 4-hydroxybiphenyl, (c) paracetamol, benzo(a)pyrene-3,6-quinol, 4-methylumbeliferone and 1-naphtol (Bock and Bock-Hennig, 1987). Glucuronidation of the widely used analgesic drug paracetamol is increased in smokers (Bock et al., 1987), suggesting induction by MC-type inducers. It was therefore of interest to investigate which of the two purified human liver GT isozymes (Irshaid and Tephly 1987), enzyme 1 (estriol-GT) or enzyme 2 (4-aminobiphenyl-GT) is increased in smokers. The two isozymes were partially separated by chromatofocusing of solubilized microsomes from 5 human liver samples. Table 2 lists GT activities measured in a representative liver sample without pathological findings from an adult male subject. Similar data were obtained with the other human liver samples. Although GT activities were stabilized by addition of phosphatidylcholine to column fractions and GT assay mixtures (Irshaid and Tephly 1987) it was not possible to overcome partial inactivation of the enzyme. Nevertheless ratios of enzyme 2/enzyme 1 suggest that GT activities towards paracetamol and benzo(a)pyrene-3,6-quinol are mostly associated with enzyme 2. It is therefore conceivable that enzyme 2 represents a MC-inducible GT. This suggestion was supported by immunoblot analysis showing that anti-rat GT_{MC} antibodies clearly bound to enzyme 2 (Mr 54000) after isolation by chromatofocusing, confirming preliminary studies of Coffman et al., 1987. The strongest reaction was found in the liver of a heavy smoker (unpublished results). Although enzyme 2 may be considered as a human GT_{MC} it has to be kept in mind that the inducibility of this enzyme by MC-type inducers in man appears to be much lower than that of rat GT_{MC}.

ACKNOWLEDGEMENTS

The authors wish to thank Dr. Thomas R. Tephly, University of Iowa, U.S.A., for providing anti-rat GT_{MC} antibodies, Dr. Lennard C. Eriksson, Huddinge Hospital, Sweden, for providing liver nodules and hepatocellular carcinomas, Dr. Gorig Brunner, Medizinische Hochschule Hannover, FRG and Dr. Urs A. Meyer, Biocenter Basel, Switzerland, for providing human liver samples and the Deutsche Forschungsgemeinschaft for financial support.

REFERENCES

Blanckaert, N., Gollan, J. and Schmid, R. (1979): Bilirubin diglucuronide synthesis by a UDP-glucuronic acid-dependent enzyme system in rat liver microsomes. Proc. Natl. Acad. Sci. USA 76, 2037-2041.

Bock, K.W., Fröhling, W., Remmer, H. and Rexer, B. (1973): Effects of phenobarbital and 3-methylcholanthrene on substrate specificity of rat liver microsomal UDP-glucuronyltransferase. Biochim. Biophys. Acta 327, 46-56.

Bock, K.W., Josting, D., Lilienblum, W. and Pfeil, H. (1979): Purification of rat liver microsomal UDP-glucuronyltransferase. Separation of two enzyme forms inducible by 3-methylcholanthrene or phenobarbital. Eur. J. Biochem. 98, 19-26.

Bock, K.W., Clausbruch von, U.C., Kaufmann, R. Lilienblum, W., Oesch, F., Pfeil, H. and Platt, K.L. (1980): Functional heterogeneity of UDP-glucuronyltransferase. Biochem. Pharmacol. 29, 495-500.

Bock, K.W., Lilienblum, W., Ullrich, D. and Eriksson, L.C. (1982): Increased UDP-glucuronyltransferase activity in preneoplastic liver nodules and Morris hepatomas. Cancer Res. 42, 3747-3752.

Bock, K.W. and Bock-Hennig, B.S. (1987): Differential induction of human liver UDP-glucuronosyltransferase activities by phenobarbital-type inducers. Biochem. Pharmacol. 36, 4137-4143.

Bock, K.W., Wiltfang, J., Blume, R., Ullrich, D. and Bircher, J. (1987): Paracetamol as a test drug to determine glucuronide formation in man. Effects of inducers and of smoking. Eur. J. Clin. Pharmacol. 31, 677-683.

Bock, K.W., Schirmer, G., Green, M.D. and Tephly, T.R. (1988a): Properties of a 3-methylcholanthrene-inducible phenol UDP-glucuronosyltransferase from rat liver. Biochem. Pharmacol., in press.

Bock, K.W., Schirmer, G. and Eriksson, L.C. (1988b): UDP-glucuronosyltransferase: Adaptive responses and permanent alterations in preneoplastic liver. Microsomes and Drug Oxidations. 7th International Symposium Adelaide 1987, Birkett et al., eds. London: Taylor and Francis, in press.

Burchell, B. and Blanckaert, N. (1984): Bilirubin mono- and diglucuronide formation by purified rat liver microsomal bilirubin UDP-glucuronyltransferase. Biochem. J. 223, 461-465.

Coffman, B.L., Green, M.D., Irshaid, M. and Tephly, T.R. (1987): Characterization of antibodies to rat and rabbit liver UDP-glucuronosyltransferases. Fed. Proc. 46, 883.

Coughtrie, M.W.H., Burchell, B. and Bend, J.R. (1987): Purification and properties of rat kidney UDP-glucuronosyltransferase. Biochem. Pharmacol. 36, 245-251.

Dutton, G.J. (1980): Glucuronidation of drugs and other compounds. Boca Raton, Florida: CRC Press.

Falany, C.N. and Tephly, T.R. (1983): Arch. Biochem. Biophys. 227, 248-258.

Farber, E. (1984): Cellular biochemistry of the stepwise development of cancer with chemicals. Cancer Res. 44, 5463-5474.

Fischer, G., Ullrich, D. and Bock, K.W. (1985): Effects of N-nitrosomorpholine and phenobarbital on UDP-glucuronyltransferase in putative preneoplastic foci of rat liver. Carcinogenesis 6, 605-609.

Irshaid, Y.M. and Tephly, T.R. (1987): Isolation and purification of two human liver UDP-glucuronosyltransferases. Mol. Pharmacol. 31, 27-34.

Iyanagi, T., Haniu, M., Sogawa, K., Fujii-Kuriyama, Y., Watanabe, S., Shively, J.E. and Anan, K.F. (1986): J. Biol. Chem. 261, 15607-15614.

Koster, A.S., Schirmer, G. and Bock, K.W. (1986): Immunochemical and functional characterization of UDP-glucuronosyltransferases from rat liver, intestine and kidney. Biochem. Pharmacol. 35, 3971-3975.

Legraverend, C., Harrison, D.E., Ruscetti, F.W. and Nebert, D.W. (1983): Bone marrow toxicity induced by oral benzo(a)pyrene: Protection resides at the level of the intestine and liver. Tox. Appl. Pharmacol. 70, 390-401.

Lilienblum W., Bock-Hennig, B.S. and Bock, K.W. (1985): Protection against toxic redox-cycles between benzo(a)pyrene-3,6-quinone and its quinol by 3-methylcholanthrene-inducible formation of the quinol mono- and diglucuronide. Mol. Pharmacol. 27, 451-458.

Lilienblum, W., Platt, K.L, Schirmer, G., Oesch, F. and Bock, K.W. (1987): Regioselectivity of rat liver microsomal UDP-glucuronosyltransferase activities towards phenols of benzo(a)pyrene and dibenz(a,h)anthracene. Mol. Pharmacol. 32, 173-177.

Nebert, D.W. and Gonzalez, F.J. (1987): P450 genes: Structure, evolution, and regulation. Ann. Rev. Biochem. 56, 945-993.

Owens, I.S. (1977): Genetic regulation of UDP-glucuronosyltransferase induction by polycyclic aromatic compounds in mice. J. Biol. Chem. 252, 2827-2833.

Pantuck, E.J., Pantuck, C.B., Anderson, K.E., Wattenberg, L.W., Conney, A.H. and Kappas, A. (1984): Effect of brussels sprouts and cabbage on drug conjugation. Clin. Pharm. Ther. 35, 161-169.

Peters, W.H.M., Jansen, P.L.M. and Hauta, H. (1984): The molecular weights of UDP-glucuronyltransferase determined with radiation-inactivation analysis. J. Biol. Chem. 259, 11701-11705.

Rao G.S., Haueter, G., Rao, M.L. and Breuer, H. (1976): An improved assay for steroid glucuronyltransferase in rat liver microsomes. Anal. Biochem. 74, 35-40.

Segura-Aquilar, J.E., Barreiro, V. and Lind, C. (1986): Dicoumarol-sensitive glucuronidation of benzo(a)pyrene metabolites in rat liver microsomes. Arch. Biochem. Biophys. 251, 266-275.

Sogawa, K., Fujisawa-Sehara, A., Yamane, M. and Fujii-Kuriyama, Y. (1986): Location of regulatory elements responsible for drug induction in the rat cytochrome P450c-gene. Proc. Natl. Acad. Sci. USA 83, 8044-8048.

Williams, J.B., Lu, A.Y.H., Cameron, R.G. and Pickett, C.B. (1986): Rat liver NAD(P)H:quinone reductase. J. Biol. Chem. 261, 5524-5528.

Wishart, G.J. (1978): Demonstration of functional heterogeneity of hepatic uridine diphosphate glucuronosyltransferase activities after administration of 3-methylcholanthrene and phenobarbital to rats. Biochem. J. 174, 671-672.

Yin, Z., Sato, K., Tsuda, H. and Ito, N. (1982): Changes in activities of uridine diphosphate-glucuronyltransferase during chemical hepatocarcinogenesis. Gann 73, 239-248.

Résumé

Des progrès ont été récemment observés concernant la purification des isoenzymes d'UDP-glucuronosyltransférase (GT) de rat. Il est couramment admis que la forme protéique (GTmc) inductible par le 3-méthylcholanthrène (MC) est induite simultanément avec les isoenzymes de cytochrome P-450. GTmc doit prendre part à l'élimination et détoxification effectives des composés aromatiques plans. Cependant certaines observations sont difficilement compatibles avec l'existence d'une seule GTmc.

a) La formation du monoglucuronide du benzo(a)pyrène-3,6-quinol (QMG) ainsi que celle du diglucuronide (QDG) sont augmentées de façon importante après traitement des rats au 3MC. Cependant le rapport QDG/QMG est augmenté après induction bien que les deux réactions soient catalysées par la GTmc fortement purifiée (PM du monomère, 55000).

b) Les rapports QDG/QMG varient dans les différents organes comme le rein et le foie et chez les différentes espèces.

c) GTmc est augmentée de façon permanente après initiation de l'hépatocarcinogénèse. Dans les nodules hépatiques de rats et dans les carcinomes hépatocellulaires différenciés les rapports QDG/QMG sont augmentés. Cependant l'analyse par immunoblot suggère qu'une GTmc immunoréactive de plus petit poids moléculaire (PM 53000) est augmentée préférentiellement dans les nodules hépatiques.

La glucuronoconjugaison du paracétamol est augmentée chez les gros fumeurs, ce qui indique que l'isoenzyme Gt responsable est induite par les inducteurs de type MC. La séparation des isoenzymes GT humaines par chromatofocalisation suggère que la glucuronoconjugaison du paracétamol est catalysée surtout par une enzyme non spécifique (PM 54000) qui conjugue préférentiellement le 4-aminobiphényle.

Inter-individual variability and induction of cytochromes P-450 and UDP-glucuronosyl transferases in human liver microsomes and primary cultures of human hepatocytes

Jean-Paul Cano*, Gérard Fabre*, Patrick Maurel**, Nicole Bichet*, Yves Berger* and Patrice Vic*

*Sanofi Recherche, 32 rue du Professeur J. Blayac, 34082 Montpellier Cedex, France
** INSERM U128, Site du CNRS, Route de Mende 34033 Montpellier Cedex, France

ABSTRACT

A study on the inter- and intra-individual variabilities in phase I (cytochrome P-450) and phase II (UDP-glucuronosyl transferase) reactions has been undertaken with liver microsomal preparation from 20 organ donors. Data demonstrate an important inter-individual variability for both phase I and phase II-dependent reactions. Erythromycin (ER) N-demethylation and nifedipine (NIF) oxidation were highly correlated in all livers ($p < 0.001$). Four other activities also exhibited significant degrees of correlation : benzphetamine (BZ) and aminopyrine (AMP) N-demethylation, 7-ethoxyresorufine-O-deethylation (EROD) and acetanilide (ACET) hydroxylation. Among UDP-GT reactions tested, only p-nitrophenol and 1-naphthol glucuronidations correlated with $p < 0.002$. Finally ER demethylation and NIF oxidation exhibited significant correlation with valproic acid glucuronidation ($p < 0.002$).

Human hepatocytes obtained after collagenase-dissociation of either whole liver (organ donors) or resected lobes (patients with secondary liver cancer), were maintained over 120 hr in primary culture, in serum-free medium, in the absence or the presence of inducers including phenobarbital (PB), rifampycin (RIF), dexamethasone (DEX), 3-methylcholanthrene (3MC) and ß-naphthoflavone (ßNF). Microsomes prepared from these cultures were analyzed in Western blots developed with either anti-P450IIIA3 or -P450IA2 antibodies and assayed for cyt P-450 and UDP-GT reactions. RIF and to a lesser extent DEX and PB induced P450IIIA3 and related monooxygenase activities, NIF oxidation, as observed in vivo. ßNF and 3MC induced P450IA2 as well as EROD which is known to be related to P-450 isozymes from family P450I. Induction of 1-naphthol was observed with all inducers although at a variable extent from one culture to another.

These results directly emphasize the link between regulation of cyt P-450 and UDP-GT genes expression and the hepatic metabolism of drugs.

KEYWORDS

Cytochrome P450, UDP glucuronosyl transferase, phenotype, human liver microsomes

INTRODUCTION

Numerous lipophilic endogenous compounds and xenobiotics, including drugs, are sequentially metabolized by hepatic microsomal cytochromes P450 (cyt P-450) and UDP-glucuronosyl transferases (UDP-GT) to more polar compounds that are then eliminated. Cyt P450 and UDP-GT are both encoded by multigene families, each isozyme differing in primary structure, substrate specificity and in response to prototype inducers such as phenobarbital (PB), 3-methylcholanthrene (3MC), steroids and macrolide antibiotics. The inducibility of cyt P-450 isozymes and their activities towards various substrates have been intensively studied in primary cultures of hepatocytes from various animal species (Daujat, 1987 ; Schuetz, 1986 ; Suolinna, 1986 ; Grant, 1987) and humans (Guillouzo, 1985). In contrast, only few studies have been devoted to the behaviour of the conjugating enzymes in cultured hepatocytes (Grant, 1987 ; Suolinna, 1986 ; Schuetz, 1986). There is increasing evidence that the metabolism of xenobiotics in human tissue may be different from that in animals, so that it is essential to develop systems that can be used to measure the metabolism and to predict the toxicity of xenobiotics in man. Primary cultures of human hepatic parenchymal cells have become widely used for this purpose (Guillouzo, 1985). When considering the potential of cultured hepatocytes for drug metabolism studies, knowledge of the overall metabolism is essential since conjugation reactions are of importance, e.g. in removing reactive metabolites formed by the mixed function oxidases. Moreover since conjugating enzymes are inducible, the usefulness of hepatocyte cultures for investigating regulation of their expression should also be considered.

The present communication reports the measurement of a variety of cyt P-450 and UDP-GT activities in microsomes from (i) 20 different samples of human liver and (ii) human hepatocytes in primary cultures treated with various inducers.

MATERIALS AND METHODS

Liver donors. Twenty human liver specimens obtained from kidney transplant donors (Service de Chirurgie Urologique et de Greffe Rénale, Marseille, Pr Rampal) were kindly supplied from the Hospitalo-Universitary laboratory of pharmacokinetic in Marseilles. All liver specimens were stored at − 80°C until preparation of the microsomes. Previous studies have already demonstrated that liver storage at − 80°C has no effect on monooxygenase (Von Bahr, 1980) and UDP-GT (Schuetz, 1986) activities. Characteristics of organ donors, termed HL-1 to HL-23, have been described elsewhere (Fabre, 1988b).

Human hepatocytes obtention and primary cultures. Hepatocytes were prepared from both healthy organ donors (heart and kidneys) and resected liver lobe from patients with secondary liver cancer. Whole human liver was obtained from Lapeyronie Hospital, Montpellier, France (Service de Nephrologie, Drs. Mourad and Guiter). Donor was 30-years old male Caucasian who died from cerebral hemorrhage. Preparation was termed FH-1. Samples from patients who underwent elective resection of a hepatic angioma (patient HTL-8, 63-years old, male) or hepatic lobectomy for metastatic colorectal cancer (patient HTL-9, 45-years old, male ; patient HTL-11, 43-years old, female) were obtained at Paul Lamarque Hospital, Montpellier, France (Service de Chirurgie Abdominale ; Pr. Joyeux). The organ, or the lobe, was then perfused with a oxygenized collagenase solution (0.05 % in Hepes buffer, pH 7.6) at 37°C according to a previously reported method (Cano, 1988 ; Fabre, 1988b ; Rahmani, 1988). The viability of the purified hepatocytes, assessed by trypan blue exclusion, ranged between 85 and 95 %. Human hepatocytes ($8 \cdot 10^6$) were plated on collagen-coated 100 mm-diameter plastic dishes in 8 ml of a medium consisting of Ham F-12/Williams E (50/50) supplemented as described elsewhere (Isom, 1984). At the end of a 6-12 hours period during which hepatocytes attached to the dishes, dead cells were removed and medium was renewed in the presence of various inducers solubilized in dimethyl sulfoxide (0.1 % final) : 3MC (0.05 mM), Rifampicin (RIF ; 0.05 mM), dexamethasone (DEX ; 0.05 mM), ß-naphthoflavone (ßNF ; 0.05 mM) and PB (2 mM). Control cells were treated with dimethyl sulfoxide at a final concentration of 0.1 %. After 3-5 days, during which medium and inducers were renewed every day, hepatocytes were scrapped in 0.1 M potassium phosphate buffer (pH 7.4) and microsomes were prepared as previously reported (Daujat, 1987).

Preparation of microsomes. Human liver microsomes were prepared as previously described (Fabre, 1988a) and resuspended in potassium phosphate buffer (pH 7.4 ; 0.1 M) containing 1 mM EDTA and 20 % glycerol (v/v). They were stored as small aliquots at - 80°C. A single preparation of microsomes was used from each liver sample. Protein measurements were performed by the method of Pollard (1978) using bovine serum albumin as a standard.

Monooxygenase assays. Erythromycin (ER), d-benzphetamine (BZ) and aminopyrin (AMP) N-demethylase activities were determined by colorimetric measurement of formaldehyde formed (Nash, 1953). Hydroxylation of aniline (ANL) was determined according to the method of Mieyal (1976). The formations of the nitropyridine derivative of nifedipine (NIF) and of the hydroxylated derivative of acetanilide (ACET) were quantified by HPLC analysis according to the method of Guengerich (1986). 7-ethoxyresorufin-O-deethylation (EROD) was measured by modification of the direct fluorimetric assay described by Burke (1983). Reactions rates were determined under conditions where they were linear as a function of incubation time and protein concentration. Cyt b5 and cyt P-450 were assayed by the method of Omura (1964) using absorption coefficients of 185 cm-1.mM-1 and 91 cm-1.mM-1 respectively.

UDP-glucuronosyltransferase assays. Enzyme activities towards various substrates were assayed according to previously described methods : 4-nitrophenol (pNP)(Isselbacher, 1962), testosterone (TEST)(Rao, 1976), valproic acid (VPA)(Gregus, 1982 ; Watkins, 1982) and 1-naphthol (1-NP)(Miners, 1988).

Immunoblot analysis. Cyt P-450 HLp (P450IIIA3) and LM4 (P450IA2) were quantitated by immunoblot analysis of electrophoretically separated microsomal proteins (Daujat, 1987). Usually, 5 µg of microsomal proteins were submitted to electrophoresis and the immunoblots were developed in the presence of 0.1 mg/ml of specific IgG as described previously (Daujat, 1987).

Preparation for transmission electron microscopic examination. HTL-8 and HTL-11 control and treated human hepatocytes cultures were prepared for electron microscopic examination as follows : the cell pellet was fixed with glutaraldehyde and then with osmium tetroxide ; after dehydration it was embedded in Epon and sectionned with the ultramicrotome Reichert. After staining with uranyl acetate and lead acetate, the grids were examined in a Jeol 100S electron microscope. The Thiery (1967) histochemical reaction was used to stain the glycoproteins in granules.

RESULTS

Cytochromes P-450 and b5 content of human liver microsomes. Cyt P450 and cyt b5 specific contents in liver microsomes were 0.37 ± 0.13 and 0.55 ± 0.09 nmol/mg prot respectively. These contents did not differ with the sex of the donor and fell within the range of previously reported values (Kremers, 1981 ; Beaune, 1986).

Monooxygenase activities in human liver microsomes. Several monooxygenase activities were measured and are illustrated in fig 1.

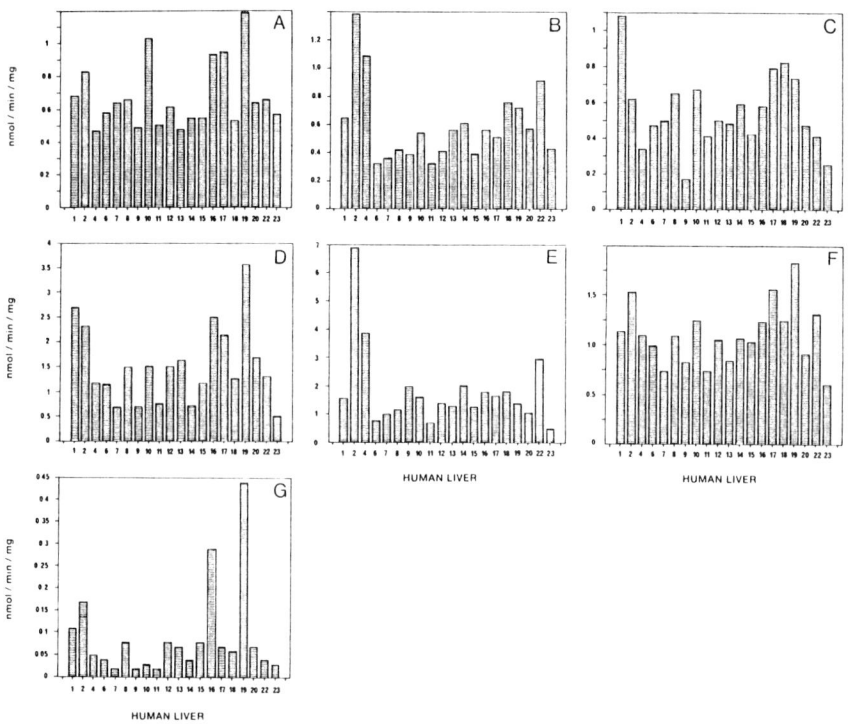

Figure 1 : Intersubject variabilities in the oxidation of various substrates by cyt P450 using human liver microsomes : A, BZ ; B, ER ; C, ANL ; D, ACET ; E, NIF ; F, AMP and G, EROD

Large interindividual variabilities in the metabolism of the standard drugs were demonstrated but could not be related to cyt P-450 and/or cyt b5 specific contents as reported by others (Kremers, 1981 ; Beaune, 1986).

Various monooxygenase activities have been extensibely compared. We observed a high correlation ($p < 0.001$) between ER N-demethylase and NIF oxidase activities. BZ and AMP N-demethylations, ACET hydroxylation and EROD activities also correlated with $p < 0.001$. This suggested that in humans both NIF and ER are metabolized by a single cyt P-450 isozyme, in agreement with recent reports of Guengerich (1986) and Combalbert (1988).

UDP-glucuronosyltransferases activities in human liver microsomes. Various drugs have been used for the study of UDP-GT activities, i.e. pNP, TEST, 1-NP and VPA. Results are illustrated in fig 2. They illustrate both the large inter-individual variability in drug metabolism and the specificity of various substrates.

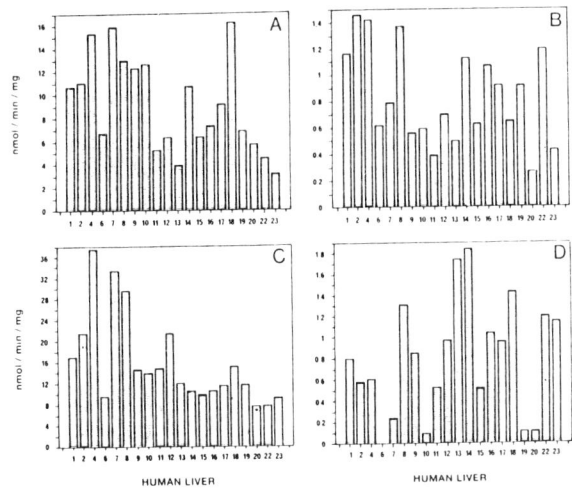

Figure 2 : Intersubject variabilities in the glucuronidation of various substrates by UDP-GT using human liver microsomes : A, pNP ; B, VPA ; C, 1-NP and D, TEST

We also determined the extent of relation between the various UDP-GT activities. 1-NP and pNP UDP-GT activities correlated with $p < 0.002$ suggesting that at least a same UDP-GT isozyme was involved in their metabolism. Studies investigated in rats already showed that these two UDP-GT activities were inducible by 3MC and characterized the GT1 isozyme (Grant, 1987 ; Miners, 1988).

A key property of cyt P-450 and UDP-GT and a basis for the classification of these enzymes is their specific inducibility, in animals, by xenobiotics and their specificity substrate (Schuetz, 1986). We therefore searched for correlation between monooxygenase and UDP-GT activities. A correlation of about $p < 0.002$ was found between VPA glucuronidation and NIF oxidation but also with ER N-demethylation, two cyt P-450-dependent reactions highly correlated. Such observation suggests that VPA conjugation and NIF oxidation exhibit similar polymorphism among individual humans.

Observation on electron microscopy. Preparation of control human hepatocytes confirmed the good viability of the hepatocytes sampled and the integrity of the cell organelles. Nevertheless, the presence of lipids and lipofuscins was observed, as well as unusual and inconstant areas of smooth endoplasmic reticulum in the human hepatocytes. When the hepatocytes were treated with 3MC, concentric or parallel arrays of smooth endoplasmic reticulum associated with moderately osmophilic granules (more or less circular and of middle size (400A) were systematically observed (figure 3). The granules were slightly positive in Thiery's reaction ; so that, their nature could be not precisely defined. The other organelles were constant with a few areas of smooth endoplasmic reticulum. The preparation of hepatocytes treated with DEX showed organelles similar to those observed in controls, with slightly increased areas containing smooth reticulum.

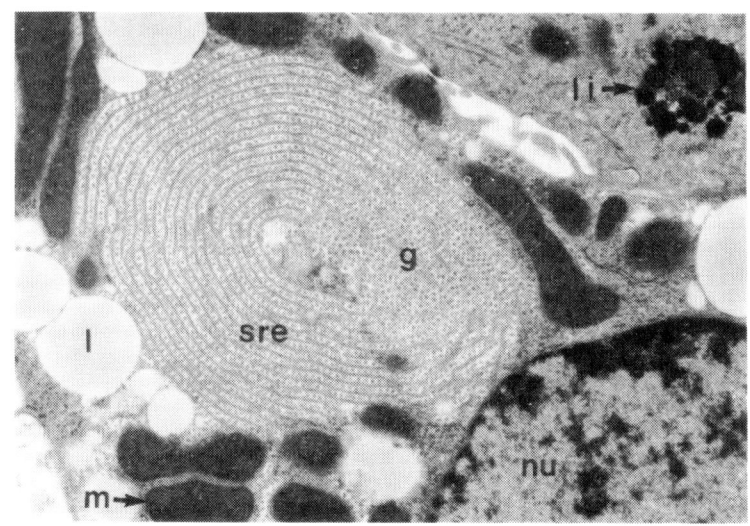

Figure 3. Human hepatocytes (treated with 3MC) with concentric smooth endoplasmic reticulum (sre) with granules (g) Nucleus (nu) Lipids (l) Mitochondria (m) Lipofuscin (li) : EM x 8000

In vitro induction of cytochromes P450IIIA3 and IA2 in primary cultures of human hepatocytes. Microsomes prepared from cultures treated for 4 days with various inducers, were analyzed by Western blots. When immunoblots were developed with a polyclonal antibody directed against LM3c (P450IIIA4), a glucocorticoïd and macrolide antibiotic-inducible cyt P-450 orthologous to the human isozyme P-450 HLp (P450IIIA3), a single protein was visualized co-migrating with authentic purified HLp (figure 4A). Quantitative analysis of these blots indicated that hepatocytes pretreated with RIF had the highest amount of HLp, whereas DEX and PB are moderate inducers. Hepatocytes pretreated with 3MC or ßNF exhibited low immunoreactive HLp as in control cultures.

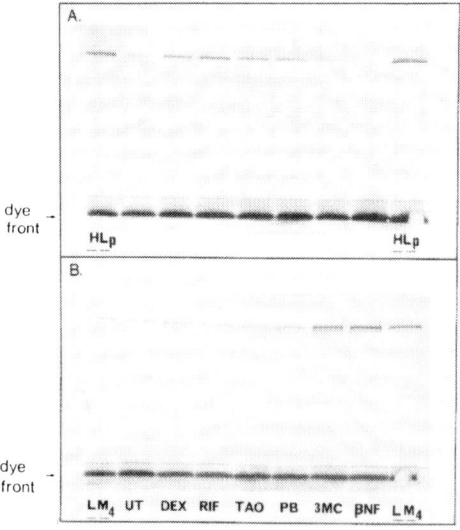

Figure 4 : Immunoblot analyses of microsomes prepared from primary cultures of human hepatocytes (FH-1) pretreated for 5 days with various inducers as described. Blots were developed with anti-LM3c (P450IIIA3) IgG (A) or with anti-LM4 (P450IA2) IgG (B)

In contrast, when these same microsomes were assayed in Western blot developed with a monoclonal antibody directed against cyt P-450 LM4 (P450IA2), a cyt P-450 isoenzyme inducible by 3MC and ßNF in rabbits, only 3MC- and ßNF-pretreated human hepatocytes exhibited a major band co-migrating with authentic rabbit liver isozyme LM4 (fig 4B). This immunoreactive isozyme was only slightly detectable in control hepatocytes or those pretreated with DEX, RIF or PB.
Monooxygenase activities of these microsomes towards various substrates were also determined. Results are reported in Tables I and II for the NIF oxidase and the EROD microsomal activities respectively.

Table I. Nifedipine oxidase activity in microsomes from human hepatocytes pretreated with various inducers. Results are expressed in nmole of metabolites formed/minute/mg of proteins

Patient	Control	RIF	DEX	PB	3MC	ßNF
FH-1	0.063	1.452	0.790	0.534	0.063	0.063
HTL-8	0.471	ND	1.291	ND	0.070	ND
HTL-9	0.359	1.646	0.700	0.490	0.113	ND
HTL-11	0.085	0.624	ND	0.260	0.039	0.052

ND = Not determined

Table II. EROD activity in microsomes from human hepatocytes pretreated with various inducers. Results are expressed in pmole of metabolites formed/minute/mg of proteins

Patient	Control	RIF	DEX	PB	3MC	ßNF
FH-1	UD	UD	7.8	6.5	35.2	83.6
HTL-8	2.1	ND	2.7	ND	0.4	ND
HTL-9	3.2	0.2	2.6	5.2	8.6	ND
HTL-11	0.4	0.5	ND	2.1	1.3	3.6

ND = Not determined ; UD = Undetectable

These data demonstrate that NIF oxidase activity was strongly and specifically increased in human hepatocytes pretreated with RIF and DEX while EROD activity was increased only following treatment with polycyclic aromatic hydrocarbons (3MC and ßNF). There was a closed relationship between the immunoreactives HLp and LM4 and their enzymatic activity towards NIF and EROD following induction of hepatocytes with RIF-DEX and 3MC-ßNF respectively. These data are in complete agreement with those reported in vivo (Maurel, 1986 ; Watkins, 1985) which demonstrated that cyt P-450 HLp was specifically induced in microsomes prepared from liver of patients pretreated with RIF or PB.

UDP-glucuronosyl transferase activities in human hepatocytes induced in vitro
Various UDP-GT activities have been investigated in control and inducer-treated primary cultures of human hepatocytes. Metabolism of 1-NP has been specially studied since it is a preferential substrate for the 3MC-inducible transferase in rats (Grant, 1987). Suolinna et al (1986) already demonstrated the inducibility of pNP activity following 3MC-treatment of primary-cultures of rat hepatocytes. The rates of 1-NP glucuronidation in microsomes prepared from control and pretreated human hepatocytes are reported in Table VI.

Table III. 1-Naphthol glucuronidation in microsomes prepared from human hepatocytes. Results are expressed in nmoles of glucuronides formed/minute/mg proteins

Patient	Control t = 0	Control t = 5d	3MC	RIF	PB	ßNF	DEX
FH-1	ND	9.3	17.5	18.3	11.1	22.0	17.1
HTL-8	51.5	40.3	23.1	ND	ND	ND	38.2
HTL-9	34.2	23.7	34.8	33.0	35.4	ND	29.9
HTL-11	14.9	13.5	19.5	16.9	18.9	9.3	ND

ND = not determined ; UD undetectable

1-NP glucuronidation appears to be a very stable activity over time. Indeed activity in 5 days culture was about 78-91 % of that determined at day 0 (when hepatocytes were just attached to the collagen-coated plastic dishes). However and of particular interest are the observations that this activity can be inducible by various agents (DEX, RIF, PB, ßNF, 3MC) and that large variabilities exist between the various cultures. Although only few studies have been carried out on conjugating enzymes in cultured hepatocytes, Suolinna (1986) demonstrated in rats that induction of UDP-GT1 (towards pNP) by 3MC showed a dependence on the age of the culture. The time dependence of 1-NP activity in 3MC-treated cultures is actually under furter investigation.

DISCUSSION

Routinely observed interindividual variability on monooxygenases and UDP-GT is likely to result from at least two distinct contributions acting either separately or concomittantly. One of these is genetic, the other is of environmental origin. The finding that some activities are significantly correlated when analyzed on a number of patients indicates accordingly that they are catalyzed either by the same enzyme or by distinct but closely regulated enzymes. In this respect the high correlation found between ER demethylase and NIF oxidase is definitely to be ascribed to the fact that both substrates are oxidized by the same form of P-450 (P450IIIA3) as recently demonstrated (Combalbert, 1988). On the other hand it is known mainly from animal studies that EROD and ACET hydroxylase are more specifically supported by P450IA1 and P450IA2, respectively. These proteins which exhibit, in rat, rabbit and human, aminoacid sequence homology of 65 to 72 % appear to be closely regulated and co-induced in animal species by a number of chemicals including 3MC and ßNF. Outfinding that these activities are significantly correlated in 20 patients is therefore an indication that P450IA1 and IA2 could also be closely regulated in man. In contrast, absence of correlation between two activities should indicate that they are catalyzed by two (or more) distinct enzymes, differently regulated. This is the case for example with ANL hydroxylase and ER demethylase or EROD. From animal studies it is clearly established that these activities are supported by different forms of P-450 belonging to three different families, P450IIE1, P450IIIA3 and P450IA1, respectively. This approach has also been verified for UDP-GT activities. Indeed 1-NP and pNP glucuronidations which correlated to p 0.002 are known to be co-induced by 3MC in rats in vivo and are also catalyzed by isozyme UDP-GT1. However it is now well known that UDP-GT substrate specificities generally exhibit partial overlapping, though there is a strict specificity with regard to endogenous substrates, particularly bilirubin and steroids (Siest, 1987). Hence pNP was metabolized by two UDP-GT isozymes purified from human liver microsomes (Irshaid, 1987). The observation that ER demethylase and NIF oxidase are closely correlated with VPA glucuronidation suggests that both P450IIIA3 and UDP-GT (VPA) genes could be coregulated and located on the same locus. From a pharmacological point of view these observations might help in defining different groups of drugs whose metabolism should not interfere when administered in association.

Except for special occasion (Leroux, 1986 ; Bock, 1987a ; Bock, 1987b , Boobis, 1980 ; Maurel, 1986 ; Pelkonen, 1986) and for obvious ethical reasons it has not been possible to directly study the contribution of P450 or UDP-GT induction on the hepatic metabolism of xenobiotics in human. As previously mentioned, however, this is a very critical aspect of the pharmacological and clinical implications of cyt P-450 and UDP-GT. Indeed, as reported in this communication, primary cultures of human hepatocytes and the use of specific antibodies provide an invaluable way to investigate this phenomenon in man. As previously shown from in vivo studies (Maurel, 1986 ; Combalbert, 1988) P450IIIA3 was strongly induced by RIF and to a lesser extent by DEX and PB in primary cultures of human hepatocytes. Interestingly similar observation was recently made on the rabbit orthologue P450IIIA4 (Daujat, 1987). P450IA2 was induced by both ßNF and 3MC, here again as observed for the rat and rabbit orthologues, both in vivo and in primary cultures. In both cases increase in specific monooxygenase activities accompanied P450 induction, ER demethylase and NF oxidase (P450IIIA3) and EROD (P450IA2), indicating that not only the apoprotein (quantitated in Western blot) but the functional cytochrome was present in the cultures. Results on 1-NP glucuronidation in human hepatocytes induced with various compounds are more difficult to be interpreted. Most likely reasons are as follows : the relative unsensitivity of UDP-GTs, aside from their activation, to phenomena of binding and rapid regulation and the absence of receptors and (ii) the weak inducibility of UDP-GT both in vivo and in vitro (Siest, 1987). Although these results are only preliminary they clearly demonstrate the potentiality of this approach to investigate and characterize the contribution of cytochromes P-450 (and other enzymes like UDP-GT) induction in human hepatic metabolism on both fundamental and pharmacological levels.

BIBLIOGRAPHY

Beaune, P.H., Kremers, P.G., Kaminsky, L.S., de Graeve, J., Albert, A., and Guengerich, F.P. (1986) : Comparison of monooxygenase activities and cytochrome P-450 isozyme concentrations in human liver microsomes. Drug Metab. Dispos. 14, 437-442

Bock, K.W., Witfang, J., Blume, R. Ullrich, D., and Bircher, J. (1987a) : Paracetamol as a test drug to determine glucuronide formation in man. Effects of Inducers and of smoking. Eur. J. Clin. Pharmacol. 31, 677-683

Bock, K.W., and Bock-Henning, B.S. (1987b) : Differential induction of numan liver UDP-glucuronosyltransferase activities by phenobarbital-type inducers. Biochem. Pharmacol. 36, 4137-4143

Boobis, A.R., Brodie, M.J. Kahn, G.C., Fletcher, D.R., Saunders, J.H. and Davies D.S. (1980) : Monooxygenase activity of human liver in microsomal fractions of needle biosy specimens. Br. J. Clin. Pharmac. 9, 11-19.

Burke, M.D., and Mayer, R.T. (1983) : Differential effects of phenobarbitone and 3-methylcholanthrene induction on the hepatic microsomal metabolism and cytochrome P-450 binding of phenoxazone and homologous series of its n alkyl ethers (alkoly resorufins). Chem. Biol. Interact. 45, 243-247

Cano, J.P., Rahmani, R., Fabre, G., Richard, B., Lacarelle, B, Bore, P., Bertault-Peres, P., De Sousa, G., Fabre, I., Placidi, M., Coulange, C, Ducros, M., and Rampal, M. (1988) : Human hepatocytes as an alternative model to the use of animal in experiments. in : Editions INSERM, ed. Guillouzo, A., in press

Combalbert, J. Fabre, I., Fabre, G., Dalet-Beluche, I., Devancourt, J., Cano, J.P., and Maurel, P. (1988) Metabolism of Cyclosporin A : IV. Purification and identification of the rifampicin-inducible human liver cytochrome P-450 (Cyclosporin A oxidase) as a product of P450IIIA gene subfamily. Drug Metab. Dispos. (submitted)

Daujat, M., Pichard, L., Dalet, C., Larroque, C., Bonfils, C., Pompon, D., Li, D., Guzelian, P.S. and Maurel, P. (1987) : Expression of five forms of microsomal cytochrome P-450 in primary cultures of rabbit hepatocytes treated with various classes of inducers. Biochem. Pharmacol. 36 : 3597-3607

Dragacci, S., Hamar-Hansen, C., Fournel-Gigleux, S., Lafaurie, C., Magdalou, J., and Siest, G. (1987) : Comparative study of clofibric acid and bilirubin glucuronidation in human liver microsomes. Biochem. Pharmacol. 36, 3923-3927

Fabre G., Crevat-Pisano, P., Dragna, S., Covo, J., Barra, Y., and Cano, J.P. (1988a) : Involvement of the macrolide antibiotic inducible cytochrome P-450 LM3c in the metabolism of midazolam by microsomal fractions prepared from rabbit liver. Biochem. Pharmacol. 37, 1947-1953

Fabre, G., Rahmani, R., Placidi, M., Combalbert, J., Covo, J., Cano, J.P., Coulange C., Ducros, M., and Rampal, M. (1988b) : Characterization of midazolam metabolism using human hepatic microsomal fractions and hepatocytes in suspension obtained by perfusing whole human livers. Biochem. Pharmacol. in press

Grant, M.J., Burke, D., Hawksworth, G.M., Duthie, S.J., Engeset, J., and Petrie J.C. (1987) : Human adult hepatocytes in primary monolayer culture. Maintenance of mixed function oxidase and conjugation pathways of drug metabolism. Biochem. Pharmacol. 36, 2311-2316

Gregus, Z., Watkins, J.B., Thompson, T.N. and Klaassen, C.D. (1982) : Resistance of some phase II biotransformation pathways to hepatotoxins. J. Pharm. Exp. Ther. 222, 471-479

Guengerich, F.P., Martin, M.V., Beaune, P.H., Kremers, P. Wolff, T. and Waxman, D.J. (1986) : Characterization of rat and human liver microsomal cytochrome P-450 forms involved in nifedipine oxidation, a prototype for genetic polymorphism in oxidative drug metabolism. J. Biol. Chem. 261, 5051-5060

Guillouzo, A., Beaune, P., Gascoin, M.N., Begue, J.M., Campion, J.P., Guengerich, F.P. and Guguen-Guillauzo, C. (1985) : Maintenance of cytochrome P-450 in cultured adult human hepatocytes. Biochem. Pharmacol. 34, 2991-2995

Irshaid, M.Y. and Tephly, T.R. (1987) : Isolation and purification of two human liver UDP-glucuronosyl transferases. Mol. Pharmacol. 31 : 27-34

Isom, H.C. and Georgoff, I. (1984) : Quantitative assay for albumin-producing liver cells after simian virus 40 transformation of rat hepatocytes maintained in chemically defined medium. Proc. Natl. Acad. U.S.A. 81, 6378-6382

Isselbacher, K.J., Chrabas, M.F., and Quinn, R.C. (1962) : The solubilization and partial purification of a glucuronyl transferase from rabbit liver microsomes. J. Biol. Chem. 237, 3033-3038.

Kremers, P., Beaune, P., Cresteil, T., de Graeve, J., Columelli, S. Leroux, J.P. and Gielen, J.E. (1981) : Cytochrome P-450 monooxygenase activities in human and rat liver microsomes. Eur. J. Biochem. 118, 599-606

Leroux, J.P., Beaune, P., Cresteil, T. and Flinois, J.P. (1986) : Isolation and characterization of different cytochrome P-450 isoenzymes in human liver : in Hepatotoxicity of drugs (eds : J.P. Fillastre) pp 305-309

Maurel, P., Dalet-Beluche, I., Dalet, C., Bonfils, C., Bories, P., Bauret, P. and Michel, H. (1986): Activités enzymatiques et dosage immunologique d'une forme de cytochrome P-450 microsomal dans des biopsies hépatiques à l'aiguille : in Hepatotoxicity of drugs (eds : J.P. Fillastre) pp 289-304

Mieyal, J.J. and Blumer, J.L. (1976) : Acceleration of the autooxidation of human oxy hemoglobin by aniline and its relation to hemoglobin-catalyzed aniline hydroxylation. J. Biol. Chem. 251, 3442-3446

Miners, J.O., Lillywhite, K.J., Matthews, A.P., Jones, N.E., and Birkett, D.J. (1988) : Kinetic and inhibitor studies of 4-methylumbelliferone and 1-naphthol glucuronidation in human liver microsomes. Biochem. Pharmacol. 37, 665-671

Nash, T. (1953) : The colorimetric estimation of formaldehyde by means of the Hantzsch reaction. Biochem. J. 55, 416-421.

Omura, T. and Sato, R. (1964) : the carbon-monooxide binding pigment of liver microsomes J. Biol. Chem. 239 : 2370-2378

Pelkonen, O., Pasanen, M., Kuha, M., Gachalyi, B.j Kairaluoma, M., Sotaniemi, E.A., Park, S.S., Friedman, F.K., and Gelboin, H.V. (1986) : The effect of cigarette smoking on 7-ethoxyresorufin O-deethylase and other monooxygenase activities in human liver : analyses with monoclonal antibodies. Br. J. Clin. Pharmacol. 22, 125-134.

Pollard, H.B., Menard, R., Brandt, H.A., Pazoles, C.J., Creutz, C.E. and Ramu, A. (1978) : Application of Bradford's protein assay to adrenal gland subcellular fractions. Anal. Biochem. 86 : 761-763

Rahmani, R., Richard, B., Fabre, G. and Cano, J.P. (1988) : Extrapolation of preclinical pharmacokinetic data to therapeutic drug use. Xenobiotica 18, 71-86.

Rao, S.G., Haueter, G., Rao, M.L., and Breur, H. (1976) : An improved assay for steroid glucuronyltransferase in liver microsomes. Anal. Biochem. 74, 35-40.

Schuetz, E.G., Hazelton, G.A., Hall, J., Watkins, P.B., Klassen, C.D., and Guzelian, P.S. (1986) : Induction of digitoxigenin monodigitoxoside UDP-glucuronosyltransferase activity by glucocorticoïds and other inducers of cytochrome P-450p in primary monolayer cultures of adult rat hepatocytes and in human liver. J. Biol. Chem. 261-18, 8270-8275

Siest, G., Antoine, B., Fournel, S., Magadlou, J. and Thomassin, J. (1987) : the glucuronosyl/transferases : what progress can pharmacologist expect from molecular biology and cellular enzymology ? Biochem. Pharmacol. 36 : 983-989

Suolinna, E.M., and Pitkäranta, T. (1986) : Effect of culture age on drug metabolizing enzymes and their induction in primary cultures of rat hepatocytes. Biochem. Pharmacol. 35, 2241-2245

Thiery, J.P. (1967) : Mise en évidence de polysaccharides sur coupes fines en microscope électronique, J. Microscop., (Paris) 6 : 967-1018

Von Bahr, C , Groth, C.G., Jansonn, H., Lundgren, G., Lind, K. and Glaumann, H. (1980) : Drug metabolism in human liver in vitro : establishment of a human liver bank. Clin. Pharmacol. Ther. 27, 711-725

Watkins, P.B., Klaassen, C.D. (1982) : Effet of inducers and inhibitors of glucuronidation on the biliary excretion and choleretic action of valproïc acid in the rat. J. Pharmacol. Exp. Ther. 220, 305-310

Watkins, P.B., Wrington, S.A., Maurel, P., Schuetz, E.G., Mendez-Picon, G., Parker, G.A. and Guzelian, P.S. (1985) : Identification of an inducible form of cytochrome P-450 in human liver. Proc. Natl. Acad. Sci. U.S.A. 82, 6310-6314

ACKNOWLEDGEMENTS

We are grateful to Pr. Rampal and Dimarino from Marseille Hospitals and Pr. Joyeux and Mion and Dr Mourad from Montpellier Hospitals for providing human liver samples. We wisk to acknowledge Mrs Bourrié and Mr Eric Marti for their excellent cooperation. We thank Mrs Patricia Lopez for her skilled collaboration and Mrs Catherine Foucault for her excellent secretarial assistance.

Résumé

Une étude des variabilités inter- et intra-individuelles des processus de Phase I (cytochromes P-450) et de Phase II (UDP-glucuronosyltransferases) a été réalisée sur des microsomes préparés à partir de 20 foies de donneurs. Les résultats mettent en évidence une importante variabilité inter-individuelle des réactions enzymatiques mettant en jeu les processus de Phase I et de Phase II.

Les réactions de N-déméthylation de l'érythromycine (ER) et d'oxydation de la Nifédipine (NIF) sont très fortement corrélées ($p < 0.001$). Quatre autres activités enzymatiques (N-déméthylations de la Benzphétamine (BZ) et de l'aminopyrine (AMP), la O-dééthylation de la 7-éthoxyrésorufine (EROD) et l'hydroxylation de l'acétanilide (ACET)) sont aussi corrélées à $p\ 0.001$.

Parmi les réactions de glucuronoconjugaison étudiées, seules celles mettant en jeu le 1-naphthol (1-NP) et le p-nitrophénol (pNP) sont corrélées à $p\ 0.002$). Enfin une corrélation de $p < 0.002$ a été démontrée entre l'oxydation de l'ER ou de la NIF et la conjugaison de l'acide valproïque.

Des hépatocytes humains obtenus après la dissociation à la collagénase d'un foie entier (donneurs d'organes) ou de lobes de foies (patients présentant des métastases hépatiques) ont été maintenus pendant 5 jours en culture primaire en l'absence ou en présence de divers inducteurs enzymatiques dont le phénobarbital (PB), la rifampycine (RIF), la dexaméthasone (DEX), le 3-méthylcholanthrène (3MC) et la ß-naphtoflavone (ßNF). Les microsomes préparés à partir de ces cultures ont été analysés par la technique du Western blot au moyen d'anticorps spécifiquement dirigés contre les isozymes P450IIIA3 et P450IA2. Leur capacité de métabolisation dépendant des Phases I et II a été aussi étudiée vis-à-vis de divers substrats (NIF, EROD, 1-NP). RIF, et à un degré moindre DEX et PB, induisent la forme P450IIIA3 et l'oxydation de la NIF. ßNF et 3MC induisent d'une part l'isozyme(s) P450IA2 mais aussi l'EROD, une activité enzymatique reliée aux isoenzymes de la famille P450I.

L'inductibilité de la glucuronoconjugaison du 1-Naphthol a été observée avec tous les inducteurs étudiés bien qu'elle soit variable d'une préparation à l'autre.

Ces études démontrent les relations étroites entre la régulation de l'expression des gènes des cytochromes P-450 et des UDP-glucuronosyl transférases et le métabolisme hépatique des médicaments.

Acyl migration and covalent binding of drug glucuronides — potential toxicity mediators

Leslie Z. Benet and Hildegard Spahn

Department of Pharmacy, University of California, San Francisco, California 94143-0446, USA

ABSTRACT

Reports from several laboratories have documented irreversible binding of carboxylic acids to proteins via their acyl glucuronide metabolites. We have demonstrated that such binding occurs in vivo in humans as well as in vitro for the non-steroidal anti-inflammatory drugs (NSAIDs) zomepirac, tolmetin and carprofen. We have also shown different formation rates as well as different stabilities for the acyl glucuronides of R and S enantiomers of racemic NSAIDs such as carprofen, benoxaprofen and flunoxaprofen. We hypothesize that the potential for toxicity can be predicted on the basis of: the ability of the corresponding acyl glucuronide to form irreversible bonds with proteins in vitro, the plasma concentration time profile of the acyl glucuronide and the in vivo stability of the formed adduct. The exact nature of the mechanism for irreversible binding has not yet been clearly elucidated. A direct nucleophilic displacement mechanism was proposed. We favor irreversible binding of acyl glucuronides to proteins via formation of an imine between the glucuronic acid moiety of an isomeric metabolite, formed by acyl migration, and the protein. As yet no relationship can be established between the irreversible binding of drugs to proteins, as found in our studies, and the incidence of immunologic reactions observed in humans. However, a correlation between the ability to form adducts with proteins and an immunogenic sensitizing ability is generally accepted.

KEY WORDS

Acyl migration, glucuronides, non-steroidal anti-inflammatory drugs, irreversible binding, reactive metabolites, drug hypersensitivity

INTRODUCTION

Drug conjugates with D-glucuronic acid are hydrophilic metabolites, which were previously assumed to be 'inactive' and rapidly excreted so that measurable plasma concentrations of the glucuronide conjugate were not expected. For acyl glucuronides, however, this is not absolutely true. Acyl glucuronides of several drugs and of bilirubin were found to yield measurable glucuronide concentrations, to form isomers via acyl migration and to irreversibly bind to plasma proteins under physiological conditions. Acyl migration is the rearrangement of the conjugate by intramolecular transesterification at the hydroxyl groups of the glucuronic acid moiety and leads to the formation of β-glucuronidase-resistant glucuronides (Faed, 1984), exhibiting chromatographic properties different from those of the β-1-glucuronide (Langendijk et al., 1984; Hyneck et al., 1987). This phenomenon was first described in drug metabolism for clofibric acid by Faed and McQueen in 1978. Furthermore, the β-1-glucuronide and the isomers are known to be labile to hydrolysis, both during in vitro biological sample workup and also under the pH and temperature conditions found in vivo. The instability of ester glucuronides to acyl migration and hydrolysis was reviewed by Faed in 1984 and has been more recently described in the literature for a number of compounds known to form acyl glucuronides in vivo including zomepirac (Smith et al., 1985a), diflunisal (Musson et al., 1985), tolmetin (Hyneck et al., 1988a), valproic acid (Dickinson et al., 1985), furosemide (Rachmel et al., 1985) and oxaprozin (Ruelius et al., 1986). Compounds exhibiting these properties with respect to their glucuronide metabolite are primarily from the aryl alkanoic class of non-steroidal anti-inflammatory drugs (NSAIDs) and a number of drugs from this class have been withdrawn from the market due to severe side-effects, e.g. zomepirac and benoxaprofen. For zomepirac, the well-known toxicities of gastric irritation, nephritis and acute renal failure (Clive and Stoff, 1984) were not responsible for its withdrawal from the market, which resulted rather from a high incidence of immunologic and anaphylactic reactions. Case-reports have also described anaphylactic and anaphylactoid reactions for the structurally related tolmetin (Moore and Goldsmith, 1980; Bretza and Novey, 1985). A current explanation for drug hypersensitivity reactions ("hapten hypothesis") suggests that covalent binding of a drug or its metabolite to a macromolecule yields an adduct, which can act as an immunogen or antigen and stimulate an immune response against the drug (Park et al., 1987). The extent of exposure to the potential immunogen is one possible determinant of the occurrence or non-occurrence of adverse reactions as depicted in Fig. 1.

We describe here different aspects of formation and stability of the glucuronides, reversible and irreversible binding in vitro and in vivo, including the exposure to acyl glucuronides after drug dosage and the resulting irreversible binding to plasma proteins. Since many NSAIDs are racemic mixtures, we have also investigated the above properties with the R and S enantiomers.

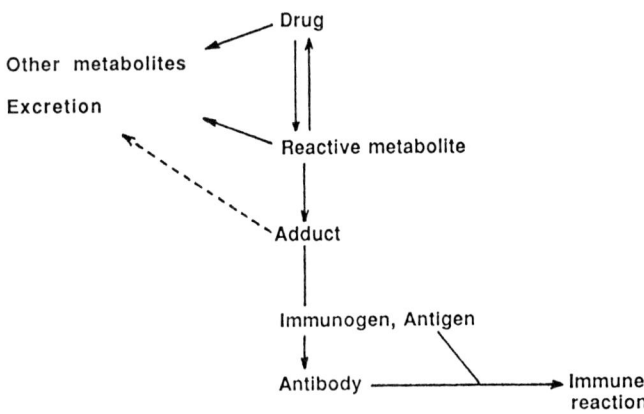

Figure 1. Interrelationship between immune response and disposition of the drug

FORMATION AND STABILITY OF ACYL GLUCURONIDES, "ACYL MIGRATION"

Formation of acyl glucuronides can take place in various organs and is subject to high interspecies variability. Advances in defining the in vivo disposition of acyl glucuronides occurred when analytical methods were developed to directly measure the metabolites (e.g., Langendijk et al., 1984; Hyneck et al., 1987) rather than measure parent drug before and after conjugate hydrolysis. We have also developed such direct assay methods for chiral NSAID substrates as depicted in Fig. 2 for benoxaprofen and carprofen.

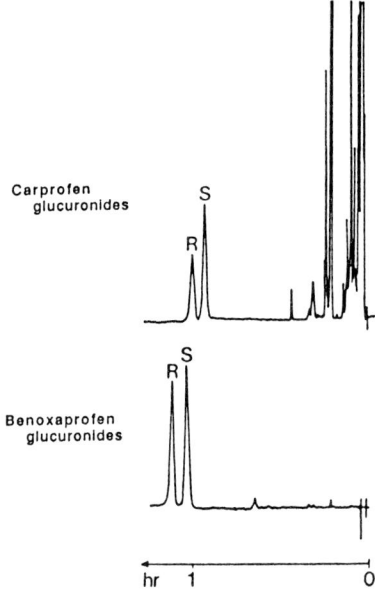

Figure 2. Direct separation of diastereomeric glucuronides of carprofen and benoxaprofen in urine samples [6-8 hr (carprofen) or 0-2 hr (benoxaprofen) after p.o. administration] (Spahn et al., submitted)

With direct assay methods it is possible to accurately quantitate the instability of acyl glucuronides under physiological conditions as represented in Table 1, where the degradation half-lives for several NSAIDs in pH 7.4 phosphate buffer at 37 °C are listed. Interestingly, there is also a difference in the degradation half-lives between the diastereomeric glucuronides of chiral compounds, such as carprofen or benoxaprofen (Spahn et al., submitted), where the glucuronide of the R-enantiomer disappears more rapidly. Hydrolysis of the glucuronide to the parent compound does not totally account for the glucuronide loss, due to the formation of structural isomers of the glucuronides. The stabilities of the conjugates are highly pH-dependent. Therefore, biological samples must be acid pH-stabilized and handled at low temperatures, in order to obtain reliable pharmacokinetic data with respect to metabolite kinetics.

Earlier studies not employing correct sample stabilization procedures yielded inaccurate measures of the pharmacokinetics of the carboxylic acid drugs and their glucuronide conjugates. With stabilized samples, significant concentrations of acyl glucuronides were detectable for zomepirac, tolmetin and the optically active carprofen, for which the R/S ratio for parent drug (<1) was less than that for the conjugates (=1 or >1). Stereochemical aspects of the formation of glucuronides on the subcellular level were included in recent investigations (el Mouelhi et al., 1987; Spahn and Benet, 1988; Caldwell et al., 1988). We found a high substrate specificity for several 2-arylpropionic acids when investigating the properties of UDPGTs from rat liver microsomes. The R/S ratio for the initial rate of glucuronide formation, however, was highly variable between the compounds (naproxen: 0.7, flunoxaprofen: 1.9, carprofen: 2.3, benoxaprofen: 2.6). Additional studies with sheep liver microsomes (R/S for flunoxaprofen: 1.1, with K_m and V_{max} being almost the same for both enantiomers) indicate the high interspecies variability, which was already described by others (Caldwell et al., 1988).

Table 1. Degradation half-lives of various β-1-acyl glucuronides at pH 7.4 (37°C)

Compound	Half-life in hours
Zomepirac	0.52
Tolmetin	0.39
Furosemide	4.40
R/S-Benoxaprofen	2.0(R), 4.1(S)
R/S-Flunoxaprofen	4.5(R), 8.0(S)
R/S-Carprofen	1.7(R), 2.9(S)

Rates of acyl migration for different compounds are quite variable and influenced by many factors. Hasegawa et al. (1982) described an apparent first order pH dependent degradation of zomepirac glucuronide with minimal isomerization occurring at pH < 5, similar to that reported for valproic acid (Dickinson et al., 1985) and furosemide (Rachmel et al., 1985). Smith et al. (1985b) demonstrated that the stability of zomepirac acyl glucuronides was affected by temperature and the nature of the solution (buffer, organic solvents, plasma, blood, urine). The disappearance of zomepirac β-1-glucuronide and the formation of isomers and parent zomepirac in vitro at pH 7.4 and 37 °C are depicted in Fig. 3. Structural assignments of the isomers were possible using high field ^{1}H-NMR, which also indicated that the isomers are present as their α/β anomeric mixtures (Smith and Benet, 1986). For tolmetin a rapid degradation of the β-1-glucuronide was found ($t_{1/2}$ = 23.7 min), which resulted mainly in the formation of isomeric conjugates, which were found to be far more stable than the β-1-glucuronide (Hyneck et al.,

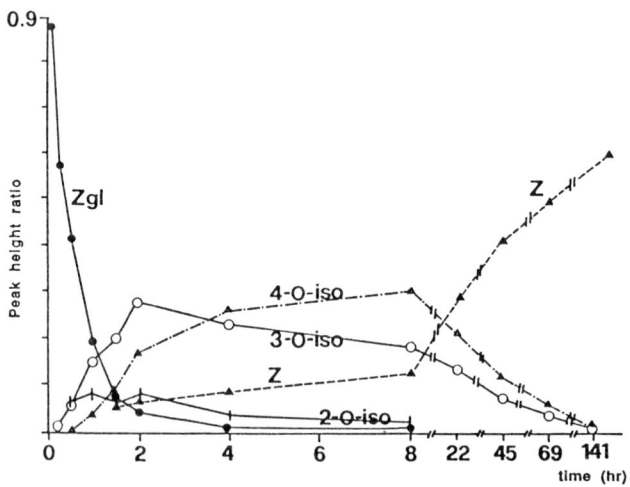

Figure 3. Time-dependent degradation of zomepirac glucuronide (Zgl) to its isomeric conjugates (2-, 3-, 4-O-iso) and hydrolysis to zomepirac (Z) in 0.1 M phosphate buffer, pH 7.4, 37 °C. [2-, 3- and 4-iso represents the α/β-2-O-, α/β-3-O- and α/β-4-O-acyl isomers] (modified from Hasegawa et al. (1982)]

1988a). In contrast to the results at pH 7.4, a very low extent of acyl migration and hydrolysis was observed at pH 3. Faed (1984) suggests that the mechanism underlying the migration phenomenon is a base-catalyzed intramolecular transesterification via an ortho acid ester intermediate.

BINDING OF ACYL GLUCURONIDES TO PROTEINS

A correlation between reversible binding and irreversible binding to plasma proteins, with reversible binding acting as a preliminary or intermediate step, was discussed by Wells et al. (1987). Data about reversible plasma protein binding of glucuronides, however, are rare. With respect to acyl glucuronides, the lack of data mainly results from experimental problems, since the studies need to be carried out at physiologic pH. By rapid ultrafiltration a comparison of the extent of binding between the R- and the S-carprofen glucuronide was possible (Iwakawa et al., submitted). Both glucuronides bind to human serum albumin, with the S-glucuronide (8% unbound at 1 μM) having a higher affinity than the R-glucuronide (14 % unbound). However, the role of reversible binding with respect to the mechanism of irreversible binding of acyl glucuronides to proteins is still unclear, as is true for the mechanism itself.

We have demonstrated irreversible binding for the glucuronides of zomepirac (Smith et al., 1986), tolmetin (Hyneck et al., 1988b) and carprofen (Iwakawa et al., submitted) to human serum albumin under in vitro conditions and following a single dose of the drug to human volunteers. The extent of binding of zomepirac glucuronide with albumin in vitro was found to be clearly time and pH dependent (Smith et al., 1986). The isomeric conjugates, but not the parent unconjugated zomepirac, were found to bind irreversibly to protein as well.

Two different mechanisms to explain irreversible binding to proteins have been proposed. The first suggests direct nucleophilic displacement of the glucuronic acid moiety (Fig. 4).

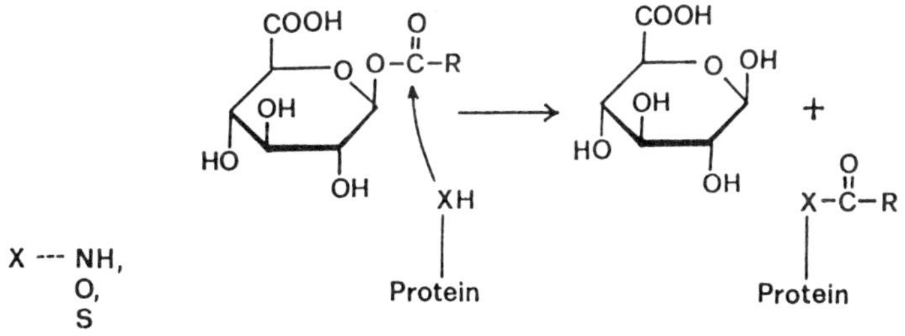

Figure 4. Postulated mechanisms for the irreversible binding of carboxylic acids to proteins via their acyl glucuronides. I. Nucleophilic displacement

This mechanism, initially proposed by van Breemen and Fenselau (1985), involves the reaction of a cysteine thiol of albumin. However, not all binding of flufenamic acid glucuronide could be prevented by blocking cysteine, and no effect on the extent of binding of zomepirac glucuronide was observed when thiols were blocked with p-hydroxymercuribenzoate (Smith et al., submitted). Ruelius et al. (1986) have implicated tyrosine in albumin for oxaprozin glucuronide. This mechanism is supported by studies with oxaprozin glucuronide labeled either in the oxaprozin or in the glucuronic acid portion. The 2-O-acyl isomer of oxaprozin glucuronide did not lead to covalent binding to albumin, however, all isomeric conjugates were found to react with albumin in the case of zomepirac glucuronide (Smith et al., 1986).

A second mechanism for the irreversible binding of acyl glucuronides was proposed by our laboratory (Smith et al., 1986), in which it is suggested that the observed irreversible binding of the isomeric conjugates of zomepirac glucuronide occurs via imine formation between the free aldehyde of the open-chain glucuronic acid and a nucleophil, possibly lysine, in the albumin molecule (Fig. 5). This step is reversible, but it is then followed by an Amadori rearrangement of the imino sugar to the more stable 1-amino-2-keto product. In preliminary binding studies with zomepirac glucuronide in our laboratory, imine trapping reagents (NaCN, NaCNBH$_3$) increased the extent of irreversible binding significantly. Furthermore, isomeric glucuronide conjugates were released after extensive washing and subsequent acid treatment giving evidence that the glucuronic acid moiety is part of the adduct.

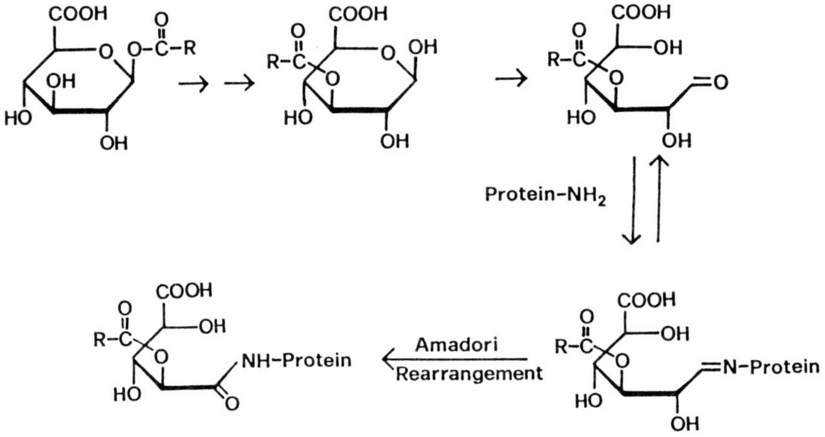

Figure 5. Postulated mechanism for the irreversible binding of carboxylic acids to proteins via their acyl glucuronides: II. Imine formation and Amadori rearrangement (acid-catalyzed)

After single dose human studies adduct concentrations were relatively low, however, it can be assumed from our in vitro and in vivo data, that with increasing concentration of the 'reactive' metabolite and with increasing exposure time, the extent of covalent binding should increase. Increased adduct formation can thus be expected during chronic dosage or with decreased clearance of the glucuronide as in renal failure or for drug-drug interactions. Indeed, adduct concentrations in an elderly patient currently treated with tolmetin were significantly higher than those in the control group of elderly patients given a single dose (Munafo et al., submitted).

The influence of probenecid on the pharmacokinetics with respect to glucuronide formation and elimination was investigated for zomepirac (Smith et al., 1985a) and for carprofen (Spahn et al., 1988). For both compounds, the renal clearance of the glucuronide was significantly lower and the AUC significantly higher than in the controls (Table 2). Thus the exposure to reactive metabolite is increased. For zomepirac, the extent of covalent binding was also investigated. A good positive correlation was found between the AUC of the glucuronide and the concentration of adduct (Smith et al., 1986).

If the scheme depicted in Fig. 1 does explain the toxicity of aryl alkanoic NSAIDs, three determinants of the potential for toxicity can be hypothesized:
1) ability of acyl glucuronides to lead to irreversible binding with proteins. This can be determined under in vitro conditions, and we believe, in terms of the imine mechanism we favor, can be predicted upon the tendency for acyl migration to occur.
2) the plasma concentration-time profile of the acyl glucuronides. This should be determined in the species of interest, man. If plasma glucuronide concentrations are found, irreversible binding should occur. Increases in glucuronide concentrations, as in our concurrent probenecid dosing studies (Smith et al., 1985a; Spahn et al., 1988) lead to increased binding. However, the extent of irreversible bin-

Table 2. Influence of probenecid on the area under the plasma concentration-time curve (AUC) and the renal clearance (CL_R) in clinical studies with zomepirac (100 mg) and R/S-carprofen (150 mg) with and without probenecid [Zomepirac glucuronide = Zgl, carprofen glucuronide = Cgl] (from Smith et al.,1985b; Spahn et al.,1988)

	Zomepirac	Zomepirac/probenecid
AUC_{Zgl} [µg x min/ml]	180 ± 57	499 ± 134
$CL_{R(Zgl)}$ [ml/min]	406 ± 110	115 ± 32
	S-carprofen	S-carprofen/probenecid
AUC_{Cgl} [µg x min/ml]	1638 ± 168	3348 ± 1656
$CL_{R(Cgl)}$ [ml/min]	35.6 ± 5.1	3.4 ± 2.8
	R-carprofen	R-carprofen/probenecid
AUC_{Cgl} [µg x min/ml]	2076 ± 324	3774 ± 2076
$CL_{R(Cgl)}$ [ml/min]	26.4 ± 5.0	3.6 ± 3.0

ding observed for different drugs will be a function of both determinants 1 and 2. For example, following a 400 mg single dose of tolmetin, the mean area under the curve (AUC) for tolmetin glucuronide concentrations was less than one-fourth the AUC for zomepirac glucuronide concentrations following a 100 mg zomepirac dose (Hyneck et al., 1988b). However, the epitope density (defined as the number of moles bound per mole of protein) for tolmetin ($2.77 \pm 1.54 \times 10^{-4}$) slightly exceeds that for zomepirac ($2.33 \pm 0.45 \times 10^{-4}$) in two groups of healthy volunteers. Our recent studies with carprofen (25 and 50 mg doses) yield comparable epitope densities.
3) the stability of the in vivo adduct. Estimated half-lives for the zomepirac and tolmetin adducts exceed the 24 - 48 hr sampling times.

Finally an understanding of adduct formation is not just of academic interest. Since cross reactivities towards several NSAIDs have been reported, either a complex immune reaction or a common immunologic determinant could be an explanation. The mechanism depicted in Fig. 5 leads to an identical functional group in the hapten, i.e., the glucuronic acid moiety, which may be consistent with the immunologic cross reactivity observed.

It is difficult to test the scheme depicted in Fig. 1, due to the lack of a suitable animal model for immunologic studies, since the extent of exposure to glucuronides is usually small in rodents after dosage of the drug or even the acyl glucuronide. Further immunologic studies using human serum and in animals dosed with esterase inhibitors are now ongoing.

ACKNOWLEDGEMENTS

This work was supported by National Institutes of Health grant GM 36633.

REFERENCES

Bretza, J.A., H.S. Novey (1985): Anaphylactoid reactions to tolmetin after interrupted dosage. Western J. Med. 143, 55-59.
Caldwell J., A.J. Hutt, S. Fournel-Gigleux (1988): The metabolic chiral inversion and dispositional enantioselectivity of the 2-arylpropionic acids and their biological consequences. Biochem. Pharmacol. 37, 105-114.
Clive, D.M., J.F. Stoff (1984): Renal syndromes associated with non-steroidal an-

ti-inflammatory drugs. N. Engl. J. Med. 310, 563-572.

Dickinson, R.G., W.D. Hooper, M.J. Eadie (1985): pH-Dependent rearrangement of the biosynthetic ester glucuronide of valproic acid to β-glucuronidase-resistant forms. Drug Metab. Dispos. 12, 247-252.

El Mouelhi, M., H.W. Ruelius, C. Fenselau, D.M. Dulik (1987): Species-dependent enantioselective glucuronidation of three 2-arylpropionic acids. Naproxen, ibuprofen, benoxaprofen. Drug Metab. Dispos. 15, 767-772.

Faed, E.M. (1984): Properties of acyl glucuronides: Implications for studies of the pharmacokinetics and metabolism of acidic drugs. Drug Metab. Rev. 15, 1213-1249.

Faed, E.M., E.G. McQueen (1978): Separation of two conjugates of clofibric acid (CPIB) found in the urine of subjects taking clofibrate. Clin. Exp. Pharmacol. Physiol. 5, 195-198.

Hasegawa J., P.C. Smith, L.Z. Benet (1982): Apparent intramolecular acyl migration of zomepirac glucuronide. Drug Metab. Dispos. 10, 469-473.

Hyneck, M.L., P.C. Smith, E. Unseld, L.Z. Benet (1987): High-performance liquid chromatographic determination of tolmetin, tolmetin glucuronide and its isomeric conjugates in plasma and urine. J. Chromatogr. 420, 349-356.

Hyneck, M.L., A. Munafo, L.Z. Benet (1988a): Effect of pH on acyl migration and hydrolysis of tolmetin glucuronide. Drug Metab. Dispos. 16, 322-324.

Hyneck, M.L., P.C. Smith, A. Munafo, A.F. McDonagh, L.Z. Benet (1988b): Disposition and irreversible protein binding of tolmetin in humans. Clin. Pharmacol. Ther. 43, in press.

Langendijk, P.N.J., P.C. Smith, J. Hasegawa, L.Z. Benet (1984): Simultaneous determination of zomepirac and its major metabolite zomepirac glucuronide in human plasma and urine. J. Chromatogr. 307, 371-379.

Moore, M.E., D.P. Goldsmith (1980): Non-steroidal anti-inflammatory intolerance: Anaphylactic reaction to tolmetin. Arch. Int. Med. 140, 1105-1106.

Musson, D.G., J.H. Lin, K.A. Lyon, D.J. Tocco, K.C. Yeh (1985): Assay methodology for quantification of ester and ether glucuronide conjugates of diflunisal in human urine. J. Chromatogr. 337, 363-378.

Park B.K., J.W. Coleman, N.R. Kitteringham (1987): Drug disposition and drug hypersensitivity. Biochem. Pharmacol. 36, 581-590.

Rachmel, A, G.A. Hazelton, A.L. Yergey, D.J. Liberato (1985): Furosemide 1-O-acyl glucuronides. In vitro biosynthesis and pH-dependent isomerization to β-glucuronidase-resistant forms. Drug Metab. Dispos. 13, 705-710.

Ruelius, H.W., S.K. Kirkham, E.M. Young, F.W. Janssen (1986): Reactions of oxaprozin-1-O-acyl glucuronide in solutions of human plasma and albumin. Adv. Exp. Med. Biol. 197, 431-441.

Smith, P.C., P.N.J. Langendijk, J. Hasegawa, L.Z. Benet (1985a): Effect of probenecid on the formation and elimination of acyl glucuonides: Studies with zomepirac. Clin. Pharmacol. Ther. 38, 121-127.

Smith, P.C., J. Hasegawa, L.Z. Benet (1985b): Stability of acyl glucuronides in blood, plasma and urine. Studies with zomepirac. Drug Metab. Dispos. 13, 110-112.

Smith, P.C., L.Z. Benet (1986): Characterization of the isomeric esters of zomepirac glucuronide by proton NMR. Drug Metab. Dispos. 14, 503-505.

Smith, P.C., A.F. McDonagh, L.Z. Benet (1986): Irreversible binding of zomepirac to plasma protein in vitro and in vivo. J. Clin. Invest. 77, 934-939.

Spahn H., L.Z. Benet (1988): Enantioselectivity of hepatic UDP-glucuronyltransferase in rat liver microsomes towards 2-arylpropionic acids: Glucuronidation of naproxen enantiomers. Proc. 3rd Eur. Congr. Biopharm. Pharmacokinet., Freiburg 1987, in press.

Spahn, H., I. Spahn, L.Z. Benet (1988): Probenecid-induced changes in the clearance of carprofen enantiomers - A preliminary study. Clin. Pharmacol. Ther., in press.

van Breemen, R.B., C. Fenselau (1985): Acylation of albumin by 1-O-acyl glucuronides. Drug Metab. Dispos. 13, 318-320.

Wells, D.S., F.W. Janssen, H.W. Ruelius (1987): Interactions between oxaprozin glucuronide and albumin. Xenobiotica 17, 1437-1449.

Résumé

Des travaux de divers laboratoires nous ont fourni des renseignements sur les liaisons irréversibles se formant entre les acyl glucuronides d'acides carboxyliques et les protéines. Dans l'étude d'anti-inflammatoires non stéroïdiens (AINS) [zomepirac, tolmetine et carprofène], nous avons montré que de telles liaisons apparaissent chez l'homme aussi bien *in vivo* qu'*in vitro*.

Nous avons également montré que les acyl glucuronides provenant d'énantiomères R et S d'un mélange racémique d'AINS tels que le carprofène, le benoxaprofène et le fluroxaprofène, présentaient des stabilités différentes, entraînant des taux de formation différents.

Nous avons émis l'hypothèse que la capacité de toxicité pouvait être prédite sur les bases suivantes :
- la capacité des acyl glucuronides à former des liaisons irréversibles avec les protéines, *in vitro*.
- la concentration plasmatique du glucuronide en fonction du temps (demi-vie) et la stabilité *in vivo* du complexe formé.

La nature exacte du mécanisme de formation de cette liaison irréversible n'a pas encore été clairement élucidée. Un mécanisme d'attaque nucléophile a été proposé. Nous préférons la formation d'une liaison irréversible entre acyl glucuronides et protéines par la formation d'imine entre la partie de l'acide glucuronique d'un isomère métabolite, formé par une migration de la fonction acyl, et la protéine.

Aucune relation ne peut être établie entre la liaison irréversible de médicaments aux protéines, mise en évidence dans nos travaux, et l'incidence des réactions immunologiques observées chez l'homme. Toutefois, une corrélation entre la capacité à former des complexes avec les protéines et une capacité de sensibilité immunologique est généralement acceptée.

Acyl-glucuronidation of ponalrestat in the rat *in vivo* and its role in the sex difference in urinary excretion of the drug

Gérard J. Mulder*, Frank C.J. Wierckx*, Peter L.M. Jansen** and Alan Warrander**

*. Division of Toxicology, Center for Bio-Pharmaceutical Sciences, University of Leiden, Leiden, The Netherlands.
**. Department of Internal Medicine, Division of Gastroenterology, University of Amsterdam, Amsterdam, The Netherlands.
***. Department of Drug Metabolism, ICI Pharmaceuticals, Macclesfield, UK

ABSTRACT

The drug Ponalrestat (ICI 128,436; STATIL[R]) contains a carboxylic group that is glucuronidated; in the rat this glucuronide is the main metabolite. The rat demonstrates a marked sex difference with regard to excretion of ponalrestat: both after oral and intravenous administration only 5% of the dose is excreted in urine in males, but up to 85% in females. In both sexes the initial route of excretion of [^{14}C]-ponalrestat is as glucuronide in bile. When ponalrestat was infused into the duodenum directly, the sex difference in urinary excretion was again observed. The same was the case after i.v. administration of the glucuronide, which was initially excreted mainly in bile. The biliary excretion after intravenous administration of ponalrestat or its glucuronide was similar in both sexes. There was no difference in the uptake of the glucuronide from the intestinal loop preparation in both sexes. In a mutant strain with a deficiency in biliary excretion of many cholephilic compounds the biliary excretion of ponalrestat was also deficient; the sex difference in urinary excretion disappeared to a large extent in this strain. The localization of the sex difference is discussed.

KEY WORDS

Ponalrestat, acyl glucuronidation, biliary excretion, sex difference.

INTRODUCTION

Ponalrestat is an aldose reductase inhibitor, which is undergoing clinical trials in insulin-treated diabetics. It reduces some of the complications of the disease caused by sorbitol accumulation. The structure is shown in Fig. 1. The metabolism of ponalrestat has been studied in rat, mouse, rabbit, dog and man (Suker et al, 1987). In all the species studied, the major route of metabolism was conjugation of the carboxyl group with glucuronic acid.

Many drugs containing a carboxyl group are extensively glucuronidated in the rat and man; well investigated examples are valproic acid, clofibric acid and iopanoic acid (Cooke and Cooke, 1983; Watkins and Klaassen, 1982; Baldwin et al, 1980).

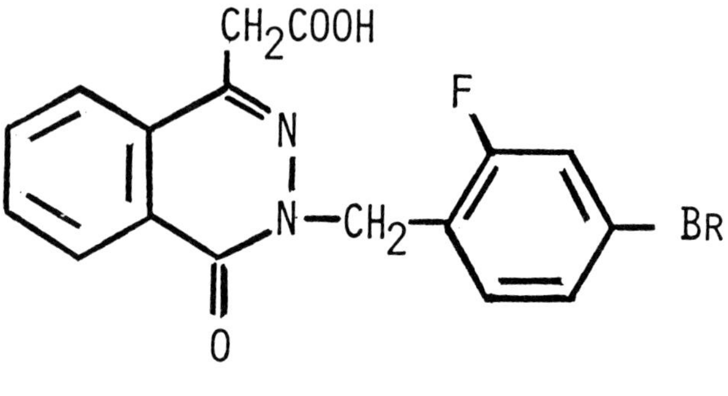

Fig. 1. Structure of ponalrestat.

Bilirubin presents an important endogenous substrate of that type of glucuronidation (see elsewhere in this volume).

Ester glucuronides are rather labile, certainly at alkaline pH. The acyl group may migrate from the 1- to the 2- and 3-positions of the pyranose ring. These glucuronides then become resistant to β-glucuronidase activity and, therefore, their identification presents problems. Such shifts have first been noted for bilirubin conjugates (Compernolle et al, 1978; Faed, 1984).

In general only minor sex differences in glucuronidation have been found (see Mulder 1986 for a review). Usually the published results are highly variable and sometimes conflicting. There seems to be a tendency for higher glucuronidation of phenols in male than in female liver, while for steroids the opposite trend is observed. We now report a pronounced sex difference in the elimination of ponalrestat after its glucuronidation; as yet the exact localization of the sex difference has not been identified.

MATERIALS AND METHODS

[^{14}C]-Labeled Ponalrestat and the unlabeled compound (Statil^R, ICI 128,436) were obtained from ICI Pharmaceuticals. The glucuronide had been synthesized by the immobilized enzyme technique (Lehman et al, 1981; Pallante et al, 1986). The radiolabel was in the phthalazinone ring (C3 and C8 positions). The specific radioactivity of ponalrestat was 2.5 µCi/µmol at a radiochemical purity of over 98%. That of ponalrestat glucuronide was 0.35 µCi/mg; it contained also the isomers in which the acyl group had shifted. Male and female rats of the Wistar strain of the Sylvius Laboratories, University of Leiden were used. They had free access to food and water, and were kept on a 12 hr dark-light schedule. The body weight was between 180 and 240 g. In some experiments we have used a mutant rat strain which is deficient in the biliary excretion of a number of cholephilic compounds. It is Wistar-derived strain which has been well characterized (Jansen et al, 1985a, 1985b, 1987; Huber et al, 1987). The main mutation seems to be a loss of carrier-systems for these compounds; as a result they are jaundiced, because they cannot excrete bilirubin conjugates. Their bile production is somewhat reduced, to approx. 60% of normal.

Ponalrestat was administered in an alkaline solution; the dose was in most experiments 25 mg/kg, or 64 µmol/kg (and 2.5 µCi/kg). It was administered in a lateral tail vein under diethyl ether anaesthesia when the animals were subsequently kept in a metabolism cage. In other experiments rats were anaesthetized with pentobarbital, and bile duct and urine bladder were catheterized as described elsewhere; an infusion of mannitol was given to ensure sufficient urine production (Mulder et al, 1981). The body temperature of the rats was kept between 37.5 and 38.5 °C. during the experiment. Bile and urine were collected in fractions and radioactivity in urine was determined by scintillation counting; in some cases urine or bile samples were analysed by hplc (see below). When the absorption of ponalrestat metabolites from the intestinal tract was determined, this was done either in vivo or in vitro. In the in vivo experiment, a bile sample containing ponalrestat and its metabolite (it consisted mainly of ponalrestat glucuronide) was injected directly into the duodenum, after which the rats were put in a metabolism cage. Alternatively, in situ gut loops were studied, with instillation of ponalrestat glucuronide into the jejunum after this had been rinsed out with saline. After 15 minutes the radio-activity that remained either in the lumen, or was in the gut preparation was counted. This was subtracted from the radioactivity originally introduced, to calculate the percentage absorbed.

Analysis Of Bile And Urine
Samples of urine or bile were counted after addition of Hydrocount scintillation medium. Radioactivity present in faeces was counted after addition of water to the faeces so that a slurry resulted. Bile and urine samples were injected directly onto the hplc column, Spherisorb ODS II 5 µm (15 x 0.3 cm).
Elution was by a linear gradient of water-methanol from 0 to 100% methanol in 20 or 30 minutes. Flow rate was 0.45 ml/min. Detection was by UV absorbance at 254 nm or by on-line radioactivity monitoring.

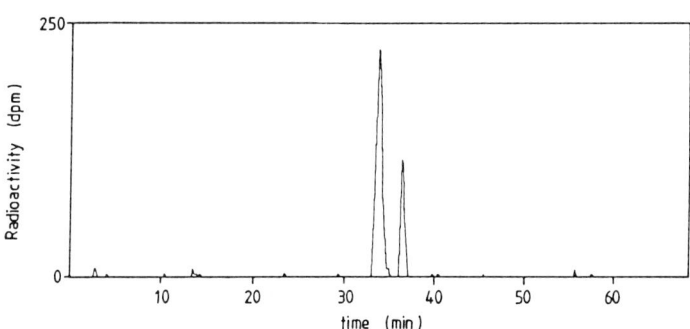

Fig. 2: Hplc profile of a bile sample containing [^{14}C]labeled ponalrestat (retention time 36 min) and its glucuronide (r.t. 33 min) obtained from a rat treated with 25 mg/kg ponalrestat i.v.

RESULTS

Metabolites Of Ponalrestat In Urine And Bile.
When urine or bile samples of rats that had been dosed with ponalrestat (64 μmol/kg o were analysed they contained only two peaks of radioactivity. In bile Fig.2 almost exclusively ponalrestat glucuronide was observed (Fig. 2), while in urine most of the radioactivity was the unchanged compound. However, when the rats had been pretreated with ammonium chloride so that their urine became slightly acidic in stead of the regular pH of around 8.5, only the glucuronide conjugate was observed. This was taken to indicate that under the slightly alkaline conditions in urine already a rapid break down of the glucuronide takes place. Over 95% of the radioactivity in bile and urine could be accounted
for in the form of the glucuronide or the unchanged compound.

Excretion Of Radioactivity In Urine In Male And Female Rats After Oral Or Intravenous Administration Of Ponalrestat.
When the urinary excretion of radioactivity of [^{14}C]-labeled ponalrestat was measured in male and female rats, there was a very marked difference: only some 4% of the radioactivity was excreted in male rats, while in females this was approx. 80% after 72 hours (Fig. 3). This was the same after oral and intravenous

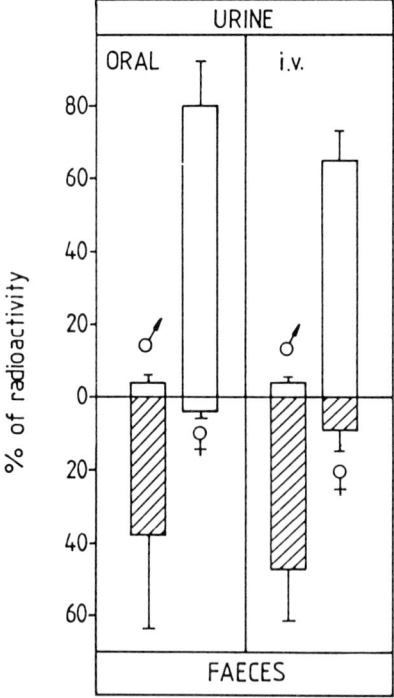

Fig. 3: Percentage of radioactivity in urine or faeces after administration of [^{14}C]-ponalrestat either orally or i.v. to male and female rats. Urine and faeces were collected during 72 hrs (n=4 in each group); means ± SD are given.

administration. Part of the difference was reflected in an opposite sex difference in the amount of radioactivity in faeces: some 40-50% of the radio activity was in the faeces of male rats, while only 5-10% was recovered in female faeces. This suggested the possibility of a difference in biliary excretion, as has been demonstrated for the glucuronide of 1-hydroxynitrotoluenes (Rickert et al, 1987).

Biliary Excretion Of Ponalrestat In Male And Female Wistar And Mutant Rats.
In rats with a catheter in the bile duct and in the urine bladder, the excretion of ponalrestat after intravenous injection was followed. The biliary excretion is plotted cumulatively in Fig. 4. Clearly the females excreted ponalrestat more slowly than the males. However, still more than 33% of the radioactivity had been excreted in bile in the females after 4 hours, and the excretion was not yet complete after this period. In addition only 3% of the radioactivity had been excreted in urine over that period. This is lower than anticipated, based on the 24-hrs urinary excretion in the intact animal. Therefore, it seems that the initial route of elimination also in female rats is mainly biliary excretion of the glucuronide and the sex difference seems to develop later in the excretory process. This was confirmed in rats with a mutation in their biliary excretion of cholephilic compounds: in this case the sex difference in urinary excretion had disappeared to a large extent. In the mutants biliary excretion was severely impaired: it had decreased to only 3% of the dose in 2 hours.

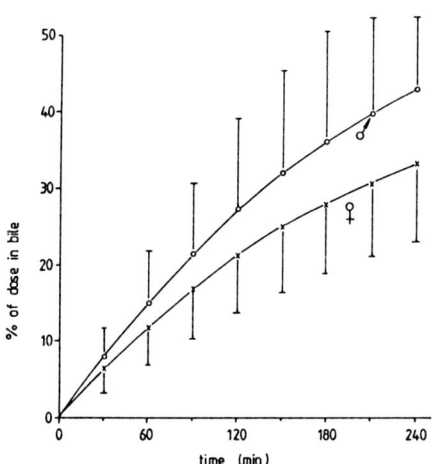

Fig. 4: Cumulative excretion of radioactivity in bile after i.v. administration of ponalrestat (25 mg/kg) to male and female rats under pentobarbital anesthesia (n=4).

Intraduodenal Administration Of Ponalrestat Glucuronide.
When in normal rats the biliary excretion was bypassed by injection of a bile sample containing ponalrestat glucuronide, in female and male rats, we still

observed the sex difference in urinary excretion (Fig. 5). The bile sample was derived from a rat that had received a high dose of radioactive ponalrestat.

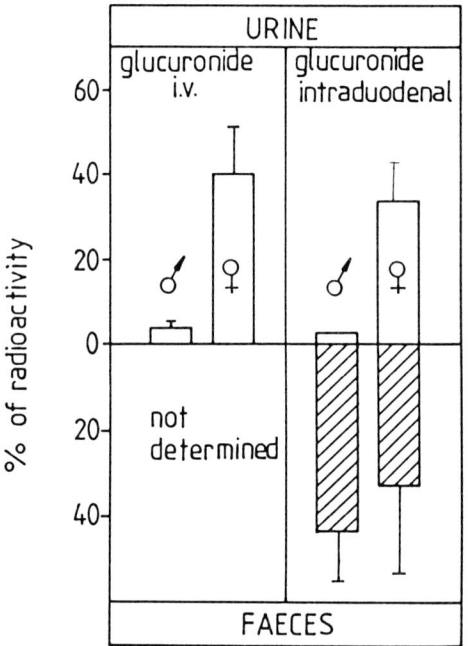

Fig. 5: Excretion of radioactivity in urine or faeces in rats receiving either [^{14}C]labeled ponalrestat glucuronide i.v., or a bile sample containing [^{14}C]ponalrestat glucuronide intraduodenally. (n=3 in each group). Urine and faeces were collected for 72 hrs.

The sex difference might, therefore, be at the level of reabsorption of the glucuronide in the gut. This was investigated in the gut loop preparation in which a solution of ponalrestat glucuronide was instilled in the lumen. After 15 minutes the loop was taken out and the contents of the loop were analysed for radioactivity. In such loop preparations from both sexes approx. 30% of the added radioactivity had been absorbed, indicating that at that level there was no sex difference.

Excretion Of Intravenously Administered Ponalrestat Glucuronide.
It also appeared possible that ponalrestat in blood might show a sex difference in elimination. We have injected the glucuronide intravenously but also in this case we observed the sex difference in urinary excretion. Moreover, the females excreted the glucuronide even more extensively in bile than the males (Fig. 5).

Effect of gut decontamination.
In a number of rats the gut flora was killed by oral treatment with a antibiotic cocktail. However, when ponalrestat was administered orally in these rats, still the same sex difference was observed, suggesting that the gut flora was not responsible.

DISCUSSION

In the rat, both the male and the female, glucuronidation of ponalrestat to form an ester glucuronide is the almost exclusive route of metabolism. The initial route of excretion is into bile. It seems that there is no difference in handling of the glucuronide at that level. Moreover, the glucuronide that is present in blood is rapidly excreted in bile, also in female rats. The only simple explanation for the high urinary excretion of the glucuronide in female rats therefore seems the possibility that there is a pronounced sex difference in kidney glucuronidation of ponalrestat. Because the in vitro rate of glucuronidation by rat kidney and liver microsomes was extremely low, we have not yet been able to get evidence for this. However, a sex difference in glucuronidation of phenols by GT-1 in the kidney has been noted: Rush et al (1983) and Tremaine et al (1985) have demonstrated that in female rats upto 22% of the total body glucuronidation capacity for p-nitrophenol is in the kidney, and only 11% in males. If the same, applies in a more pronounced form to ponalrestat, that might be the reason for the sex difference in its urinary excretion in the rat.

REFERENCES

Baldwin, J.R., Witiak, D.T., Fellers, D.R. (1980): Disposition of clofibrate in the rat. Biochem. Pharmacol. 29, 3143-3154.
Compernolle, F., Van Hees, G.P., Blanckaert, N., Heirweght, K.P.M. (1978): Glucuronic acid conjugates of bilirubin-IXα in normal bile compared with postobstructive bile. Transformation of the 1-O-acylglucuronide into 2-, 3- and 4-O-acylglucuronides. Biochem. J. 171, 185-201.
Cook, W.J., Cooke, L.M. (1983): Effects of anesthetics on the hepatic metabolism and biliary secretion of lopanoic acid enantiomers in rat. J. Pharmacol. Exp. Ther. 225, 85-93.
Faed, J. (1984): Properties of acyl glucuronides: implications for studies of the pharmacokinetics and metabolism of acidic drugs. Drug Metab. Revs 15, 1213-1249.
Hubert, M., Guhlmann, A., Jansen, P.L.M., Keppler, D. (1987): Hereditary defect of hepatobiliary cysteinyl leucotriene elimination in mutant rats with defective hepatic anion excretion. Hepatology 7, 224-228.
Jansen, P.L.M., Peters, W.H.M., Lamers, W.H. (1985a): Hereditary chronic conjugated hyperbilirubinemia in mutant rats caused by defective hepatic anion transport. Hepatology 5, 573-579.
Jansen, P.L.M., Groothuis, G.M.M., Buscher, H.P., Peters, W.H.M., Fricker, G., Müller, M., Nolte, A., Gerok, W., Kurz, G., Meijer, D.K.F. (1985b): Defective hepatic canalicular transport in mutant rats with conjugated hyperbilirubinemia. Hepatology 5, 954-
Jansen, P.L.M., Groothuis, G.M.M., Peters, W.H.M., Meijer, D.K.F. (1987): Selective defect in the hepatobiliary transport of organic compounds in mutant rats with hereditary conjugated hyperbilirubinemia. Heterogeneity of hepatobiliary transport. Hepatology 7, 71-76.
Lehman, J.P., Ferrin, L., Fenselau, C., Yost, G.S. (1981): Simultaenous immobilisation of cytochrome P450 and glucuronyl transferase for synthesis of drug metabolites. Drug Metab. Disp. 9, 15-18.

Mulder, G.J., Scholtens, E., Meijer, D.K.F. (1981): Collection of metabolites in urine and bile in the rat in vivo. In Methods in Enzymology, Vol 77: Detoxication and Drug Metabolism: Conjugation and Related Systems, ed W.B. Jakoby, pp. 21-30. New York: Academic Press.

Mulder, G.J. (1986): Sex differences in drug conjugation and their consequences for drug toxicity. Sulfation, glucuronidation and glutathione conjugation. Chem. Biol. Interact. 57, 1-15.

Pallante, S.L., Lisck, C.A., Dulik, D.M., Fenselau, C. (1986): Immobilised Enzyme synthesis and characterisation by FAB-Mass Spectrometry. Drug Metab. Disp. 14, 313-318.

Rickert, D.E. (1987): Metabolism of nitroaromatic compounds. Drug Metab. Revs. 18, 23-53.

Rush, G.F., Newton, J.F., Hook, J.B. (1983): Sex differences in the Excretion of glucuronide conjugates: the role of intrarenal glucurondation. J. Pharmacol. Exp. Ther. 227, 658-662.

Shuker, B., Warrander, A., Bastain, W., Perkins, C.M., Crampton, W. (1987): The dispostion of [^{14}C]-ICI 128,436 in man. Excepta Medica Int. Congress Series no. 760.

Tremaine, L.M., Diamond, G.L., Quebbemann, A.J. (1985): Quantitative determination of organ contribution to excretory metabolis. J. Pharmacol. Methods 13, 9-35.

Watkins, J.B., Klaassen, C.D. (1982): Effect of inducers and inhibitors of glucuronidation on the biliary excretion and choleretic action of valproic acid in the rat. J. Pharmacol. Exp. Ther. 220, 305-310.

Résumé

Le médicament Ponalrestat (ICI 128,436 ; STATIL^r) contient un groupement carboxylique qui est glucuronoconjugué ; et chez le rat, ce glucuronide est le principal métabolite. Le rat montre une différence inter-sexe très marquée quand on regarde l'excrétion du ponalrestat : quelle que soit la voie d'administration (orale ou intraveineuse), seulement 5 % de la dose sont excrétés dans les urines chez les mâles, alors que ce pourcentage excède 85 % chez les femelles. Chez les 2 sexes, le (^{14}C)-ponalrestat est excrété initialement sous forme de glucuronide dans la bile. Quand le ponalrestat est injecté directement dans le duodénum, la même différence inter-sexe est observée dans les urines. Le même phénomène est observé après administration par voie i.v. du glucuronide, lequel est excrété tout d'abord en quantité importante dans la bile. L'excrétion biliaire de ponalrestat après administration i.v. ou celle de son glucuronide est similaire dans les deux sexes. Pas de différence entre deux sexes est observée dans la formation du glucuronide au niveau de l'anse intestinale. Chez une souche mutante ayant une déficience de l'excrétion biliaire de nombreux composés cholephiles, l'excrétion biliaire du ponalrestat est aussi absente, la variation inter-sexe concernant l'excrétion urinaire disparaît dans une large population de cette souche. La localisation de cette différence inter-sexe est discutée.

Effects of drugs and of bilirubinostasis on glucuronidation of bilirubin

J. Fevery, V. Mesa, M. Muraca and W. Van Steenbergen

Hepatology, Department of Medical Research, University of Leuven, B-3000 Leuven, Belgium

ABSTRACT

The conjugation of bilirubin-IXα was studied in vivo in rats treated with drugs decreasing or enhancing the microsomal enzyme UDP-glucuronosyltransferase. These results were compared with assays in vitro of the enzyme activity in liver homogenates. The transferase activity seems the major determinant for the biliary excretion of unconjugated and conjugated bilirubins and for the plasma levels of the bile pigments. At low enzyme levels, relatively more unconjugated and monoconjugated pigment is present in serum, liver and bile. The ratios of mono- to diconjugates obtained in these 3 compartments correlated with each other. Conditions of bilirubinostasis promote diconjugate formation.

Keywords

Bilirubin, Conjugation, UDP-glucuronosyltransferase.

INTRODUCTION

Unconjugated bilirubin-IXα, the predominant breakdown product of haem is released in plasma after its formation by reticuloendothelial cells in liver, spleen and bone marrow (Blanckaert & Schmid, 1981; Berthelot et al., 1983). It is extensively bound to serum albumin and is taken up by the hepatocyte, freed from albumin. The uptake seems to involve a dissociation-limited diffusion together with a transmembranous transport catalyzed by a specific membrane-localized "organic anion-binding" protein. The latter is distinct from binding proteins operative in hepatocellular uptake of bile acids or fatty acids (Sorrentino et al., 1987). Once in the liver cell, the pigment is bound to intracellular carrier proteins and undergoes conjugation (mainly glucuronidation) at one or two of its propionic acid side chains. The mono- and diconjugates formed are efficiently secreted in bile by mechanisms as yet undefined. A small fraction of the conjugates refluxes to plasma (Muraca et al., 1987). Previously it had been shown that up to 40% of the intracellular unconjugated pigment also refluxes back to plasma. The conjugation is carried out by a microsomal UDP-glucuronosyltransferase system utilizing UDP-glucuronic acid, -glucose or -xylose as donor substrates.

We will review a series of studies performed mainly in the Wistar rat in vivo to more clearly define the role of the microsomal UDP-glucuronosyltransferase activity (GTa). The aim of these studies was to obtain more insight in the mechanisms leading to alteration of the serum and biliary bilirubin levels.

SERUM BILE PIGMENTS

Preceding studies (Fevery et al., 1977, 1979; Goresky et al., 1978) had shown that patients and neonates with unconjugated hyperbilirubinaemia and decreased GT levels excreted more mono- and less diglucuronidated bilirubin in bile. The development of a sensitive method that allowed to specifically measure mono- and diconjugates in serum by alkaline methanolysis (Blanckaert, 1980) followed by reverse-phase HPLC (Muraca & Blanckaert, 1983) allowed to document that mono- and diconjugates are present also in plasma of normals. The relative amount of diconjugates is decreased in conditions characterized by low GTa such as Gilbert syndrome and Crigler-Najjar disease (Muraca et al., 1987) (Table 1). In normal Wistar rat serum, mono-and diconjugates can also be detected. The overall hepatic transport of bilirubin was thus modified to encompass reflux of conjugates in normal conditions (Fig. 1).

Table 1.

Adults

	Healthy controls n = 42	Gilbert syndrome n = 22	Haemolysis n = 14
UCB µmol/l	1.8-14.9	18.1-58.3*	17.4-35.2*
CB	0.06-0.48	0.10-0.56	0.20-1.80*
CB/TB %	3.6±2.1	0.9±0.4*	4.0±2.3
Diconj/CB %	51±15	33±9*	36±10*
TSBA µmol/l	1-8	2-8	

*p<0.01

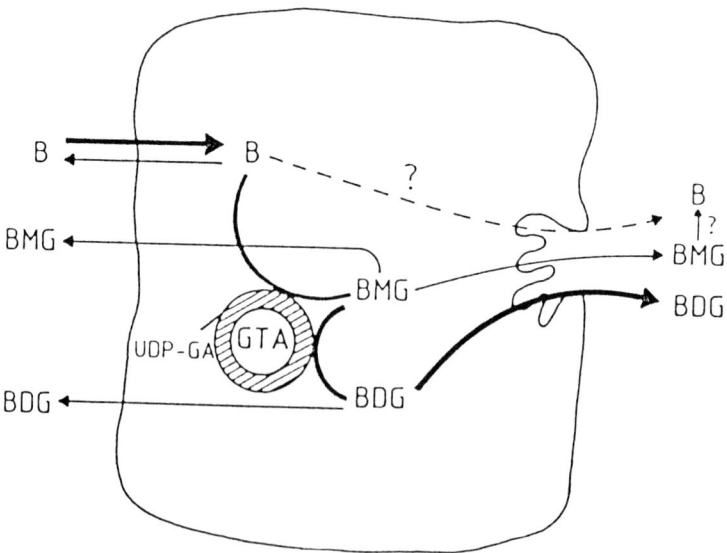

Fig. 1. Schematic representation of bilirubin metabolism.

EFFECTS OF BILIRUBINOSTASIS ON BILE PIGMENT COMPOSITION

In a first approach, the secretion of the conjugates was hampered by infusion of rats with substances competing for the biliary secretory process of bilirubin conjugates. They include ioglycamide, a biliary contrast agent, BSP, ICG and bromcresolgreen. All agents, except ICG, were given at dosages resulting in saturation of their own biliary excretion. The biliary bilirubin output dropped but this was more pronounced for unconjugated and monoconjugated pigment than for the diglucuronide. This resulted in a marked increase in the ratio of di- to monoconjugate in bile as well as in serum, and resulted in a conjugated hyperbilirubinaemia (Mesa et al., 1985, 1987). As changes in bile acid metabolism do not occur in these conditions, we prefer here to use the term bilirubinostasis rather than cholestasis. Similar results were observed by Jansen et al. (1985) in a mutant Wistar rat strain characterized by a defective biliary excretion of bilirubin conjugates and of related organic anions. Temporary mechanical obstruction of the common bile duct also leads to an enhanced ratio of di- to monoconjugates in bile and serum. This was even the most rapid event to be noted, long before alterations in serum transaminases, bile acids, alkaline phosphatase etc. occurred (Mesa et al., 1987).

Interference with the biliary secretion of conjugates thus produces an enhanced ratio of di- to monoconjugates presumably because the monoconjugated pigment is longer restraint within the cell and has a prolonged contact with the GT. This allows further transformation to the diglucuronidated pigment. The higher intracellular concentration of conjugates also leads to enhanced reflux to plasma.

MODULATION OF GLUCURONOSYLTRANSFERASE ACTIVITY AND OF THE PIGMENT LOAD TO THE LIVER

A mild increase of the pigment load to the liver can be produced by intraperitoneal or intravenous administration of unconjugated bilirubin, and occurs in conditions of mild haemolysis such as induced by injection of taurocholate or of red cell lysate. In these conditions, the concentration of all 3 pigment classes (unconjugated, mono- and di-) went up in parallel in bile as well as in serum; the ratio between the pigments thus remained constant. These results again point to "equilibration" between the liver, plasma and bile compartments, thus making analyses of serum representative of intracellular and biliary events. Prolonged infusions of high amounts (above 150 nmoles/min/100 g) lead to decreased ratios of di- to monoconjugate in bile.

The activity of the hepatic bilirubin UDP-glucuronosyltransferase was decreased by treatment of rats with L-thyroxin (6.26 or 12.52 nmoles/day/100 g b.wt. for 5 days) and increased by treatment with enzyme inducing agents such as glutethimide, phenobarbitone, clofibrate and spironolactone. Some of the pretreated rats were infused with unconjugated bilirubin (256 nmoles/min/100 g body wt. after a single bolus of 3.42 µmoles/100 g body wt. for 60 min) to saturate the overall hepatic transport. They were killed after 60 min and blood, liver and bile was analyzed for bile pigments. In addition GT activity was measured in digitonin activated liver homogenate both with low (10-15 µM) and high (164 µM) bilirubin substrate concentration. The former system allows to monitor in vitro formation of mono-and diglucuronides whereas the latter assays the so-called maximal conjugating activity obtained in vitro.

The results obtained show that decreasing the GTa leads to enhanced relative amounts of UCB and monoconjugates in bile whereas enhancing the GTa results in lowering of these pigment fractions with an augmented biliary excretion of diglucuronides. Similar alterations were documented in liver tissue and in plasma. Indeed, the ratio of di- to monoconjugates obtained in bile correlated with that in liver homogenate and with that of serum in the various animal groups. The ratio di- to monoconjugate whether obtained in serum, liver or bile was thus related to the in vitro measured GT activity. Furthermore, the ratio of di- to monoglucuronide present in vivo correlated very well with the ratios obtained after incubation of liver homogenates in vitro with low concentrations of bilirubin substrate (Van Steenbergen, 1987).

The amount of bilirubin excreted in bile by the animals loaded with bilirubin over the 60 min period was clearly related to the GT activity measured. This is in agreement with the concept that conjugation of bilirubin is a near-absolute requirement for its biliary secretion. The latter increased in a presumably hyperbolic fashion with enhancing GT activity. The last part of the hyperbolic curve suggests that at very high concentrations the conjugates may have an inhibiting effect on their own excretion. Such phenomena have been observed with other substances such as BSP (Dhumeaux et al., 1970), ioglycamide (Mesa, 1985) and even with taurocholate (Herz et al., 1975).

CONCLUSIONS

The investigations reported stress the importance of bilirubin UDP-glucuronosyltransferase activity in regulating the concentrations and composition of unconjugated, mono- and diconjugated bilirubins in serum, bile and liver tissue in normal situations and in conditions whereby a high "saturating" load of bilirubin was presented to the liver.

REFERENCES

Berthelot, P., Duvaldestin, Ph., Fevery, J. (1982): pp. 173-214: Physiology and disorders of human bilirubin metabolism. In Bilirubin (Heirwegh, K.P.M. & Braun, S.B., Eds.) CRC Press, Boca Raton, Florida.

Blanckaert, N. (1980): Analysis of bilirubin and bilirubin mono- and diconjugates. Determination of their relative amounts in biological samples. Biochem. J. 185, 115-128.

Blanckaert, N., Schmid, R. (1982): pp. 246-296: Physiology and pathophysiology of bilirubin metabolism. In Hepatology: A Textbook of Liver Disease (Zakim, D. & Boyer, T., Eds.) W.B. Saunders Co., Philadelphia.

Dhumeaux, D., Berthelot, P., Préaux, A.M. et al. (1970): A critical study of the concept of maximal biliary transport of sulfobromophthalein (BSP) in the Wistar rat. Rev. Europ. Et. Clin. Biol. 15, 279-286.

Fevery, J., Blanckaert, N., Berthelot, P., Heirwegh, K.P.M. (1979): pp. 251-266: Bilirubin metabolism in neonatal life. In Neonatal Hepatitis and Biliary Atresia (Javitt, B.N., Ed.).

Fevery, J., Blanckaert, N., Heirwegh, K.P.M., Préaux, A.-M., Berthelot, P. (1977): Unconjugated bilirubin and an increased proportion of bilirubin monoconjugates in the bile of patients with Gilbert's syndrome and Crigler-Najjar disease disease. J. Clin. Invest. 60, 970-979.

Goresky, C.A., Gordon, E.R., Schaffer, E.A., Paré, P., Carassavas, D., Aronoff, A. (1978): Definition of a conjugation dysfunction in Gilbert's syndrome: Studies on the handling of bilirubin loads and of the pattern of bilirubin conjugates secreted in bile. Clin. Sci. Mol. Med. 55, 63-71.

Herz, R., Paumgartner, G., Preisig, R. (1975): Inhibition of bile formation by high doses of taurocholate in the perfused rat liver. Scand. J. Gastroent. 11, 741-746.

Jansen, P.L.M., Peters, W.H., Lamers, W.H. (1985): Hereditary chronic unconjugated hyperbilirubinemia in mutant rats caused by defective hepatic anion transport. Hepatology 5, 573-579.

Mesa, V.A. (1985): Effect of organic anions on hepatic transport of bilirubin. Ph. D. Thesis, University of Leuven, Belgium.

Mesa, V.A., De Vos, R., De Groote, J., Fevery, J. (1987): Increase in the ratio of bilirubin di-to monoconjugates (BDC:BMC) in bile and serum constitutes a sensitive marker of cholestasis in rats. J. Hepatol. 5, S168.

Mesa, V.A., Fevery, J., Heirwegh, K.P.M., De Groote, J. (1985): Effects of ioglycamide on the hepatic transport of bilirubin and its mono- and diconjugates in the rat. Hepatology 5, 600-606.

Muraca, M., Blanckaert, N. (1983): Liquid-chromatographic assay and identification of mono-and diester conjugates of bilirubin in normal serum. Clin. Chem. 29, 1767-1771.

Muraca, M., Fevery, J., Blanckaert, N. (1987): Relationships between serum bilirubins and production and conjugation of bilirubin. Studies in Gilbert's syndrome, Crigler-Najjar disease, hemolytic disorders, and rat models. Gastroenterology 92, 309-317.

Sorrentino, D., Stremmel, W., Berk, P.D. (1987): The hepatocellular uptake of bilirubin: Current concepts and controversies. Molec. Aspects Med. 9, 405-428.

Van Steenbergen, W. (1987): Effect of UDP-glucuronosyltransferase and of bile flow on hepatic transport of bilirubin: in vivo and in vitro study in the rat. Ph.D. Thesis, University of Leuven, Belgium.

Résumé

Nous avons étudié la conjugaison *in vivo* de la bilirubine-IX α chez des rats traités avec des xénobiotiques qui diminuent ou augmentent l'UDP-glucuronosyltransférase microsomale. Les résultats obtenus sont comparés à ceux d'essais *in vitro* pour l'activité enzymatique d'homogénats de foie. L'activité transférase semble êtrele facteur déterminant pour l'excrétion biliaire des bilirubines conjuguées ou non et pour le taux plasmatique en pigments biliaires. A de faibles activités enzymatiques, il y a dans le sérum, foie et bile, relativement plus de pigments monoconjugués et non conjugués. Les rapports mono-sur diconjugués obtenus dans ces trois compartiments sont corrélés entre eux. Les conditions de stase bilirubine favorisent la formation de diconjugués.

Effects of an experimental hepatitis induced by D-galactosamine on the metabolism and toxicity of chlorpropham : *in vivo* and *in vitro* studies

G. Carrera, S. Forgues, J. Alary and H. Lapontarique

INSERM U87, 2 Rue François Magendi, 31400 Toulouse, France

ABSTRACT

The metabolism and toxicity of chlorpropham (CIPC) are strongly modidied by galactosamine as well in vitro as in vivo. The inhibition of sulfo and glucuronoconjugation gives an increase of free 4-OH CIPC yielding a decrease of ATP levels and an increase of the Na^+/K^+ ratio. These results show that the biotransformation and the toxicity of xenobiotics can be strongly influenced in pathology associated with acute liver injury.

KEY WORDS

Chlorpropham, biotransformation, toxicity, D-galactosamine, in vivo, in vitro.

INTRODUCTION

In the presence of nutritional and pathological states leading to serious hepatic injuries the metabolism and toxicity of xenobiotics may be strongly modified (Rajpurohit et coll., 1985 ; Dudley et Klaassen, 1984 ; Kamdem et coll., 1983). The aim of this study was to investigate the influence of an hepatic injury on the metabolism and toxicity of chlorpropham (CIPC). This herbicide is metabolised by liver into 3 chloroaniline, which is further acetylated and into 4 hydroxy chlorpropham (90%) excreted as sulfo (60%) and glucuroconjugates (40%) (Alary et coll., 1986 ; Fang et coll., 1973). Several studies have shown that D-galactosamine inhibits glucuronoconjugation (Ullrich and Bock, 1984 ; Watkins and Klaassen, 1982) and induces cellular lesions in rat liver similar to those observed in human viral hepatitis (Tran-Thi et coll., 1985 ; Keppler et coll., 1970).

MATERIAL AND METHODS.

In vitro study

Isolated rat hepatocyte suspensions were incubated during 2 hours at 37°C in absence of any treatment, in presence of D-galactosamine (4 mM) or of CIPC (0.1 mM) or of both. At the end of the incubation, CIPC and its metabolites have been determined by HPLC in hepatocytes and in extracellular medium (Alary et coll., 1986). The cytolysis has been estimated by the percentages of extracellular LDH and proteins. The functional state of the membrane by the intracellular Na/k ratio and the energy metabolism by the ATP level in the hepatocyte.

In vivo study

First, the inhibition kinetics of conjugation reactions by D-galactosamine have been determined in male wistar rats receiving p-nitrophenol intragastrically (5 mg/kg) and D-galactosamine (an intraperitoneal injection of 400 mg/kg or 2 injections of 200 mg/kg each at a 4 hours interval). Then a LD50 study was carried out on 2 rat groups receiving intragastrically CIPC, one group receiving 2 intraperitoneal injections of D-galactosamine (200 mg/kg) 30 min and 4h30 after administration of CIPC.

Statistical analysis

Variance analysis on 2 factorial experiments (18 repetitions) was used to evaluate the effect of CIPC, D-galactosamine and of any interaction between them. Finney's method (1971) was used for the LD50 study.

RESULTS

In vitro study

	CIP unmetabolised	3 chloro-aniline	3 chloro-acetanilide	Free	4 OH-CIPC conjugates	
					Sulfo	Glucurono
CIPC MEDIUM	20±2.6(a)	1.5±0.38	3.4±0.47	9±1.5	37±2.7	18±2.1
CIPC + D-GAL	14±1.5	2.4±0.54	4.1±0.86	32±3.1	25±1.6	6±0.8
CIPC CELLS	13±1.9	ND (b)	0.7±0.18	4±0.38	ND	ND
CIPC + D-GAL	10±0,9	ND	1.3±0.19	6.5±0.73	ND	ND

Means ± SEM of 11 determinations except for conjugates (n = 8) (a)
(b) ND = Not detectable.

Table I : CIPC metabolites (% of CIPC).

CIPC metabolites are shown in table I. In presence of D-galactosamine sulfate conjugation of 4-OH CIPC is inhibited by 32.4 % and glucuronoconjugation by 66.6%. The statistical analysis of the results in table II shows that CIPC has a specific significant effect on LDH (F=34.4***) and protein (F=7.99***), percentages, on intracellular ATP level (F=14.07***) and Na/K ratio in hepatocytes (F=15.49***). D-galactosamine has no specific significant effect on cytolisis (LDH, F=1.34 ; proteins, F < 1) but significantly decreases ATP (F = 19.2***) and increases Na/K intracellular ratio (F = 13.06***). Analyses of intertactions show that the effect of CIPC on cytolysis is not potentialized by addition of D-galactosamine. Its effects on the cellular energy metabolism (ATP, F = 2.92*) and on the functional state of the membrane (Na/K = 6.3**) are highly potentialized by D-galactosamine.

	LDH (a)	Proteins	ATP (b)	Na/K
Control	27.83±0.32 (c)	10.25±0.971	14.22±0,942	2.90±0.114
CIPC	40.76±1.338	14.72±1.161	11.69±0,801	3.31±0.152
Control + D-GAL	30.05±0.998	11.22±0.962	10.90±0,666	3.21±0.151
CIPC + D-GAL	43.81±1.746	17.18±1.152	4.12±0,286	5.05±0.222

Table II : CIPC cytotoxicity : (a) LDH % or protein % in the extracellular medium with respect to total (LDH extra + LDH intracellular) (b) nmol/mg prot. (c) means ± SEM of 18 determinations.

In vivo study

The results in table III show that the longest and most important inhibition of conjugation reactions by D-galactosamine is obtained by 2 intraperitoneal injections of 200 mg/kg at 4 hours interval. In absence of D-galactosamine the LD50 of CIPC is 7.2 ± 1.65 mg/kg. In D-galactosamine treated rats 30 min and 4h30 hours after the administration of CIPC, the LD50 is of 4.3 ± 1.03 g/kg.

D-GAL treatment	4h		8h		12h	
	S	G	S	G	S	G
1 injection IP 400 mg/kg	-80.0	-72.2	+ 8.3	+36.3	+3.53	+17.00
2 injections IP 200 mg/kg	-78.7	-77.7	-35.3	-10.2	-7.87	+ 7.35

Table III : Uninary excretion of sulfate (S) and glucurono (G) conjugates of p-nitrophenol as a function of time : results are expressed in percentage of change with respect to control.

DISCUSSION

In standard conditions, 55 % of CIPC is metabolized as conjugates, 4-OH-CIPC sulfate conjugation being the major pathway. The presence of D-galactosamine strongly disturbs CIPC metabolism. The consequence of the inhibition of conjugation is an important increase of free 4-OH-CIPC, in the extracellular medium and to a lesser extend in hepatocytes, which leads to an increased toxicity (Carrera et coll., 1986). The study of ATP and Na/K intracellular ratio, a more sensitive test than LDH or proteins (Klaassen and Stacey, 1982), show that the CIPC toxicity is highly potentialized by D-galactosamine. Acute galactosamine hepatitis can be induced either by a single dose of 400 mg or by 6 injections of 250 mg/kg within 24 h. (Keppler et coll., 1970). Plasma level of CIPC after oral administration being maximum after 1h30 (Somda, 1986) hence for the CIPC acute toxicity study we have chosen 2 intraperitoneal injections of D-galactosamine (200 mg/kg) 30 min and 4h30 after the CIPC administration in order to avoid the pathology of hepatitis. In these conditions, acute CIPC toxicity is increased by 40 %. This confirms the results of the in vitro study.

This study shows that the D-galactosamine by its effects on the conjugation reactions, can potentialize the CICP toxicity in vivo as well as in vitro. From these results, it can be expected that, as from many other xenobiotics (Kamdem et coll., 1982 ; Mulder, 1981), people with hepatic diseases leading to enzyme detoxication deficiency can be considered as a particularly sensitive group towards this xenobiotic.

REFERENCES.

Alary, J. ; Carrera, G. ; Bergon, M. ; Periquet, A. ; Vandaele, J. (1986) : High performance liquid chromatography determination of chlorpropham and its metabolites in isolated rat hepatocytes incubations. J. Liquid Chromato. 9, 3597-3606.
Carrera, G. ; Periquet, A. ; Alary, J. (1986) : Détermination et toxicité des métabolites du chlorphophame après une modulation des enzymes de conjugaison. C.R.G.F. Pest 16, 9-13.
Dudley, R.E., Klaassen, C.D. (1984) : Changes in hepatic glutathione concentration modify cadmium-induced hepatotoxicity. Toxicol. Appl. Pharmacol. 72, 530-236.
Fang, S.C. ; Fallin, E. ; Montgomery, M.L. ; Freed, V.H. (1973) : Metabolic studies of ^{14}C labelled propham and chlorpropham in the female rat. Pest. Biochem. Physiol. 4, 1-11.
Finney, D.J. (1964) : Assays based on quantal responses. In Statistical method in biological assay, Hafner Ed., New-York, pp 471-472.
Kamdem, L. ; Magdalou, J. ; Siest, G. ; Ban, G. ; Zissu, D. (1983). Induced hepatotoxicity in Female rats by aflatoxin B_1 and ethylnylestradiol interaction. Toxicol. Appl. Pharmacol. 67, 26-40.
Kamdem, L. ; Siest, G. ; Magdalou, J. (1982) : Differential toxicity of aflatoxin B_1 in male and female rats : relationship with hepatic drug-metabolizing enzymes. Biochem. Pharmacol., 31, 3057-3062.
Keppler, D. ; Rudigier, J. ; Bischoff, E. ; Decker, K. (1970) : The tropping of uridine - phosphates by D-galactosamine, D-glucosamine and 2-deoxy-D-galactose. A study on the mechanism of galactosamine hepatitis. Eur. J. Biochem. 17, 246-253.
Klaassen, C.D. ; Stacey, N.H. (1982) : Use fof isolated hepatocytes in toxicity assessment. In Toxicology of the Liver, Plaa, G. and William, R. eds, Raven Press, New-York, 147-179.
Mulder, G.J. (1981) : Sulfation in vivo and in isolated intact cell preparations. In Sulfation of Drugs and Related Compounds. Mulder, G. ed., CRC Press, Boca Raton pp 131-185.
Rajpurohit, R. ; Kalamegham, R. ; Chary, A.K. ; Krishnaswamy, K. (1985) : Hepatic drug metabolising enzymes in undernourished man. Toxicol. 37, 259-266.
Somda, J.C. (1986) : Toxicocinétique du chlorpropname et défense métabolique liée à sa détoxication. Thèse, Université Paul Sabatier, Toulouse pp33-60.
Tran-Thi, T.A.; Phillips, J.; Falk, H.; Decker, K. (1985) : Toxicity of D-galactosamine for rat hepatocytes in monolayer culture. Exp. Mol. Pathol. 42, 89-116.
Ullrich, D. ; Bock, K.W. (1984) : Inhibition of glucuronide formation by D-galactosone or D-galactosamine lin isolated hepatocytes. Biochem. Pharmacol. 33, 1827-1830.
Watkins, J.B. ; Klaassen, C.D. (1982) : Effect of inducers and inhibitors of glucuronidation on the biliary excretion and choleretic action of Valpoic Acid in the rat. J. Pharmacol. Exp. Therap. 220, 305-310.

Résumé

Le métabolisme et la toxicité du chlorpropname sont fortement modifiés par un traitement à la D-galactosamine tant in vitro qu'in vivo. L'inhibition de la sulfo et de la glucuronoconjugaison par la D-galactosamine provoque une augmentation de la forme libre du 4-hydroxychlorpropname entraînant une diminution du taux d'ATP intracellulaire et une augmentatin du rapport Na/K dans l'hépatocyte. Ces résultats montrent que la biotransformation et la toxicité des xénobiotiques peuvent être fortement modifiés au cours de pathologies entrainant des atteintes hépatiques graves.

Hepatic drug-metabolizing enzymes and prenatal exposure to clofibrate

C. Celier, S. Marie, T. Cresteil and J.-P. Leroux

INSERM U 75, 156 rue de Vaugirard, 75730 Paris Cedex 15, France

ABSTRACT

In adult rats, clofibrate specifically enhances ω hydroxylation of lauric acid and bilirubin glucuronidation. The present work is focused on the effect of clofibrate administration to pregnant mothers on the enzymatic profile of hepatic fetal and neonatal rats. In fetuses from clofibrate-treated dams a marked increase in lauric acid ω and ω-1 oxidation is observed whereas bilirubin conjugation is unaffected. When treated with phenobarbital, no modification of either activities is noticed. In an attempt to putatively correlate enzymatic activities with modification of mRNA concentration the hepatic content in P-450 b/e and UDPGTr2 mRNAs was examined. Both are increased by PB whereas Clo fails to or marginally modify their concentration in fetal liver. Data are discussed in regard to the substrate specificity of enzymes reported elsewhere.

KEY WORDS.

Development, cytochrome P-450, glucuronosyltransferase, clofibrate, induction.

INTRODUCTION

The study of drug-metabolizing enzymes in both fetuses and newborns is important for understanding the influence of drug administration during this period of life. The spontaneous ontogenesis of some cytochrome P-450-dependent monooxygenases and bilirubin UDP-glucuronosyltransferase (B-GT) exhibits similar patterns: present at an extremely low or low level in fetal liver these activities readily increase after birth (Cresteil et al. 1986, Wishart 1978). Transplacental induction of monooxygenases by phenobarbital is now well documented in regard to the enhancement of enzymatic activities (Cresteil et al. 1981), isoenzyme content (Cresteil et al. 1982) or P-450b and e accumulation of mRNAs estimated by synthetic oligonucleotides (Giachelli and Omiecinski 1986). However, bilirubin conjugation remains refractory to any induction by barbiturates (Cresteil et al. 1981)

Clofibrate a hypolipidaemic drug, is known to induce specifically the
ω-hydroxylation of lauric acid and B-GT in adult rats (Gibson et al. 1982;
Foliot et al. 1977). The aim of the present work was to evaluate the inductive
effect of clofibrate on fetal hepatic monooxygenase and bilirubin conjugating
activities after maternal treatment, in order to get insights in the induction
mechanism undertaken by clofibrate.

MATERIAL AND METHODS.

Clofibrate (200 mg/kg) in corn oil was administered i.p. twice a day for 4 days
to pregnant rats either at days 14,15,16 and 17 or at days 18,19,20 and 21 of
gestation. Phenobarbital (80 mg/kg/day) in saline was administered i.p. to
pregnant rats at days 19, 20 and 21 of gestation. Livers of fetuses (18 and 22
days of gestation) and newborns (2 and 6 days) were excised and used for
microsomal preparation. Cytochrome P-450 content, lauric acid and benzo(a)pyrene
hydroxylations were assayed as previously described (Cresteil et al. 1986).
Bilirubin glucuronosyltransferase was measured on Triton X 100-activated
microsomes according to Van Roy and Heirwegh (1968).
For mRNA examination a single injection of inducer was given at day 21 of
gestation. Fetuses were killed 16 h later and livers were immediately frozen in
liquid N2 and kept at -80°C until used within three weeks. RNA was isolated from
frozen livers according to Chirgwin et al.(1979). 5 to 10 ug of total RNA were
applied to nitrocellulose with a Schleicher and Schull Minifold II apparatus and
hybridizations conducted as recommended by the manufacturer. Membranes were
washed with 0.1x SSC, 0.1% SDS at 52°C and finally with 0.1x SSC at 45°C. Films
were exposed for various periods of time and scanned at 600 nm. ^{32}P-cDNA
probes (nick translation kit from Amersham) are: PB7 (1.7kbp long insert, 3'end
of P-450b/e cDNA) from Dr. Anderson (Quebec)(Affolter et al, 1986) and UDPGTr2 a
3' non translated fragment (0.2 kbp long) from a cDNA coding for a phenobarbital
-inducible UDP-GT (MacKenzie, 1986). Reference is actin, probed by a genomic
clone (7.5 kbp long) obtained from Dr. Batthula (NCI, Bethesda). All results of
mRNA quantitation by slot blots were standardized to actin mRNA concentration.

RESULTS AND DISCUSSION.

The effect of treatment of pregnant rats by clofibrate and phenobarbital on
drug-metabolizing enzymes in 22 day-old fetuses are shown in Table I.
In fetuses from PB-treated mothers, an increase in benzopyrene hydroxylation
was noticed as previously reported (Cresteil et al 1986) whereas laurate
hydroxylase was unchanged. Clofibrate treatment provoked a considerable increase
in laurate hydroxylation in ωposition (and to a lesser extent in ω-1)
without modification of benzopyrene hydroxylase activity. Such an increase is
also observed in 18-day-old fetuses where hydroxylation rises from 0.062 to
0.467 nmol. min^{-1}.mg^{-1} prot. Bilirubin-GT activity was unchanged whatever was
the pretreatment of the animals. After birth, bilirubin-GT remains unchanged by
a prenatal treatment of mothers by clofibrate: 0.27 versus 0.26 in 2-day-old and
0.47 versus 0.44 in 6-day-old newborns. These results indicate that no delayed
or long-term effect of clofibrate appeared since a treatment of the pregnant
rats does not induce B-GT activity either in fetuses or newborns.
To go further in the elucidation of Clo induction, we have investigated the role
of maternal Clo administration on the P-450 b/e mRNA and UDPGTr2 mRNA content of
fetal and neonatal rat liver (Fig. 1).

Table I: Drug-metabolizing activities in 22 day-old fetuses

	Untreated	Clo-treated	PB-treated
Cytochrome P-450 (nmol.mg^{-1} prot)	0.12 + 0.01	0.16 + 0.02	0.13 + 0.01
Benzopyrene hydroxylase (nmol.min^{-1}.mg^{-1} prot)	0.052 + 0.005	0.062 + 0.040	0.096 + 0.005
Laurate hydroxylase (nmol.min^{-1}.mg^{-1} prot.)			
ω -1	0.048 + 0.005	0.390 + 0.005	0.041 + 0.004
ω	0.063 + 0.006	1.300 + 0.025	0.053 + 0.006
Bilirubin GT (nmol.min^{-1}.mg^{-1} prot.)	0.025 + 0.002	0.020 + 0.002	0.014 + 0.002

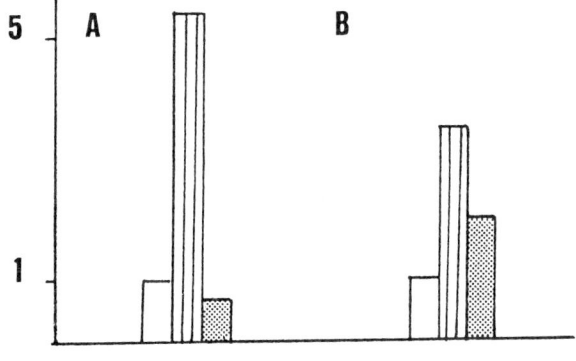

Figure 1: Expression of mRNA P-450b/e (panel A) and UDPGTr2 (panel B) in 22-day-old fetuses from pretreated mothers
☐ untreated rats
▥ PB-treated rats
▨ Clo-treated rats
The ratio of mRNA to actin is considered as 1 in untreated animals.

As expected, P-450b/e mRNA accumulates in liver from PB-treated fetus, as well as UDPGTr2 mRNA. This enhancement is in agreement with the concomittant increase of cytochrome P-450b/e isozyme estimated by enzymatic determination and by immunoquantitation of apoprotein that we have previously demonstrated. Treatment with clofibrate did not result in a modification of P-450b/e expression. This conclusion was expected since in adults clofibrate stimulates the synthesis of a specific P-450 species but not P-450b/e. On the other hand, clofibrate does not affect the expression of UDPGTr2 in fetal liver, neither in adult liver (data not shown). This could indicate that although inducible by PB in rat liver, UDPGTr2 cDNA does not code for a bilirubin conjugating enzyme. Actually, when expressed in COS cells, UDPGTr2 directed the synthesis of a protein conjugating 4-methylumbelliferone, testosterone and β-estradiol (Mackenzie 1987). No informations are available about conjugation of bilirubin. Alternatively we can hypothetize that PB and Clo induce different bilirubin-GT isozymes.

Our results show that PB and Clo cross the placental barrier and are able to activate several genes. A differential effect was observed with glucuronosyl transferase: the accumulation of UDPGT mRNA in response to PB administration was not accompanied by a simultaneous enhancement of enzymatic activity, likely due to a lag period required for protein synthesis. The exact nature of the mechanism of the apparent lack of induction of B-GT remains to be elucidated: multiplicity of B-GT isozymes, delayed regulation (via a trans-acting element?).

REFERENCES.

Affolter, M., Labbe, D., Jean, A., Raymond, M., Noel, D., Labelle, Y., Parent Vaugeois, C., Lambert, M., Bojanowski, R., Anderson, A. (1986). cDNA clones for liver cytochrome P-450s from individual Aroclor-treated rats: constitutive expression of a new P-450 gene related to phenobarbital-inducible forms. DNA, 58 209-218.

Chirgwin, J.M., Przybyla, A.E., MacDonald, R.J., Rutter, W.J. (1979) Isolation of biologically active ribonucleic acid from sources enriched in ribonuclease. Biochemistry, 18, 5294-5299.

Cresteil, T., Mahu, J.L., Beaune, P., Columelli, S., Leroux J.P. (1981). Comparison of the effects of phenobarbital and its hydroxylated metabolites on drug-metabolizing enzymes during ontogenesis. Ped. Pharmacol, 1, 331-340.

Cresteil, T., LeProvost, E., Flinois, J.P., Leroux, J.P. (1982). Enzymatic and immunological evidences that phenobarbital induces cytochrome P-450 in fetal and neonatal rat liver. Biochem. Biophys. Res. Commun. 106, 823-830.

Cresteil, T., Beaune, P., Celier, C., Leroux, J.P., Guengerich, F.P. (1986). Cytochrome P-450 isoenzyme content and monooxygenase activities in rat liver: effect of ontogenesis and pretreatment by phenobarbital and 3-methylcholanthrene J. Pharmacol. Exp. Ther. 236, 269-276.

Cresteil, T., Jaiswal, A.K., Eisen, H.J. (1987) Transcriptional control of human cytochrome P1-450 gene expression by 2,3,7,8-tetrachlorodibenzo-p-dioxin in human tissue culture cell lines. Arch. Biochem. Biophys. 253, 233-240.

Foliot, A., Drocourt, J.L., Etienne, J.P., Housset, E., Fiessinger, J.N., Christoforov, B. (1977). Increase in the hepatic glucuronidation and clearance of bilirubin in clofibrate-treated rats. Biochem. Pharmacol. 26, 547-549.

Giachelli, C.M., Omiecinski, C.J. (1986) Regulation of cytochrome P-450b and P-450e mRNA expression in the developing rat. Hybridization to synthetic oligodeoxyribonucleotide probes. J. Biol. Chem. 261, 1359-1363.

Gibson, G.G., Orton, T.C., Tamburini, P.P. (1982) Cytochrome P-450 induction by clofibrate. Biochem. J. 203, 161-168.

MacKenzie, P.I. (1986). Rat liver UDP-glucuronosyltransferase. Sequence and expression of a cDNA encoding a phenobarbital-inducible form. J. Biol. Chem. 261, 6119-6125.

MacKenzie, P.I. (1987). Rat liver UDP-glucuronosyltransferase. Identification of cDNAs encoding two enzymes which glucuronidate testosterone, dihydrotestosterone and β-estradiol. J. Biol. Chem. 262, 9744-9749.

Van Roy, F.P., Heirwegh, K.P.M. (1968). Determination of bilirubin glucuronide and assay of glucuronyltransferase with bilirubin as acceptor. Biochem. J. 107, 507-518.

Wishart, G.J. (1978) Functional heterogeneity of UDP-glucuronosyltransferase as indicated by its differential development and inducibility by glucocorticoids. Biochem. J. 174, 485-489.

Résumé

Chez le rat adulte, l'administration de clo provoque l'augmentation des activités d'hydroxylation de l'acide laurique et bilirubine-GT. Les résultats montrent que l'administration de clo à des rattes gestantes se traduit chez le foetus par une augmentation de l'hydroxylation en ω de l'acide laurique sans modification de la B-GT. L'administration de PB aux femelles gestantes, sans effet sur la B-GT provoque cependant une accumulation chez le foetus d'ARNm spécifiques des cytochromes P-450b/e et d'une forme d'UDPGT inductible par le PB.

Study of UDPG-transferases in the carp, *Cyprinus carpio*

Alain Devaux and Jean-Louis Rivière

Institut National de la Recherche Agronomique Laboratoire d'Ecotoxicologie INRA-ENVL, Ecole Nationale Vétérinaire de Lyon BP31, 69752, Charbonnières Cedex, France

ABSTRACT

UDPGA-transferase (UDPGT) activity towards p-nitrophenol and 1-naphthol was studied on microsomes from untreated carp (Cyprinus carpio). The following parameters were investigated : effects of detergent, concentrations of substrate and UDPGA, and temperature. The properties of the fish enzyme show some interesting differences when compared to those of rat liver enzyme.

KEYWORDS

UDPG-transferase; enzyme; liver; fish.

INTRODUCTION

In the field of environmental toxicology, a particular interest is focused on aquatic ecosystems for several reasons. First, the possible toxicity of many xenobiotic compounds (pesticides, industrial wastes, oil spills, heavy metals, PCBs,...) to fish. Second, the above compounds being potent inducers/inhibitors of hepatic cytochrome P-450-dependent activities in fish, there is a growing interest in the use of these activities as biochemical indicators of pollution (Payne et al.,1987). Third, fish as human food are possible sources of residues of toxic substances or their metabolites .
Most studies have emphasized investigations on phase I enzymes such as cytochromes P-450 (Monod et al.,1987), but data on functioning and role of UDPG-transferases (UDPGT) are still scarce. We investigated here the in vitro activity of UDPGT in microsomes from untreated immature carp towards p-nitrophenol and 1-naphthol as substrates.

MATERIALS AND METHODS

Immature carps (Cyprinus carpio) weighing ca 400 g were supplied by local fisheries. They were maintained in flowing tap water at 18°C and were fed trout pellets ad libitum.
UDPGA and DTT (dithiotreitol) were obtained from Boehringer, France. 1-Naphthyl-β-D-glucuronic acid, sodium salt was from Sigma, France. All other chemical reagents used in the enzyme assays were of the highest commercial quality available.
Fish liver microsomes were prepared as previously described (Monod et al.,1987). UDPGT activity with 4-nitrophenol as a substrate was assayed according to Frei (1966). Incubation mixtures contained 1.0 mg microsomal protein, 100 mM Tris-HCl (pH 7.4), 5 mM $MgCl_2$, 0.105 mM 4-nitrophenol, 4mg/mg protein Triton X-100 and 2 mM UDPGA in a final volume of 1.0 ml. After activation of enzyme (5 min, 0°C) by Triton, reaction rate was measured directly by following the decrease in absorbance at 405 nm. Incubation was performed in a thermostated spectrophotometer. Kinetic assay for UDPGT using 1-naphthol as a substrate was realised according to MacKenzie and Hänninen (1980). Incubation medium contained 300 μg of protein, 50 mM phosphate buffer, pH 7.4, 4 mM $MgCl_2$, 0.1 mM 1-naphthol, 0.25 mg/mg of protein Triton and 2 mM UDPGA. Incubation was performed in a thermostated fluorometer (excitation wavelength : 293 nm; emission wavelength : 335 nm) and activity was measured by monitoring continuously the formation of the conjugate, with 25 nmole of 1-naphthylglucuronide as an external standard. Incubations were performed at 25°C under conditions which result in linearity over the 2-3 min that the reactions were followed. Microsomal protein was determined by the method of Hartree (1972) using bovine serum albumin as a standard.

RESULTS AND DISCUSSION

In the present study, levels of p-nitrophenol activity found in carps were higher than those previously reported for the same species; however, they are reasonably close to those of other species of fish and lower than in rat (Table 1). These results are obviously due to species differences, but it seems possible to obtain higher values for UDPGT activities in lower vertebrates by improving substantially experimental conditions.

Table 1. UDPGT activity towards p-nitrophenol in various species

Species	Specific activity (nmole/mg/min)	Ref.
male rat	28	Bock et al. (1983)
carp	0.16-0.50	this study
"	0.08	Sivarajah et al. (1978)
"	0.07	Kobayashi et al. (1987)
rainbow trout	0.38	Lindström-Seppa et al. (1981)
"	0.08	Castrén and Oikari (1983)
"	1.23	Förlin and Haux (1985)
"	0.29	Andersson and Koivusaari (1985)
roach	0.11	Lindström-Seppa et al. (1981)
vendace	0.07	"
perch	0.09	"

Activities were assayed in the activated state using Triton X-100. A concentration

Fig 1. Effect of concentration of detergent (Triton X-100; A), concentration of substrate (B), concentration of UDPGA (C), and temperature (D), on UDPGT activity in hepatic microsomes from untreated carp. Open circles and closed circles refer to 1-naphthol and 4-nitrophenol as substrates, respectively. Values are expressed as per cent of maximal activity.

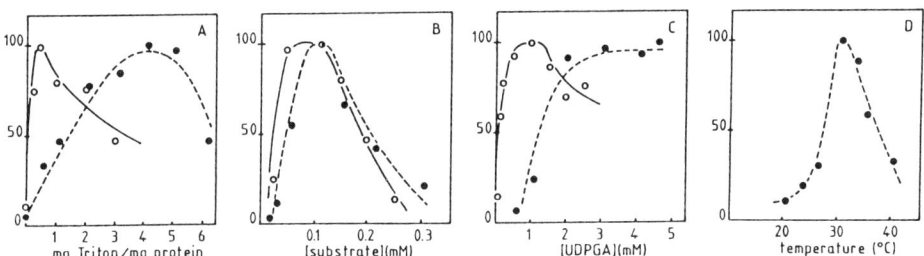

of detergent of about 0.5 mg/mg of protein was found optimal with 1-naphthol as a substrate, but activity towards p-nitrophenol required higher concentrations (5 mg/mg of protein; Fig. 1A). A concentration of detergent in the range 0.2-0.6 mg/mg of protein was shown to be optimal in activating microsomes from rat, mice and guinea pig (Winsnes, 1969; Bock et al.,1983; Boutin et al.,1987), man (Dragacci et al.,1987), and bluegill and channel catfish (Ankley and Agosin, 1987). Thus, p-nitrophenol activity in carp represents a striking difference from the generally observed pattern. A concentration of substrate of 0.1 mM was found optimal with both 1-naphthol and p-nitrophenol (Fig. 1B). Lower or higher values resulted in drastic loss of activities. A strong inhibition by excess of substrate was also shown by Castrén and Oikari (1983) with microsomes from rainbow trout. The optimal concentration of UDPGA was 1 mM (1-naphthol) or 3 mM (p-nitrophenol), closely related to values found with other species (Fig. 1C). Maximal activation was found after 5 min at 0°C (data not shown). Maximal activity was found at 30°C, but in sharp contrast with the results of Castrén and Oikari from rainbow trout (1983), a strong dependency on temperature was shown in microsomes from carp. A ±5°C difference from the optimal temperature results in a 40-60% loss in activity (Fig. 1D). We suggest that some UDPGT of fish are deeply embedded in the phospholipid bilayer. We also strongly emphasize the fact that fish are poikilothermic animals, whose hepatic metabolizing activities are highly dependent on temperature. The question arises of the real activity inside the fish cells at environmental temperatures, but the very low UDPGT activities of fish do not allow measurements at low temperatures.

The effect of pH was not assayed, but previous data with rainbow trout have shown that the reaction rate varies little in the range 7.0-7.8 (Dutton and Montgomery, 1958, Castrén and Oikari, 1983).

CONCLUSIONS

Our results and previous data show that carps possess hepatic UDPGT activities indicating that they are capable of conjugating xenobiotics with UDPGA. However, some striking differences from usual conditions in assaying the in vitro activity are clearly shown in our experiments, and point out the need for careful determination of experimental conditions with each substrate studied, because inappropriate conditions could result in failing to detect activity.

REFERENCES

Andersson, T. and Koivusaari, U. (1985) : Influence of environmental temperature on the induction of xenobiotic metabolism by β-naphthoflavone in rainbow trout, Salmo gairdneri. Toxicol. Appl. Pharmacol. 80, 43-50.

Ankley, G.T. and Agosin, M. (1987) : Comparative aspects of hepatic UDP-glucuronosyltransferases and glutathione S-transferases in bluegil and channel catfish. Comp. Biochem. Physiol. 87B, 671-673.

Bock, K.W., Burchell, B., Dutton, G.J., Hänninen, O., Mulder, G.J., Owens, I.S., Siest, G. and Tephly, T. (1983) : UDP-glucuronosyltransferase activities. Guidelines for consistent interim terminology and assay conditions. Biochem. Pharmacol. 32, 953-955.

Boutin, J.A., Antoine, B., Fournel, S. and Siest, G. (1987) : Heterogeneity of hepatic microsomal UDP-glucuronosyltransferase activities : use and comparison of differential inductions in some mammalian species. Comp. Biochem. Physiol. 87B, 512-522.

Castrén, M. and Oikari, A. (1983) : Optimal assay conditions for liver UDP-glucuronosyltransferase from the rainbow trout, Salmo gairdneri. Comp. Biochem. Physiol. 76C, 365-369.

Dragacci, S., Thomassin, J., Magdalou, J., Souhaili-El-Amri, H., Boissel, P. and Siest, G. (1987) : Properties of human hepatic UDP-glucuronosyltransferases : relationship to other inducible enzymes in patients with cholestasis. Eur. J. Clin. Pharmacol. 32, 485-491.

Dutton, G.J. and Montgomery, J.P. (1958) : Glucuronide synthesis in fish and the influence of temperature. Biochem. J. 70,17.

Förlin, L. and Haux, C. (1985) : Increased excretion in the bile of 17β-(3H)-estradiol derived radioactivity in rainbow trout treated with β-naphthoflavone. Aquat. Toxicol. 6, 197-208.

Frei, J. (1966). Leucocytes and glucuronoconjugaison. Helv. Physiol. Pharmacol. Acta 24, 84-85.

Hartree, E.F. (1972) : Determination of protein : a modification of the Lowry method that gives a linear photometric response. Anal. Biochem. 48, 422-427.

Kobayashi K., Oshima Y., Taguchi C. and Wang Y. (1987) : Induction of drug-metabolizing enzymes by long-term administration of PCB and duration of their induced activities in carp. Nippon Susan Gakkaishi 53, 487-491.

Lindström-Seppä, P., Koivusaari, U. and Hänninen, O. (1981) : Extrahepatic xenobiotic metabolism in North-european freshwater fish. Comp. Biochem. Physiol. 69C, 259-263.

MacKenzie, P.I. and Hänninen, O. (1980) : A sensitive kinetic assay for UDPglucuronosyltransferase using 1-naphthol as substrate. Anal. Biochem. 109, 362-368.

Monod, G., Devaux, A. and Rivière, J.L. (1987) : Characterization of some monooxygenase activities and solubilization of hepatic cytochrome P-450 in two species of freshwater fish, the nase (Chondrostoma nasus) and the roach (Rutilus rutilus). Comp. Biochem. Physiol. 88C, 83-89.

Payne, J.F., Fancey, L.L., Rahimtula, A.D. and Porter, E.L. (1987) : Mixed-function oxygenases in biological monitoring programs : review of potential usage in different phyla of aquatic animals. Comp. Biochem. Physiol. 86C, 233-245

Sivarajah, K., Franklin, C.S. and Williams, W.P. (1978) : The effects of polychlorinated biphenyls on plasma steroid levels and hepatic microsomal enzymes in fish. J. Fish Biol. 13, 401-409.

Winsnes, A. (1969) : Studies on the activation in vitro of UDP-glucuronosyltransferase. Biochim. Biophys. Acta 191, 279-291

Résumé

L'activité UDPGA-transférase (UDPGT) a été mesurée dans des microsomes de foie de carpe (Cyprinus carpio) avec du p-nitrophénol et du 1-naphtol comme substrats. Les paramètres suivants ont été étudiés : concentration en détergent, en substrat, et en UDPGA et température. Les résultats montrent que les propriétés de l'enzyme de poisson sont différentes de celles du rat.

Influence of repeated administration of fengabine, a new antidepressant on its own metabolism — in vitro study with rat hepatic microsomes

A. Durand, J.-P. Thenot, G. Gillet, M. Beauvallet and P.-L. Morselli

Department of Clinical Research, Laboratoires d'Etudes et de Recherches Synthélabo (L.E.R.S.), 58, rue de la Glacière, 75013 Paris, France

ABSTRACT

The influence of the pretreatment of rats with fengabine (F), a novel antidepressant drug, on the metabolic profile of this compound was investigated in vitro using hepatic microsomes. Results indicate that 3 x 300 mg.kg^{-1} p.o. of F increase the phase I and phase II biotransformation reactions. Due to the important increase of the glucuronidation, the unconjugated phase I metabolites are not apparently increased after pretreatment of the animal with F.
Similar modifications were observed after pretreatment of the animals with phenobarbital while 20-methylcholanthrene produced little changes in the metabolic profile of F.

KEY WORDS

Fengabine, rat, hepatic microsomes, glucuronidation.

INTRODUCTION

Fengabine (F) (2-[(butylimino)(2-chlorophenyl)methyl]-4-chlorophenol) is a new benzylidene derivative with interesting antidepressive activity. In both human and animal species (rat, dog), the compound is mainly eliminated after biotransformation according to the following reactions :
- oxidation on the aliphatic side chain leading to alcohols, ketones or carboxylic acids,
- oxidation on the aromatic moiety leading to ortho diphenolic metabolites,
- hydrolysis of the imine bond with formation of benzophenone derivatives.
These phase I metabolites, together with the parent compound are glucuroconjugated prior to their elimination, mainly in the bile.
In the rat, chronic administration of F produces a significant increase in the hepatic cytochrome P-450 levels together with an important diminution of the plasma levels of the mother molecule and of its main unconjugated metabolites.

The aim of this study was to characterize, using rat hepatic microsomes, the influence of repeated administrations of F on its own metabolism and to compare the results with those obtained under similar experimental conditions with hepatic microsomes prepared from rats pretreated with classical enzymic inducers : phenobarbital and 20-methylcholanthrene.

MATERIAL AND METHODS

This study was conducted with twelve 8 week old male Sprague Dawley rats (Charles Rivers, France). The animals were grouped by three and received the following daily treatment during three days :

GROUP	TEST COMPOUND	DOSE ($mg.kg^{-1}$)	VEHICLE ($4\ ml.kg^{-1}$)	ROUTE
1	control	-	1% tween 80 in normal saline	p.o.
2	fengabine	300	1% tween 80 in normal saline	p.o.
3	phenobarbital	80	normal saline	i.p.
4	20-methylcholanthrene	40	corn oil	i.p.

The animals were sacrified 24 hours after the third administration and hepatic microsomes (100,000 g fraction) were prepared according to the conventional method (Funae et col, 1986). For each animal, 45 minutes incubations were performed with 125 ug of ^{14}C-fengabine and 25 mg of microsomal proteins after addition of cofactors including or not UDPGA. At the end of the incubations the samples were deproteinized with methanol and an H.P.L.C. separation of fengabine and its related metabolites was achieved with on line UV and radioactive detection. These compounds were quantified from the percentages of radioactivity associated to their chromatographic peaks.

RESULTS

After incubations of F with hepatic microsomes, more than 15 radioactive chromatographic peaks were detected (corresponding to at least 20 metabolites yet identified using various analytical technics). In order to facilitate the interpretation, the data were analysed according to 3 groups of compounds :
- fengabine (RT = 41.7 minutes)
- phase I metabolites (RT between 22.5 and 32.5 minutes)
- phase II metabolites (RT between 10.0 and 19.0 minutes)
  (in the latter case the nature of the metabolites was ascertained by their decrease in proportion after enzymatic hydrolysis of the samples with glucuronidase).

The results are summarized in the table below.

PRETREATMENT	CYT. P-450[1]	FENGABINE[2] *	PHASE I METABOLITES[3] *	PHASE II METABOLITES[3] *
control	0.89 ± 0.08	32.7 27.1	66.1 46.5	1.2 26.4
fengabine (3 x 300 mg.kg^{-1}) p.o.	1.71 ± 0.16	9.8 4.3	85.6 48.1	4.6 47.6
phenobarbital (3 x 80 mg.kg^{-1}) i.p.	2.80 ± 0.06	2.4 0.8	92.5 45.3	5.1 53.9
20-methylcholanthrene (3 x 40 mg.kg^{-1}) i.p.	2.12 ± 0.22	44.7 40.2	52.7 39.4	2.6 20.4

* first line values refer to incubations performed without UDPGA ; second line values refer to incubations performed after addition of UDPGA
1 nmoles.mg^{-1} of hepatic microsomal proteins
2 percent remaining in the medium at the end of the incubation
3 percent at the end of the incubation

DISCUSSION

The results of this study indicate that, in the rat, repeated administrations of F increase its biotransformation. Indeed, F, which accounted for about 30% of the initial dose, at the end of the incubations performed with control microsomes, accounted for only 4-10% of the dose when incubations were performed with microsomes prepared from F pretreated animals.
Incubations performed without UDPGA demonstrate, in the case of F pretreated rats, an enhancement of phase I metabolites (the proportion of these compounds is 85.6% versus 66.1% when incubation is performed with control microsomes). In contrast, after addition of UDPGA the proportion of these phase I metabolites is very similar with "F pretreated" or "control" microsomes (respectively 48,1 and 46,5%). On the contrary, the proportion of the conjugated metabolites in 47.6% with F pretreated microsomes and 26.4% in the case of "control" microsomes.
These results confirm and explain the data obtained in animals showing that after chronic treatment with F the circulating levels of the unchanged compound as well as the unconjugated metabolites, were lower than after single administration.
The comparison of these data with those obtained with microsomes prepared from animals pretreated with phenobarbital or 20-methylcholanthrene indicate that the modifications of the metabolic profile of F obtained after repeated administrations of fengabine is similar to that after treatment of the animals with phenobarbital while pretreatment with 20-methylcholanthrene cause little change in the metabolic profile of F.

Résumé

L'influence d'un pré-traitement de rats avec la fengabine (F), un nouveau médicament antidépresseur sur le profil métabolique de ce composé a été étudié *in vitro* avec des microsomes hépatiques. Les résultats obtenus indiquent qu'une dose orale de 3 fois 300 mg.kg^{-1} augmente les réactions de biotransformation des phases I et II. Etant donné l'augmentation importante de la glucuronoconjugaison, les métabolites non conjugués de phase I ne sont pas apparamment augmentés après un pré-traitement des animaux par F. Des modifications similaires sont observées après pré-traitement des animaux par le phénobarbital, tandis que le 20-méthylcholanthrène produit peu de changement du profil métabolique de F.

Effects of various drugs on microsomal UDP-glucuronosyltransferase activity in hamster liver

A. Foliot, A. Myara, D. Touchard and F. Trivin

Laboratoire de Biochimie, Hôpital Saint-Joseph, 75674 Paris Cedex 14, France

ABSTRACT

The effects of in vivo administration of ten xenobiotic drugs on hamster liver microsomal UDP-glucuronosyltransferase activity were compared for each of two substrates, bilirubin and 4-nitrophenol. Glucuronidation of 4-nitrophenol was increased by almost all the drugs tested whereas that of bilirubin was only enhanced by a few and was reduced by two. These results suggest that hamster liver glucuronosyltransferase activity is easily but differentially inducible by xenobiotics.

KEY-WORDS

Liver UDP-glucuronosyltransferase, bilirubin, 4-nitrophenol, drug induction, hamster.

INTRODUCTION

Phenobarbital is a potent inducer of liver enzymes involved in the biotransformation of drugs and physiological compounds in several mammalian species (Conney, 1967). Its administration to rats raises the concentration of cytochrome P 450 in the liver and the activity of related monooxygenases, as well as that of several conjugating enzymes, including UDP-glucuronosyltransferases (Bock et al, 1973) and glutathione S-transferases (Kaplowitz et al, 1975). In hamsters, however, phenobarbital is not a good inducer of cytosolic glutathione-conjugating activity (Foliot et al, 1987a). We recently showed that in hamsters, 3-methylcholanthrene enhanced liver glutathione S-transferase activity towards all the substrates used, but other drugs known to induce this activity in rat liver had no effect (Foliot et al, 1987b). We attempted to establish here whether the activity of another conjugating enzyme, UDP-glucuronosyltransferase (UDP-GT, EC 2.4.1.17) was difficult to induce in hamsters, and for this purpose tested ten xenobiotic drugs for their effects on UDP-GT activity in this species.

MATERIALS AND METHODS

Male golden Syrian hamsters weighing 100-110 g (Fichot, Ormesson, France) were injected once daily i.p. for 4 days with one of the following : phenobarbital (PB, 100 mg/kg body weight), 3-methylcholanthrene (MC, 20 mg/kg), 3,4-benzopyrene (BP, 20 mg/kg), trans-stilbene oxide (TSO, 400 mg/kg), butylated hydroxytoluene (BHT, 1 g/kg), pregnenolone-carbonitrile (PCN, 75 mg/kg), clofibrate (CL, 200 mg/kg), nafenopin (NF, 100 mg/kg) or vehicle (either saline or corn oil, 5 ml/kg). Other hamsters were given four once daily i.p. injections of 100 or 200 mg/kg rifampicin (RF) or 5 ml/kg 0.02 N HCl. Others again were given 400 or 800 mg/kg triacetyloleandomycin (TAO) or 5 ml/kg corn oil per os for 4 days. Animals were killed 24hr after the last drug dose. Livers were removed, weighed, perfused with chilled saline and homogenized in two volumes of ice-cold buffer containing 0.001 M EDTA, 0.005 M 2-mercaptoethanol, 0.03 M sodium-phosphate and 0.25 M sucrose, pH 7.4. The homogenate was centrifuged at 10,000 g for 10 min, and the resulting supernatant fraction, at 100,000 g for 60 min to give the microsomal pellet. Protein concentration was determined by the method of Lowry et al (1951). UDP-GT activity was determined with 4-nitrophenol by a kinetic method adapted from Gorski and Kasper (1977) and bilirubin, according to Black et al (1970). The microsomal fraction was activated by using 1 mg digitonin per mg of microsomal protein. The concentration of cytochrome P 450 was measured according to Omura and Sato (1964) and NADPH cytochrome c reductase activity, according to Mazel (1972).

RESULTS

Hamster UDP-GT activity was significantly modified by all ten drugs administered except TAO (Table 1). With 4-nitrophenol as substrate, glucuronidation rose by 10-56 %, the most potent inducers being PB, BHT and RF. However, with bilirubin as substrate, glucuronidation was only increased by four drugs - CL, NF, RF and PB - and was reduced by MC and TSO. Relative liver weight remained unchanged or only increased slightly after treatment with all the drugs tested, but the microsomal protein concentration was always raised (data not shown). Hamsters therefore appeared to be responsive to the drugs concerned, since the cytochrome P 450 concentration was not only enhanced by those that raised GT activity but by TAO as well. NADPH cytochrome c reductase activity was also increased by all inducers of GT activity except for MC, which reduced it (data not shown).

DISCUSSION

Hepatic microsomal UDP-GT catalyses the glucuronidation of a wide variety of endogenous and exogenous compounds. In rat, the heterogeneity of GT has been established by its substrate specificity, perinatal development, inducibility by various compounds and chromatographic purification (Dutton, 1980 ; Burchell, 1981). In this preliminary study of hamster liver GT, we measured the glucuronidation of two substrates, bilirubin and 4-nitrophenol, representing endogenous and exogenous compounds respectively. 4-nitrophenol is a standard substrate commonly used to assay GT activity. Typical microsomal activity with this substrate, reported by Bock et al (1983) for adult male Wistar rat liver, is very similar to that we found here for adult male hamster liver. The known inducers of GT activity in rat liver have been classified as inducers of GT1 enzyme forms (MC and BP), GT2 forms (PB) and other forms (PCN, TSO and CL) (Bock et al, 1973 ; Lilienblum et al, 1982 ; Mc Kenzie et al, 1982 ; Watkins et al, 1982). In addition to these inducers, we selected compounds such as TAO and RF, whose administration to rats induces bilirubin conjugation (personal observations). The data in table 1 show that hamster liver microsomal GT activity is differentially inducible by xenobiotics. As expected from the data for rats (Bock et al, 1973 ;

Mc Kenzie, 1982), PB induced both 4-nitrophenol and bilirubin conjugation in hamster, whilst MC increased 4-nitrophenol conjugation but reduced that of bilirubin. The hypolipidemic drugs CL and NF, known to induce the conjugation of bilirubin (Foliot et al, 1977) in rats but not that of 4-nitrophenol (Lilienblum et al, 1982 ; Burchell et al, 1987), enhanced the glucuronidation of both substrates in hamster. In this species, contrarily to the results published for rats (Pessayre and Mazel, 1976), RF satisfactorily induced GT activity with both substrates, in a dose-dependent manner. The other drugs (BP, TSO, BHT and PCN) only modified the GT activity towards one substrate. All these results suggest the existence of different GT isoforms in hamsters as well as rats. In conclusion, hamster liver GT activity is easily inducible by the drugs known to induce GT activity in rat liver, at least with the two substrates tested.

Table 1. Effects of ten xenobiotic drugs on UDP-glucuronosyltransferase activity and the cytochrome P 450 concentration in hamster liver microsomes.

Treatment	Cytochrome P 450 nmoles/mg protein	UDP-glucuronosyltransferase	
		4-nitrophenol	bilirubin
		nmoles/min/mg protein	
Control	1.18 ± 0.08	33.5 ± 0.8	0.67 ± 0.04
PB	2.28 ± 0.10*	51.8 ± 3.2*	1.13 ± 0,09*
MC	2.27 ± 0.10*	37.8 ± 1.5*	0.49 ± 0.03*
BP	1.75 ± 0.06*	40.2 ± 1.1*	0.72 ± 0.04
TSO	1.24 ± 0.04	31.1 ± 1.4	0.48 ± 0.04*
BHT	1.44 ± 0.03*	50.6 ± 2.9*	0.68 ± 0.03
Control	1.11 ± 0.02	29.4 ± 1.1	0.78 ± 0.04
PCN	1.10 ± 0.05	32.4 ± 0.7*	0.69 ± 0.04
Control	1.05 ± 0.03	30.6 ± 1.2	0.82 ± 0.05
RF 100	1.49 ± 0.04*	38.7 ± 1.7*	1.00 ± 0.05*
200	1.66 ± 0.14*	47.7 ± 1.0*	1.26 ± 0.11*
Control	1.11 ± 0.04	29.4 ± 1.1	0.75 ± 0.05
TAO 400	1.58 ± 0.03*	29.2 ± 1.0	0.73 ± 0.05
800	1.81 ± 0.06*	31.0 ± 1.0	0.72 ± 0.03
Control	1.10 ± 0.03	28.0 ± 1.1	0.81 ± 0.03
CL	1.53 ± 0.04*	31.8 ± 0.5*	1.13 ± 0.06*
NF	1.52 ± 0.03*	36.7 ± 0.8*	1.16 ± 0.06*

Drugs were given as indicated in Materials and methods. Results are means ± SEM for 8 animals. *Significantly different from controls, $p < 0.05$.

REFERENCES

Black, M., Billing, B.H., Heirwegh, K.P.M. (1970): Determination of bilirubin UDP-glucuronyltransferase activity in needle-biopsy specimens of human liver. Clin. Chim. Acta 29, 27-35.
Bock, K.W., Fröhling, W., Remmer, H., Rexer, B. (1973): Effects of phenobarbital and 3-methylcholanthrene on substrate specificity of rat liver microsomal UDP-glucuronyltransferase. Biochim. Biophys. Acta 327, 46-56.
Bock, K.W., Burchell, B., Dutton, G.T., Hänninen, O., Mulder, G.J., Owens, I.S., Siest, G., Tephly, T.R. (1983): UDP-glucuronosyltransferase activities : guidelines for consistent interim terminology and assay conditions. Biochem. Pharmacol. 32, 953-955.

Burchell, B. (1981): Identification and purification of multiforms of UDP-glucuronosyltransferase. Biochem. Toxicol. 3, 1-32.

Burchell, B., Coughtrie, M.W.H., Jackson, M.R., Shepherd, S.R.P., Harding, D., Hume, R. (1987): Genetic deficiency of bilirubin glucuronidation in rats and humans. Molec. Aspects Med. 9, 429-455.

Conney, A. (1967): Pharmacological implications of microsomal enzyme induction. Pharmacol. Rev. 19, 316-366.

Dutton, G.J. (1980): Glucuronidation of drugs and other compounds. CRC Press, Boca Raton, FL.

Foliot, A., Drocourt, J.L., Etienne, J.P., Housset, E., Fiessinger, J.N., Christoforov, B. (1977): Increase in the hepatic glucuronidation and clearance of bilirubin in clofibrate-treated rats. Biochem. Pharmacol. 26, 547-549.

Foliot, A., Touchard, D., Myara, A., Trivin, F., Chauffert, M. (1987a): Deficient induction of sulfobromophthalein conjugating activity by phenobarbital in hamster liver. Biochem. Pharmacol. 36, 2617-2620.

Foliot, A., Myara, A., Touchard, D. (1987b): Liver glutathione S-transferase activity : differential response to drugs in hamsters. J. Hepatol. 5, S127

Gorski, J.P., Kasper, C.B. (1977): Purification and properties of microsomal UDP-glucuronosyltransferase from rat liver. J. Biol. Chem. 252, 1336-1343.

Kaplowitz, N., Kuhlenkemp, J. Clifton, G. (1975): Drug induction of hepatic glutathione S-transferases in male and female rats. Biochem. J. 146, 351-356.

Lilienblum, W., Walli, A.K., Bock, K.W. (1982): Differential induction of rat liver microsomal UDP-glucuronosyltransferase activities by various inducing agents. Biochem. Pharmacol. 31, 907-913.

Lowry, O.H., Rosebrough, N.J., Farr, A.L., Randall, R.J. (1951): Protein measurement with the Folin-phenol reagent. J. Biol. Chem. 193, 265-275.

Mazel, P. (1972): In : Fundamentals of Drug Metabolism and Drug Disposition, pp 546-582. Ed. La Du B.N., Mandel H.G., Way E.L., Williams and Wilkins, Baltimore.

Mc Kenzie, P.I., Vaïsänen, M., Hänninen, O. (1982): Differential induction of UDP-glucuronosyltransferase activities toward various substrates after polycyclic aromatic hydrocarbon administration to rats. Toxicol. Lett. 12, 259-263.

Omura, T., Sato, R. (1964): The carbon monoxide-binding pigment of liver microsomes. 1. Evidence for its hemoprotein nature. J. Biol. Chem. 239, 2370-2378.

Pessayre, D., Mazel, P. (1976): Induction and inhibition of hepatic drug metabolizing enzymes by rifampin. Biochem. Pharmacol. 25, 943-946.

Watkins, J.B., Gregus, Z., Thompson, T.N., Klaassen, C.D. (1982): Induction studies on the functional heterogeneity of rat liver UDP-glucuronosyltransferases. Toxicol. Appl. Pharmacol. 64, 439-446.

Résumé

L'effet de l'administration de diverses drogues sur l'activité UDP-glucuronosyltransférase hépatique (UDP-GT) a été étudié chez le hamster. En effet, cette espèce est moins sensible à l'induction enzymatique que le rat, en ce qui concerne l'activité d'une autre enzyme de conjugaison, la glutathion transférase. Nous avons testé la réponse du hamster vis-à-vis de deux substrats, la bilirubine et le 4-nitrophénol. A l'exception de la triacétyloléandomycine (TAO), tous les composés administrés au hamster ont modifié l'activité UDP-GT vis-à-vis de l'un ou l'autre substrat. La conjugaison du 4-nitrophénol a été augmentée par la plupart des drogues tandis que celle de la bilirubine ne l'a été que par quatre drogues et a été diminuée par deux autres. Ces résultats montrent que l'activité UDP-GT est, comme chez le rat, inductible par de nombreuses substances chez le hamster.

Glucuronidation of perindopril by hepatic microsomes : inter-species comparison

S. Fournel-Gigleux*, J. Magdalou*, C. Lafaurie*, G. Siest*, L. Grislain**, M.H. Garnier**, J.-F. Dabé**, W. Luijten**, N. Bromet** and M. Devissaguet**

*Centre du Médicament, Faculté des Sciences Pharmaceutiques et Biologiques, UA CNRS n° 597, 30 rue Lionnois, 54000 Nancy, France.
**Bio-Pharmacie Servier, 5 rue de Bel Air, BP 2357, 45023 Orléans Cedex 1, France

SUMMARY

The glucuronidation of perindopril (S 9490), a new ACE inhibitor, was studied after incubation with liver microsomes of various animal species (mouse, rat, rabbit, dog, monkey) and man. Glucuronides were isolated and quantitated by reverse phase HPLC and TLC. Acyl glucuronide formation was confirmed by its susceptibility to be hydrolyzed by ß-glucuronidase, and by FAB ionisation, mass spectrometry. Dog, monkey and man were the most effective in conjugating S 9490, when compared to rodents (rat, mouse and rabbit). Finally, treatment by phenobarbital enhanced the formation of the acyl glucuronide, mostly in monkeys.

KEY WORDS

Acyl glucuronide, ACE inhibitor, perindopril, liver microsomes, animal species and man, phenobarbital induction, FAB ionisation, HPLC, TLC

INTRODUCTION

Perindopril (S 9490) is a new ACE inhibitor indicated for treatment of hypertention and heart failure in man. Upon administration, the molecule is cleaved by esterases into a pharmacologically active compound (S 9780), which incorporates two carboxyl groups. Analysis of urinary metabolites reveals the formation of acyl glucuronides.
Many xenobiotics and endogenous compounds with carboxylic acid functions are metabolized to acyl (or ester) glucuronides (Kuhara et al, 1986). For example, the hypolipidaemic drug clofibric acid, some non-steroid antiinflamatory compounds as well as bilirubine are substrates of UDP-glucuronosyltransferase (Dragacci et al., 1987, a; El Mouelhi et al., 1987). If glucuronidation appears, in most cases, as an elimination pathway, acyl glucuronide formation can lead to instability, isomerisation or hydrolysis of the conjugate with liberation of the aglycone from glucuronic acid (Wells et al., 1987).
Therefore it was important to characterize, in vitro, the biosynthesis of acyl glucuronide from S 9490, using liver microsomes from different species including man, as source of UDP-glucuronosyltransferase. The effect of induction by phenobarbital was also considered.

MATERIALS AND METHODS

Microsome preparation

The following male animals have been used: CBA mice, 25-30g; Wistar rats, 180-200g, (Iffa-Credo, l'Abresle, France); New-Zealand rabbits, 1.5-2.0 kg, (Elevage Scientifique des Dombes, Chatillon/Chalaronne, France); Beagle dogs, 6.7-15 kg, (Hacking and Churchill Ltd, Huntingdow, England; Centre d'Elevage du Domaine des Souches, Toucy, France), Macaque *Rhesus* monkeys, 3.5-5.0 kg, (Shamrock Ltd, Small Dole, England; Charles River France, Cléon, France). Phenobarbital, dissolved in saline, was injected *i.p.* at the daily dose of 50 mg/kg for 4 days in mice and rabbits; 80 mg/kg for 4 days in rats; 50 mg/kg for 1 day and then 25 mg/kg for 4 days in dogs and monkeys. Microsomal fraction was prepared as described by Hogeboom (1955); the protein content was measured by the technique of Lowry *et al.* (1951). Two human liver samples were obtained, *post mortem*, on patients presenting hepatic carcinoma. Human microsomes were prepared as previously described (Dragacci *et al.*, 1987, b).

Incubation conditions

Microsomal UDP-glucuronosyltransferase was activated for 30 min at 4°C by digitonin at detergent-protein weight ratios of 0.1 to 3.0. This detergent was found to be the best suitable for activation of the enzyme form involved in acyl glucuronide biosynthesis. Incubations were carried out in 150 mM Tris-HCl (pH ranged from 5.5 to 7.8), at 37°C for 0 to 60 min. The incubation medium consisted in 5 mM S 9490 and ^{14}C-S 9490 (0.5 to 2.0 Ci per assay) and 3.5 mM UDP-glucuronic acid (Boehringer, Mannheim, FRG), dissolved in the buffer. The reaction was stopped by HCl 0.2 N; the proteins were precipitated and removed by centrifugation. The supernatant was used for HPLC analysis without further work up. Control experiments were run without either UDP-glucuronic acid or S 9490. Hydrolysis of the acyl glucuronide was achieved by incubation with 3000 units of ß-glucuronidase (bovine liver, Sigma, St. Louis MO, USA) for 2 hr at 37°C. Similar experiments were performed with ^{14}C- S 9780.

Separation and identification of acyl glucuronide of S 9490

The samples were injected into a HPLC system and the metabolites separated from the parent compound using a reverse phase column LiChrosorb RP-18, Hibar RT 250-4.7 , (Merck, Darmstadt, FRG). The mobile phase consisted in acetonitrile-water-trifluoroacetic acid 24-76-0.08 v/v/v at a flow rate of 1 ml/min (Kratos pump, Spectroflow 400). The elution of the products was monitored at 220 nm using a Shimatzu SPD 2A detector coupled to a LS 400 Merck integrator. The fractions were collected and their radioactivity measured by liquid scintillation counting with a Beckman LS 801 spectrometer.
Before mass spectrometry analysis, the acyl glucuronide was extracted by two liquid/liquid extraction techniques using chloroform at pH 5 and pH 2, followed by solid/solid extraction with XAD2 resin at pH 2. Each extract was analyzed by TLC (solvant: ethylacetate 60/methanol 20/water 20/acetic acid 2) on silica plates (Merck F254). Radioactive bands were localized by autoradiography (Industrex, CX Kodak) and quantifications were performed with a TLC linear analyzer (Berthold LB 2882). Radioactive products were scraped off silica plates and extracted with methanol. Mass spectral analysis was performed on a VG Analytical 70-250S spectrometer operating in the FAB-ionisation mode. A 1µl aliquot of a solution of the acylglucuronide was loaded on a stainless steel target; 1 l of a 0.1 M HCl solution was added and finally 2 l thioglycerol was applied to the target. Xenon (8 KV, 0.1 mA) was used as the bombarding gas. The scan range was 800-100 at a scan speed of 2 seconds per decade.

RESULTS AND DISCUSSION

Incubations with dog liver microsomes were performed prior to other species because, from all the animals studied *in vivo*, the highest proportions of glucuronides was found in the dog.

Characterisation of acyl glucuronide formation by dog liver microsomes

Incubation of ^{14}C-labelled perindopril and UDP-glucuronic acid led to the formation of S 9490 glucuronide and S 9780, but not to the formation of S 9780 glucuronide (Fig.1). When microsomes were incubated with ^{14}C-9780 and UDP-glucuronic acid, no glucuronides were formed. With the HPLC conditions used in this study, the S 9490 glucuronide was eluted from the column after 13.5 min; the non conjugated aglycone presenting a retention time of about 30 min. The identity was confirmed by the mass spectrum of the sample: the protonated molecule was found at m/z 545, with a sodium adduct ion (MNa$^+$) at m/z 567 of lower intensity. Ater glucuronide hydrolysis by ß-glucuronidase or when UDP-glucuronic acid was ommitted, the HPLC chromatogram revealed no peak corresponding to the glucuronide.

The optimal experimental conditions for the formation of acyl glucuronide were determined. Upon addition of digitonin to the microsomal protein (1/1, w/w), the activity increased to about 8-fold. Optimum pH was 6.7 at 37°C, and the reaction was linear with respect to time, up to 1 hr. Determination of the kinetic constants for glucuronidation of S 9490 with dog liver microsomes led to a K_m of 2.85 mM and a V_{max} of 2.5 nmol/min/mg protein. These values were quite similar to those obtained, in rats, with other carboxylic compounds such as naphthylacetic acid or clofibric acid (Hamar-Hansen et al., 1986). In term of V_{max}, glucuronidation of carboxylic compounds proceeded at a much lower rate than hydroxylated aglycones such as naphthol or terpenes (Boutin et al., 1985).

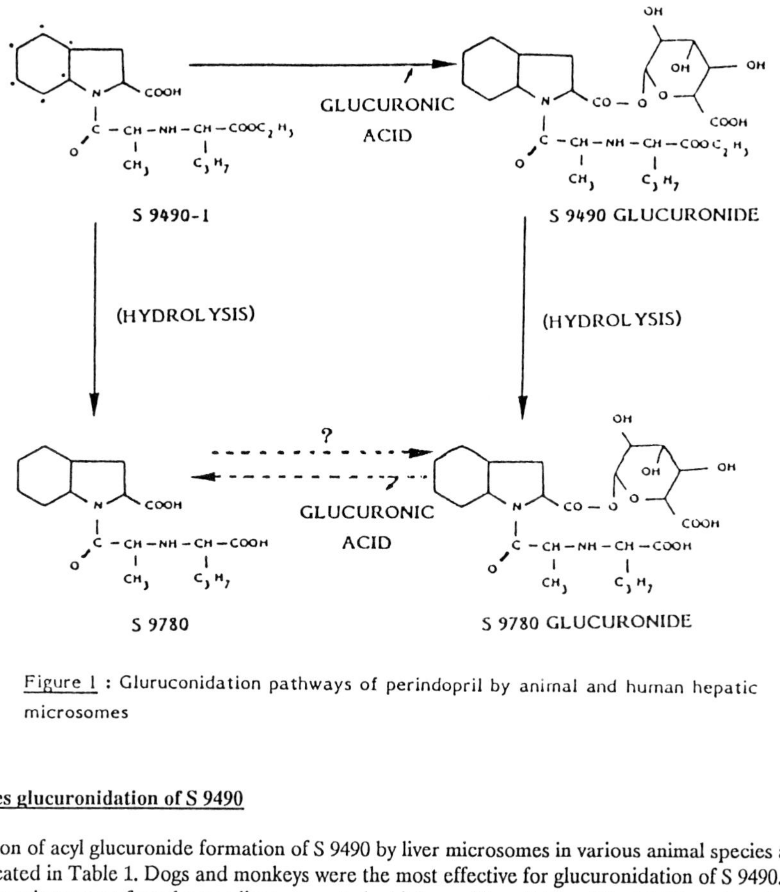

Figure 1 : Gluruconidation pathways of perindopril by animal and human hepatic microsomes

Inter-species glucuronidation of S 9490

A comparison of acyl glucuronide formation of S 9490 by liver microsomes in various animal species and in man is indicated in Table 1. Dogs and monkeys were the most effective for glucuronidation of S 9490. Interestingly, microsomes from human liver presented a high specific activity, while S 9490 conjugation in rodents was of minor importance. By contrast, conjugation in rodents was weak. The differences between these species could be due to the quick action of microsomal esterase in rodents, which, according to the chromatographic detection of S 9780, leads to the transformation of 40 to 80 % of S 9490 into S 9780, which is not a substrate for UDP-glucuronosyltransferase. By contrast the amount of this compound upon incubation with dog, monkey or man liver microsomes never exceeded 5%.

Phenobarbital is known as a non-specific inducer of drug-metabolizing enzymes. At least three isozymes of UDP-glucuronosyltransferase are induced by the antiepileptic drug. Conjugation of planar substrates (1-naphthol, 4-methylumbelliferone), bulky structures (terpenes, morphine) and bilirubin, each catalyzed by distinct forms of transferase, is increased by phenobarbital (Okulicz-Kozaryn et al., 1981). Despite their commun induction by this drug, acyl glucuronide formations from bilirubine and carboxylic compounds appear to be catalyzed by two different enzymes, as Gunn rats, which are defective in bilirubin UDP-glucuronosyltransferase, are still able to conjugate clofibric acid (Dragacci *et al.*, 1987, a; Hamar-Hansen, 1987). For S 9490 UDP-glucuronosyltransferase, from all species studied, monkeys were the most sensitive to phenobarbital induction (147%), (Table 1).

Table 1. Glucuronidation of S 9490 in liver microsomes of different species. Effect of phenobarbital

Animal	n	Specific activity*		% increase
		Control	Phenobarbital	
Dog	1	0.74	0.89	20.2
Monkey	1	0.36	0.89	147.2
Rabbit	3	0.12	0.15	25.0
Mouse	10	0.19	0.27	42.1
Rat	5	0.24	0.27	12.5
Man n°1		1.23	--	--
Man n°2		0.53	--	--

* nmoles S 9490 conjugated/min/mg protein. The results corresponded to the mean of 3 separate incubations. (n), number of animals used. The variation coefficient was less than 10%.

REFERENCES

Boutin, J. A., Thomassin, J., Siest, G. and Cartier, A. (1985): Heterogeneity of hepatic microsomal monoterpenoid aglycones in control and induced rats, and guinea pigs. Biochem. Pharmacol. 34, 2235-2249.

Dragacci, A., Hamar-Hansen, C., Fournel-Gigleux, S., Lafaurie, C., Magdalou, J. and Siest G. (1987, a): Comparative study of clofibric acid and bilirubin glucuronidation in human liver microsomes. Biochem. Pharmacol. 22, 3923-3927.

Dragacci, S., Thomassin, J., Magdalou, J., Souhaili El Amri, H. and Siest, G.(1987, b): Properties of human hepatic UDP-glucuronosyltransferases. Relationship to other inducible enzymes in patients with cholestasis. Eur. J. Clin. Pharmacol. 32, 485-491.

El Mouelhi, M., Ruelius, R. W., Fenseleau, C. and Dulik, D. M. (1987): Species dependent enantioselective glucuronidation of three 2-arylpropionic acids, naproxen, ibuprofen and benoxaprofen. Drug Met. Dispos. 15, 767-772.

Hamar-Hansen, C., Fournel, S., Magdalou, J., Boutin, J. A. and Siest, G.(1986): Liquid chromatographic assay for the measurement of glucuronidation of arylcarboxylic acids using uridine diphospho-(U-^{14}C)glucuronic acid. J. Chrom. 383, 51-60.

Hamar-Hansen, C. (1987): Glucuronoconjugaison des acides arylacétiques. PhD Thesis, University of Nancy, France.

Hogeboom, G. M. (1955): Fractionation of cell components of animals tissues: general method for the isolation of liver cell components. Meth. Enzymol.1, 16-19.

Kuhara, T., Matsumoto, I., Ohno, M. and Ohura, T. (1986): Identification and quantification of octanoyl glucuronide in the urine of children who ingested medium-chain triglycerides. Biomed. Environ. Mass Spectr. 13, 595-598.

Lowry, O. H., Rosebrough, J. N., Farr, A. L. and Randall, R. J. (1951): Protein measurement with the Folin phenol reagent. J. Biol. Chem. 226, 547-509.

Okulicz-Kozarin, I., Schaeffer, M., Batt, A. M., Siest, G. and Loppinet, V. (1981): Stereochemical heterogeneity of hepatic UDP-glucuronosyltransferase activity in rat liver microsomes. Biochem. Pharmacol. 30, 1457-1461.

Wells, D. S., Janssen, F., and Ruelius, H. W. (1987): Interactions between oxaprozine glucuronide and human serum albumin. Xenobiotica 17, 1437-1449.

Résumé

Nous avons étudié la glucuronoconjugaison du perindopril (S 9490), un nouveau médicament indiqué dans les traitements antihypertenseurs et l'insuffisance cardiaque, par des microsomes hépatiques de nombreuses espèces animales (souris, rat, lapin, chien, singe) et d'homme. Les glucuronides ont été isolés et quantifiés par HPLC en phase réverse et CCM. La formation d'un acyl glucuronide a été confirmée par la spectrométrie de masse (FAB ionisation) et la susceptibilité du métabolite d'être hydrolysé par la ß-glucuronidase. Le chien, le singe et l'homme sont les espèces qui conjuguent le mieux le S 9490 par comparaison aux rongeurs (rat, souris et lapin). Finalement, un traitement par le phénobarbital augmente la formation d'acyl glucuronide, surtout chez le singe.

Comparative induction of rat liver bilirubin UDP-glucuronosyltransferase by ciprofibrate and other hypolipidaemic agents belonging to the fibrate series: influence of the thyroid status

H. Goudonnet*, J. Mounié*, J. Magdalou**, A. Escousse* and R.C. Truchot*

*Formation de Biochimie Pharmacologique, Faculté de Médecine et Pharmacie, 7 Bd Jeanne d'Arc, 21033 Dijon, France
**Faculté des Sciences Pharmaceutiques et Biologiques, UA CNRS 597, Centre du Médicament, 30 rue Lionnois, 54000 Nancy, France

SUMMARY

The effects of equiactive doses of ciprofibrate, bezafibrate, fenofibrate and clofibrate on several forms of UDP-glucuronosyltransferases (UDPGT) measured with bilirubin, 4-nitrophenol and nopol as substrates were compared in liver microsomes of rats different in the thyroid hormonal status : control, hypothyroid, hyperthyroid animals. The results clearly showed that the thyroid status markedly modulate the response of UDPGT result to the hypolipidaemic compounds. The bilirubin UDPGT induction was increased by 50 % in hyperthyroid animals where compared to normal rats, but the hypothyroid animals were the less sensitive to induction. By contrast, glucuronidation of 4-nitrophenol was 20 to 30 % decreased whatever the thyroid status. The variations in bilirubin glucuronidation also were related to change in cytochrome P 450 content. This result emphasizes the role of hormonal control on the inducing process of drug metabolizing enzymes by xenobiotics.

KEY WORDS

Thyroid hormones - Ciprofibrate - hypolipidaemic drugs - UDP-glucuronosyltransferases - Cytochrome P 450

INTRODUCTION

It is well established that clofibrate and its structural analogues cause proliferation of hepatic peroxisomes, enlargement of the liver, concomitant increase in bilirubin glucuronidation (De Grimal, 1977 ; Reddy and al., 1971) and w-hydroxylation of lauric acid (cytochrome P 452 dependent) (Fournel and al., 1985 ; Gibson and al., 1982).

Some of these parameters are influenced by thyroid hormones such as 3,5,3'-triiodo-L-thyronine (T_3). Thyroid hormones decrease the activity of bilirubin UDPGT but increase that of 4-nitrophenol UDPGT. The reduce simultaneously the content of cytochrome P 450 (Goudonnet and al., 1980 ; Schowdhury and al., 1979). It was therefore interesting to determine in what extend the thyroid status of animals influences the inducing effect of hypolipidaemic agents structurally related to fibrate (clofibrate, fenofibrate, bezafibrate and ciprofibrate).

MATERIALS AND METHODS

Treatment of the animals (mâle Wistar rats). Each group of control rats, hypothyroid rats (after chirurgical excision of the gland) and hyperthyroïd rats (after injection of triiodothyronine 30 µg/kg/day during 8 days), received, respectively a dose of 2 and 5 mg/kg ciprofibrate, 50 mg/kg for bezafibrate or fenofibrate and 200 mg/kg clofibrate, once a day for 8 days by oral administration via gastric tubage. In addition two series of animals received two doses per day of bezafibrate or fenofibrate, because of the shorter plasma half lives of these products. (8 rats for each series)

Biochemical assays
The microsomal cytochrome P 450 was determined by the Omura and Sato method (1964). Bilirubin UDPGT activity was evaluated according to Heirwegh and al (1972) using digitonin to obtain a maximal activation. The other UDPGT activities with 4-nitrophenol or nopol were mesured by the Mulder and Van Doorn's method (1975) on a Cobas fast analyser centrifuge, after maximal activation by Triton X-100.

RESULTS

Effect on bilirubin and 4-nitrophenol UDPGT

Thyroidectomy promoted an increase of the bilirubin UDPGT activity (80 %) (fig 1,a) and a decrease of 4-nitrophenol UDPGT activity (55 %) (fig 1,b). The treatment with T_3 (hyperthyroid status) gave opposite effects. All the hypolipidaemic drug : clofibrate (200 mg/kg), ciprofibrate (2 mg/kg), bezafibrate (1 X 50 mg/kg) and fenofibrate (1 X 50 mg administrated at equiactive doses exhibited similar inducing action on bilirubin UDPGT but this induction was dependent on the hormone status of the animals. Thus, the pourcentage increase reached 200 % in hyperthyroïd animals, 150 % in normal thyroïd animals and 50 % only in hypothyroïd rat rats (fig 1,a). Higher doses in ciprofibrate (5 mg/kg), bezafibrate (2 X 50 mg/kg) or fenofibrate (2 X 50 mg/kg) emphasized these effects. By contrast, 4-nitrophenol UDPGT activity was 20 to 30 % decreased after treatment with these drugs, whatever the thyroid status (fig 1,b).

Effect on hepatic cytochrome P 450 content

The amount in cytochrome P 450 was more than 30 % increase in control rats receiving ciprofibrate 5 mg/kg/day, bezafibrate 2 X 50 mg/kg/day and fenofibrate (2 X 50 mg/kg/day). The variations were not so expensive : 15 % or 10 % in hypo or hyperthyroid animals, respectively. The hypothyroid status did not modify the amount cytochrome P 450, whereas treatment by triiodothyronine caused a 40 % loss.
    Interestingly a correlation between the content in cytochrome P 450 and the bilirubin UDPGT could be established (r = 0,82) (fig. 2).

DISCUSSION AND CONCLUSION

We showed that ciprofibrate as other hypolipidaemic agents belonging

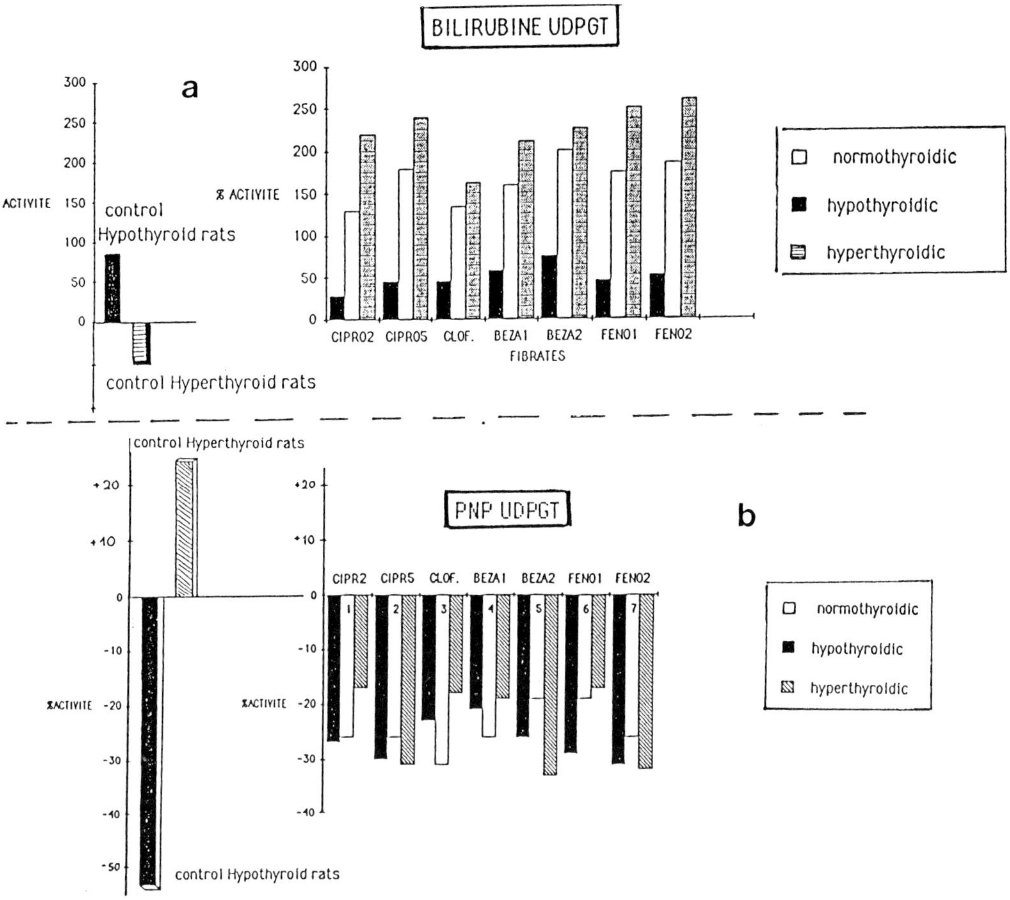

Fig. 1 - Effect of hormonal status on UDP-glucuronosyltransferase activities in hypolipidaemic drugs treated rats. The substrates used were bilirubin (fig. 1, a) and 4-nitrophenol (fig 1, b). The activities were expressed in % variations when compared to controls. For non-treated hypo- or hyperthyroid animals, the variations were calculated by reference to normal rats. The abbreviations and the daily doses used were : Cipro. 2, Cipro. 5 (2 mg and 5 mg) ; Clof. 200 mg ; Beza. 1; Beza. 2, (50 mg and 2 X 50 mg) ; Feno. 1, Feno. 2, (50 mg and 2 X 50 mg).

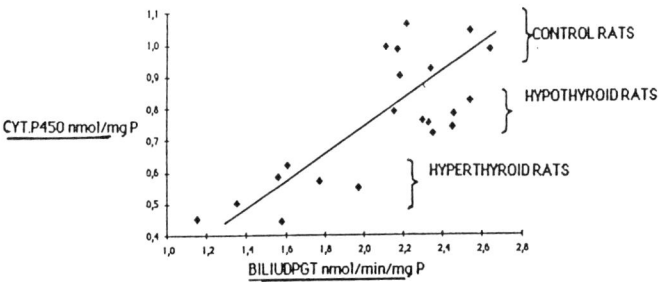

Fig. 2 - Correlation between the amount in cytochrome P 450 and the activity of bilirubin UDP-glucuronosyltransferase. Each point represent the mean obtained for each fibrate used at different doses.

to the fibrate series, administered at equiactive doses induced bilirubin UDPGT ; by contrast, conjugation of 4-nitrophenol, supported by a different form of UDPGT, was decreased. The induction of bilirubin UDPGT promoted by any fibrate responded to changes in the thyroid hormonal status, whereas 4-nitrophenol activity was not dependent : T_3 administrated at pharmacological doses to rats, exhausted the ability of fibrates to increase bilirubin UDPGT activity, whereas its own activity resulted in a decrease. This finding suggest that the bilirubin glucuronidation is regulated through different mecanisms by fibrates and thyroid hormones and emphazizes the role of hormonal control or the inducing process of drug metabolizing enzymes by xenobiotics. The correlation obtained between the amount in cytochrome P 450 and the activity in bilirubin UDPGT confirmed the possible existence of commun regulation of these two systems by hypolipidaemic drugs (Fournel and al, 1985).

REFERENCES

De Grimal, Ph., Goudonnet, H., Truchot, R.C. (1977) : Effet d'un hypolipémiant (fénofibrate) sur l'activité de diverses enzymes, en relation avec l'état thyroïdien et sur la teneur en cyt. P 450 de microsomes hépatiques chez le rat. J. Pharmacol.4, 477-485.

Fournel, S., Magdalou, J., Thomassin, J., Villoutreix, Siest,J., Caldwell, J., and André J.C. (1985) : Structure-dependent induction of bilirubin glucuronidation and lauric acid 12-hydroxylation by arylcarboxylic acids chemically related to clofibrate. BBA. 842, 202-213.

Gibson, E.E., Orton, T.C., Tamburini, P.P. (1982) : Cyt. P 450 induction by clofibrate. Purification and properties of a hepatic cyt. P 450 relatively specific for the 12 and 11-hydroxylation of dodécanoic acid (lauric acid). Biochem. J. 203, 161-168.

Goudonnet, H., Mounié, J., Truchot, R.C. (1980) : Effet de l'acide 3,5,3'-triiodothyroacétique et de la dextrothyroxine sur l'activité de diverses enzymes microsomales hépatiques induite par le phénobarbital. J. Pharmacol. 11, 245-256.

Heirwegh, K.P.M., Van de Vijver, M., Fevery, J. (1972) Biochem. J. 129, 605-618.

Mulder, G.J., Van Doorn, A.B.C. (1975) : A rapid NAD^+ linded assay for microsomal UDPGT of rat liver and some observations on substrate specificity of the enzyme. Biochem. J. 151, 131-135.

Omura, T., Sato, R. (1964) : The carbon monoxide binding pigment of liver microsomes. J. Biol. Chem. 239, 2370-2378.

Reddy, J., Chiga, M., Svoboda, D. (1971) : Biochem. Biophys. Res. Commun. 43, 318-324.

Schowdhury, J.R., Schowdhury, N.R., Moscioni, A.D., Tukey, R., Jephly, T., Arias, I.M. (1983) : Differential regulation by triiodothyronine of substrate specific UDPGT in rat liver. BBA. 761, 58-65.

ACKNOWLEDGEMENT : The "Centre de Recherche Sterling-Winthrop", Dijon, France, is acknowledged for financement and for providing the ciprofibrate use in this study.

Résumé

Les effets de doses equiactives de ciprofibrate, fenofibrate, bezafibrate et clofibrate, administrées à des rats placés dans différents états thyroïdiens, sur les activités de différentes formes microsomales hépatiques d'UDPGT ayant comme substrats respectifs : bilirubine et 4-nitrophénol ont été mesurés. Les résultats démontrent clairement l'influence de l'état hormonal thyroïdien dans la réponse des UDPGT aux hypolipidémiants quel que soit celui-ci. Par rapport à l'état normal, l'hyperthyroïdie augmente de plus de 50 % l'effet inducteur dû aux fibrates, alors que l'hypothyroïdie l'abaisse de près de 3 fois. La glucuronoconjugaison du 4-nitrophénol est au contraire abaissée de 20 à 30 % et ceci quel que soit l'état thyroïdien considéré. Par ailleurs, les variations de l'activité bilirubine UDPGT ont été comparées et mises en relation avec les variations de la teneur en cytochrome P 450 microsomal.

Induction of different forms of UDP-glucuronosyltransferases by 52028 RP, an isoquinoleine derivative

M. Totis, A.M. Batt and G. Siest

Université de Nancy-I, Centre du Médicament, UA CNRS n° 597, 30 rue Lionnois, 54000 Nancy, France

Abstract

Glucuronidation of several aglycones: 1-naphthol (GT1), morphine hydrochlorate (GT2) and bilirubin were measured in male rat liver microsomes after treatment by 52028 RP, an isoquinoleine derivative. The results have showed that the corresponding UDP-glucuronosyltransferase activities were enhanced.

Introduction

52028 RP, 1-(2-chlorophenyl)-N-methyl-(1-methylpropyl)-3-isoquinoline carboxamide (an isoquinoline derivative, previously named 11195 PK) is an antagonist from peripheral type benzodiazepine binding sites in different organs (Mestre et al.,1985). Pharmacokinetic studies have shown that 52028 RP was metabolized very rapidly in rat and human and that the rate of metabolism increased with repeated administration. This get us to study the effects of this molecule on drug metabolizing enzymes. We have demonstrated that 52028 RP is a potent inducer of different isoenzymes of cytochrome P-450: P-450b, P-450p and P-450j, with differential response depending from the sex of the animals (Totis M. et al., in preparation). As concomitant induction of cytochrome P-450 and UDP-glucuronosyltransferases (UDPGT) are known to occur, we studied the inducing effect of 52028 RP on different forms of UDPGT in male rat liver microsomes.

Materials and methods.

Animals. Male Sprague-Dawley rats (180-200g) were obtained from Iffa-Credo (St Germain/l'Arbresle-France) and allowed free access to water and a commercial available diet (U.A.R., Villemoisson, France).

Pretreatment. RP 52028, suspended in sucrose solution (700g/l), was given at a daily dose of 500 mg/kg, in 0.5 ml, for 5 days, by gastric intubation to groups of 5 male rats.
Microsomal fractions were prepared as previously described (Jayyosi et al.,1987) and stored as aliquots at -80°C until use.

Biochemical assays. Protein contents were determined with bovine serum albumin as a reference according to the method of Lowry et al. (1951). UDP-glucuronosyltransferase activities were evaluated after maximal activation for bilirubin according to Heirwegh et al. (1972) and by a modification of the Mulder and Van Doorn's method (1975) for all other substrates (1-naphthol, morphine hydrochlorate).

Results and discussion.

After treatment by 52028 RP in male rats, glucuronidation of the different aglycones measured in microsomes, was enhanced. We observed that the percentages of increase were greater for morphine and bilirubin conjugation.(Table I).

Table I: Glucuronidation of 1-naphthol (GT1), morphine hydrochlorate (GT2) and bilirubin in control and 52028 RP treated rats. The activity is expressed in nmol/min/mg protein.

Substrates	Control	52028 RP	% of increase
1-naphthol	76.9 ± 2.7	104.9 ± 7.5***	36
Morphine	3.5 ± 0.5	9.4 ± 0.6***	160
Bilirubin	0.79 ± 0.06	1.96 ± 0.09***	148

Results are expressed as mean ± standard deviation.
***: $p < 0.001$

These results show that 52028 RP was able to induce markedly distinct UDP-glucuronosyltransferases. Previous works have demonstrated that the drug was a potent inducer of different forms of cytochrome P-450, especially of cytochrome P-450b, the major form induced by phenobarbital (Guengerich et al., 1982), but also cytochrome P-450p, induced by pregnenolone 16 alpha-carbonitrile (Elchourbagy and Guzelian, 1980) and finally, cytochrome P-450j, an isoform induced by ethanol and isoniazid (Ryan et al., 1986). So the action of this drug could be compared to that of phenobarbital. We can also study the similarities between UDP-glucuronosyltransferase activities in phenobarbital and 52028 RP male treated rat liver microsomes. The glucuronoconjugation of morphine and bilirubin was stimulated by phenobarbital as much as by 52028 RP. By contrast, both drugs differ in their inducing effect toward conjugation of 1-naphthol. Indeed, phenobarbital induced little or none the glucuronidation of flat phenols (Okulicz-Kozaryn et al., 1981). A polyclic aromatic compound, 3-methylcholanthrene, is well known to stimulate the induction of the isoform active for conjugation of flat phenols (Wishart 1978a, 1978b). So, the induction of the different forms of cytochrome P-450 by 52028 RP could be compared to phenobarbital, but this drug, by contrast to phenobarbital, is able to stimulate the two different groups of UDP-glucuronosyltransferase, GT1 and GT2, generally induced by 3-methylcholanthrene and phenobarbital, respectively.

References.

Mestre M., Carriot T., Belin C., Uzan A., Renault C., Dubroeucq MC., Gueremy C., Doble A. and Le Fur G.(1985): Electrophysiological and pharmacological evidence that peripheral type benzodiazepine receptors are coupled to calcium channels in the heart. Life Sciences, 36, 391-400.

Jayyosi Z., Totis M., Souhaili H., Goulon-Ginet C., Livertoux M.H., Batt A.M. and Siest G.(1987): Induction of hepatic cytochrome P-450c-dependant monooxygenase activities by dantrolene in rat. Biochem. Pharmacol., 36, 2481-2487.

Lowry O.H., Rosenbrough N.J., Farr A.L. and Randall R.J.(1951): Protein measurement with the Folin phenol reagent. J. Biol. Chem., 193, 265-275.

Heirwegh K.P.M., Van de Vijver M. and Fevery J.(1972): Assay and properties of digitonin-activated bilirubin uridine diphosphate glucuronyltransferase from rat liver. Biochem. J., 129, 605-618.

Mulder G.J. and van Doorn A.B.D.(1975): A rapid NAD$^+$ linked assay for microsomal UDP-glucuronosyltransferase of rat liver and some observations on substrate specificity on the enzyme. Biochem. J., 151, 131-140.

Guengerich F.P., Dannan G.A., Wright S.T., Martin M.V. and Kaminsky L.S.(1982): Purification and characterization of liver microsomal cytochromes P-450: electrophoretic, spectral, catalytic and immunochemical properties and inductibility of eight isozymes isolated from rats treated with phenobarbital or ß naphtoflavone. Biochemistry, 21, 6019-6030.

Elchourbagy N.A. and Guzelian P.S.(1980): Separation, purification and characterization of a novel form of hepatic cytochrome P-450 from rats treated with pregnenolone 16-alpha carbonitrile. J. Biol. Chem., 255, 1279-1285.

Ryan D.E., Koop D.R., Thomas P.E., Coon M.J. and Levin W.(1986): Evidence that isoniazid and ethanol induce the same microsomal cytochrome P-450 in rat liver, an isozyme homologous to rabbit liver cytochrome P-450 isozyme 3a. Arch. Biochem. Biophys., 246, 633-644.

Okulicz-Kozaryn I., Schaefer M., Batt A.M., Siest G. and Loppinet V.(1981): Stereochemical heterogeneity of hepatic UDP-glucuronosyltransferase activity in rat liver microsomes. Biochem. Pharmacol., 30, 1457-1461.

Wishart G.J.(1978a): Functional heterogeneity of UDP-glucuronosyltransferase as indicated by its differential development and inducibility by glucocorticoids. Biochem. J., 174, 485-489.

Wishart G.J.(1978b): Demonstration of functional heterogeneity of hepatic UDP-glucuronosyltransferase activities after administration of 3-methylcholanthrene and phenobarbital to rats. Biochem. J., 174, 671-672.

Résumé

La glucuronoconjugaison de plusieurs aglycones: 1-naphtol (GT1), morphine (GT2) et bilirubine a été mesurée dans des microsomes de foie de rats males, après traitement par 52028 RP, un dérivé isoquinoléique. Les résultats ont montré que les activités UDP-glucuronosyltransférase correspondantes étaient augmentées.

Sulphation and glucuronidation of ethinyloestradiol in human tissues

G.M. Pacifici[1], M. Franchi[1], L. Vannucci[2] and F. Mosca[2]

Departments of [1]General Pathology and [2]Surgical Pathology, Medical School, University of Pisa, 56100 Pisa, Italy

SUMMARY

The activities of the sulpho transferase and glucuronyl transferase were measured in six human liver, intestinal mucosa, kidney and lung specimens. Tissue specimens were homogenized in 0.25 M sucrose and the microsomal and cytosolic fractions were isolated by differential centrifugation. The sulphation of ethinyloestradiol (EE2) was investigated in the cytosolic fraction whereas the glucuronidation of EE2 was studied in the microsomal fraction. Activities (mean ±SD; pmol/min/mg) of ST were 117±20 (liver); 21.8±16.1 (intestine); 5.4±1.7 (kidneys) and 9.3±5.1 (lungs). GT activities (mean ±SD; pmol/min/mg) were 174±75 (liver); 14.3±7.1 (intestine); 7.1±1.8 (kidneys) and 5.0±0.7 (lungs). The liver catalyzed the sulphation and glucuronidation of EE2 at higher rate than the other tissues. Among the non hepatic tissues, the intestinal mucosa showed the highest rate of sulphation and the glucuronidation of EE2. The balance between two methabolic pathawys is tissue dependent.

KEY WORDS

Ethinyloestradiol, sulpho transferase, glucuronyl transferase, distribution, humans.

INTRODUCTION

Ethinyloestradiol (EE2) is an oestrogen derivative molecule administered to man. Its major use is as contraceptive. It is also used in the treatment od menopausal symptoms, functional uterine bleending as well as for palliative treatment of carcinoma of the prostate and of the breast. EE2 is subjected to extensive metabolism. This molecule is hydroxylated and conjugated with sulphate and glucuronic acid. We have previously observed that "phase I" enzymes are associated with the liver whereas "phase II" enzymes have a more ubiquitous distribution in the organism (Pacifici et al. 1988 a). This prompted us to measure the activities of sulpho transfease (ST) and glucuronyl transferase (GT) with EE2 as substrate in human liver, intestinal mucosa, kidneys and lungs.

MATERIALS AND METHODS

Human liver was obtained at laparotomy from patients undergoing colecystectomy. Surplus of wedge biopsy for histological analisys was made available for our studies. All liver biopsies had normal cell architecture. Intestine, kidneys and lungs were obtained from patients undergoing the resection of the organ to remove a tumor. A normal part of the tissue next to the tumor was made available for our studies. The intestinal mucosa was isolated at room temperature after resection of the intestine. Tissue specimens were stored at -80 C.

Aliquots (0.5-2 g) of the various tissues were minced and homogenized in 4 volumes of 0.25 M sucrose by means of a glass-teflon homogenizer. Samples were centrifuged at 12,000xg for 15 min. The supernatant was centrifuged again at 105,000xg for 1 hr. The ensuing supernatants was investigated as the cytosolic fraction. The pellets were resuspended in 0.1 mM Tris-HCl (pH 7.4) contining 30% glycerol and ivestigated as the microsomal fractions.

The activities of ST and GT were measured as described by Pacifici et al. (1988b). Briefly, the incubation mixture for ST assay, final volume 0.1 ml, was as follows: 0.1 M Tris-HCl (pH 7.4), 5 mM 2-mercaptoethanol, 0.025 mM (^{3}H)EE2 (200,000 cpm), and an aliquot of cytosolic protein to give a final protein concentration varying between 1.2 and 1.9 mg/ml. The reaction was started by the addition of 0.1 mM adenosine 3'-phosphate-5'-phosphosulphate (PAPS). The incubation was carried out at 37 C for 20 min and was stopped by the addition of 0.9 ml of a mixture containing 0.4 M trichloroacetic acid (TCA) and 0.6 M glycine. The assay for GT was carried out in a final volume of 0.2 ml. The incubation mixture contained 0.1 M Tris-HCl (pH 7.4), 5 mM $MgCl_2$, 0.2 mM (^{3}H)EE2 (700,000 cpm) and an aliquot of microsomal protein to give a final protein concentration ranging between 0.6 and 0.9 mg/ml. The reaction was started by addition of 5 mM uridine 5'-diphosphoglucuronic acid (UDPGA). Incubations were carried out at 37 C for 20 min and were stopped by the addition of 0.8 ml of 0.4 M TCA and 0.6 M glycine. Following the incubation for both ST anf GT, 5 ml of water-saturated ether were added and the tubes were shaken for 20 min. Samples were centrifuged at 1500xg for 5 min, the organic layer was removed, and 0.4 ml of water phase residue was transferred into scintillation vials containing 10 ml of sintillant. The radioactivity was measured by means of a liquid scintillation spectrometry.

For both assays, each sample was assayed in duplicate and was provided of two blanks that were as the samples except that PAPS or UDPGA were replaced by water. The activities of ST and GT were measured after correction for blanks.

RESULTS

The rates of sulphation and glucuronidation of EE2 are shown in tables 1 and 2, respectively. The liver catalyzed the conjugation of EE2 with sulphate and glucuronic acid at higher rate than intestinal mucosa, kidneys and lungs. The GT activity was higher than the ST activity in liver, whereas in the intestine and lungs the ST was the predominant pathway.

Table 1. Rate of sulphation of ethinyloestradiol in human tissues.
pmol/min/mg

LIVER			INTESTINE				KIDNEYS			LUNGS		
Age	Sex		Age	Sex			Age	Sex		Age	Sex	
23	M	127	58	M	Ileum	7.9	32	F	3.6	47	M	7.4
43	F	103	58	M	Colon	5.1	56	F	6.6	54	M	18.1
45	F	96	64	M	Ileum	41.1	62	F	3.4	59	M	12.4
46	M	157	64	M	Colon	15.2	63	M	4.5	63	M	2.7
56	M	114	72	M	Ileum	46.6	69	F	6.4	64	M	4.5
70	F	106	72	M	Colon	14.8	71	M	7.9	65	M	10.7
Mean		117				21.8			5.4			9.3
±SD		20				16.1			1.7			5.1

Table 2. Rate of glucuronidation of ethinyloestradiol in human tissues
pmol/min/mg

LIVER			INTESTINE				KIDNEYS			LUNGS		
Age	Sex		Age	Sex			Age	Sex		Age	Sex	
23	M	134	58	M	Ileum	8.0	32	F	8.8	47	M	5.4
43	F	333	58	M	Colon	21.5	56	F	5.2	54	M	3.6
45	F	115	64	M	Ileum	7.9	62	F	5.6	59	M	4.9
46	M	127	64	M	Colon	16.3	63	M	9.6	63	M	5.0
56	M	148	72	M	Ileum	25.0	69	F	5.4	64	M	6.1
70	F	189	72	M	Colon	7.1	71	M	8.2	65	M	4.8
Mean		174				14.3			7.1			5.0
± SD		75				7.1			1.8			0.7

DISCUSSION

The present results show that the conjugation of EE2 with sulphate and glucuronyc acid is catalyzed by the liver, intestinal mucosa, kidneys and lungs. EE2 is a suitable model to study glucuronidation and solphation in human tissues.
The hepatic ST and GT activities are in accord with those published (Pacifici et al. 1988b). The lack of data in non-hepatic tissues does not make possible the comparison of our results. EE2 undergoes presystemic elimination in humans (Back et al. 1982), thus it is removed by the intestinal and hepatic metabolism during absorption. It is of relevance that the intestinal mucosa catalyzes the sulphation and glucuronidation of EE2 at higher rate than the other non-hepatic tissues. ST activity is higher than GT in the intestine. Such a finding is in accord with the results obtained with intact mucosa (Roger et al., 1987). ST activity is higher in ileum than colon. Such a result is consisting with that btained with 2-naphthol (unpublished results). The contribution of the kidneys and lungs to the hepatic sulphation and glucuronidation of EE2 is modest.

REFERENCES

Back, J.D., Brekenridge, A.M., MacIver, M., Orme, M.L'E., Purba H.S., Rowe, P.H., Taylor, I. (1982): The gut wall metabolism of ethinyloestrodiol and its contribution to the pre-systemic metabolism of ethinyloestradiol in humans. Br. J. Clin. Pharmacol. 13, 325-330.

Pacifici, G.M., Franchi, M., Bencini, C., Repetti, F., Di Lascio, N., Muraro, G.B. (1988a): Tissue distribution of drug-metabolizing enzymes in humans. Xenobiotioca (In Press)

Pacifici, G.M., Back, D.J. (1988b): Sulphation and glucuronidation of ethinyloestradiol in human liver in vitro. J. Steroid Biochem. (In Press)

Rogers, S.M., Back, D.J., Orme M.L'E. (1987): Intestinal metabolism of ethinyloestradiol and paracetamol in vitro: studies using Ussing chamber. Br J. Clin. Pharmacol. 23, 727-724.

Résumé

Les activités de la sulfotransférase (ST) et de la glucuronyltransférase (GT) ont été mesurées dans six échantillons humains de foie, muqueuse intestinale, rein et poumon. Ces tissus sont homogénéisés dans du saccharose 0.25 M et les fractions microsomale et cytosolique sont isolées par centrifugation différentielle. La sulfoconjugaison de l'éthinyl-oestradiol (EE2) a été mesurée dans la fraction cytosolique tandis que sa glucuronoconjugaison a été suivie dans les microsomes. Les activités de la ST (moyenne ± SD ; pmol/min/mg) sont 117 ± 20 (foie) ; 21.8 ± 16.1 (intestin) ; 5.4 ± 1.7 (reins) et 9.3 ± 5.1 (poumons). L'activité de la GT (moyenne ± SD ; pmol/min/mg) sont 174 ± 75 (foie) ; 14.3 ± 7.1 (intestin) ; 7.1 ± 1.8 (reins) et 5.0 ± 0.7 (poumons). Le foie catalyse la sulfo- et la glucuronoconjugaison de EE2 à une vitesse supérieure à celle observée dans les autres tissus. Parmi les organes extra hépatiques, la muqueuse intestinale présente la plus forte vitesse de sulfo-et glucuronoconjugaison de l'EE2. L'équilibre entre les deux voies métaboliques est tissu-dépendant.

Author Index
Index des auteurs

Alary, J. 285
André, J.C., ... 51
Antoine, B. 79, 177, 221
Armstrong, R.N. 51
Augustin, C. 229

Bagrel D. 113
Batt, A.M. 177, 311
Beauvallet, M 297
Becker, F.F. 29
Benet, L.Z. 261
Benthe, H.F. 229
Benveniste, P. 225
Berger, Y. 249
Bessems, J.G.M. 51
Bichet, N. 249
Blanckaert, N. 103
Bock, K.W. 239
Boutin, J.A. 79
Bouvier-Nave, P. 225
Bromet, N. 305
Burchell, B. 13, 43, 69
Burke, M.D. 129

Caldwell, J. 185, 233
Cano, J.P. 249
Carré, M.C. 43
Carrera, G. 285
Celier, C. 289
Chessebeuf-Padieu, M. 137
Coffman, B. 37
Coughtrie, M.W.H. 69
Cresteil, T. 289

Dabé, J.F. 305
Devaux, A. 293
Devissaguet, M. 305
Diez Ibanez, M. 137
Donn, F. 229
Doostdar, H. 129
Dragacci, F. 113
Durand, A. 297

Engeset, J. 129
Escousse, A. 311

Fabre, G. 249
Faye, B. 221
Fevery, J. 279
Foliot, A. 301
Forgues, S. 285
Fournel-Gigleux, S. 13, 43, 69, 113
                                            185, 305
Franchi, M. 93, 321

Garnier, M.H. 305
Ghersi-Egea, J.F. 169
Gillet, G. 297
Giuliani L. 93
Goldhoorn, B.G. 193
Gollan, J.L. 85
Goon, D. 159
Goudonnet, H. 311
Grant, M.H.
Green, M. 37, 129
Grislain, L. 305
Grubb, N. 185
Guichard, J.P. 233

Harding, D. 13, 43, 69
Homma, H. 59
Hume, R. 69
Hutt, A.J. 185

Iyanagi, T. 3

Jackson, M.R. 13, 43, 69
Jansen, P.L.M. 151, 193, 271
Jayyosi, Z. 177
Jongepier, U. 239

Klaassen C.D. 159
Koster, A.Sj. 151
Krull, S. 239

Lafaurie, C. 305
Lahiri, P. 29
Lapontarique, H. 285
Lefauconnier, J.M. 169
Leroux, J.P. 289
Leroy, P. 201
Luijten, W. 305

Mackenzie, P.I. 21, 29
Magdalou, J. 43, 113, 177, 221, 305, 311
Maley, M. 129
Marie, S. 289

Marschall, H.U.	141	Schulz, M.	229
Matern, H.	141	Shepherd, S.R.P.	43
Matern, S.	141	Siest, G.	43, 79, 113, 177, 221, 305, 311
Matsui, M.	59		
Maurel, P.	249	Sinclair, K.A.	185
McQueen, C.A.	121	Spahn, H.	261
Melvin, W.T.	129		
Mesa, V.	279	Tayarani, Y.	169
Minn, A.	169	Tephly, T.	37
Morselli, P.L.	297	Thenot, J.P.	297
Mosca, F.	321	Thomassin, J.	177
Mounié, J.	311	Totis, M.	311
Mulder, G.J.	271	Touchard, D.	301
Muraca, M.	279	Townsend, M.	37
Myara, A.	301	Trivin, F.	301
		Truchot, R.C.	311
Nagai, F.	59		
Nicholls, S.	185	Ullmann, P.	225
Nicolas, A.	201	Ury, A.	225
Oude Elferink, R.P.J.	151, 193	Van Breemen, R.B.	211
		Van Es H.H.G.	193
Pacifici, G.M.	93, 321	Vannucci, L.	321
Padieu, P.	137	Vanstapel, F.	103
Paul-Abrahamse, M.	193	Van Steenbergen, W.	279
Peters, W.H.M.	193	Vic, P.	249
Puig, J.	37	Von Meyerinck, L.	229
		Vries M.H. de	151
Redegeld, F.A.M.	151	Warrander, A.	271
Rivière, J.-L.	293	Weil, A.	185, 233
Roques, M.	113	Whitmer, D.I.	85
Roy Chowdhury, J.	29	Wierckx, F.C.J.	271
Roy Chowdhury, N.	29	Wietholtz, H.	141
		Williams, G.M.	121
Schirmer, G.	239	Wilson, S.	69
Schmoldt, A.	229	Wooster, R.	13

Colloques INSERM
ISSN 0768-3154

Other *Colloques* published as co-editions by John Libbey Eurotext and INSERM

133 Cardiovascular and Respiratory Physiology in the Fetus and Neonate. *Physiologie Cardiovasculaire et Respiratoire du Fœtus et du Nouveau-né.*
Scientific Committee : P. Karlberg,
A. Minkowski, W. Oh and L. Stern;
Managing Editor : M. Monset-Couchard.
ISBN : John Libbey Eurotext 0 86196 125 0
INSERM 2 85598 340 1

134 Porphyrins and Porphyrias. *Porphyrines et Porphyries.*
Edited by Y. Nordmann.
ISBN : John Libbey Eurotext 0 86196 087 4
INSERM 2 85598 281 2

137 Neo-Adjuvant Chemotherapy. *Chimiothérapie Néo-Adjuvante.*
Edited by C. Jacquillat, M. Weil and D. Khayat.
ISBN : John Libbey Eurotext 0 86196 125 0
INSERM 2 85598 340 1

139 Hormones and Cell Regulation (10th European Symposium). *Hormones et Régulation Cellulaire (10e Symposium Européen).*
Edited by J. Nunez, J.E. Dumont and R. J.B. King.
ISBN : John Libbey Eurotext 0 86196 125 0X
INSERM 2 85598 340 1

147 Modern Trends in Aging Research. *Nouvelles Perspectives de la Recherche sur le Vieillissement.*
Edited by Y. Courtois, B. Faucheux, B. Forette,
D.L. Knook and J.A. Tréton.
ISBN : John Libbey Eurotext 0 86196 125 0X
INSERM 2 85598 340 1

149 Binding Proteins of Steroid Hormones. *Protéines de liaison des Hormones Stéroïdes.*
Edited by M.G. Forest and M. Pugeat.
ISBN : John Libbey Eurotext 0 86196 125 0
INSERM 2 85598 340 1X

151 Control and Management of Parturition. *La Maîtrise de la Parturition.*
Edited by C. Sureau, P. Blot, D. Cabrol, F. Cavaillé and G. Germain.
ISBN : John Libbey Eurotext 0 86196 125 0
INSERM 2 85598 340 1

153 Hormones and Cell Regulation (11th European Symposium). *Hormones et Régulation Cellulaire (11ᵉ Symposium Européen).*
Edited by J. Nunez and J.E. Dumont
ISBN : John Libbey Eurotext 0 86196 104 8
INSERM 2 85598 324 X

158 Biochemistry and Physiopathology of Platelet Membrane. *Biochimie et Physiopathologie de la Membrane Plaquettaire.*
Edited by G. Marguerie and R.F.A.A. Zwaal.
ISBN : John Libbey Eurotext 0 86196 114 5
INSERM 2 85598 345 2

162 The Inhibitors of Hematopoiesis. *Les Inhibiteurs de l'Hématopoïèse.*
Edited by A. Najman, M. Guigon, N.-C. Gorin, and J.-Y. Mary
ISBN : John Libbey Eurotext 0 86196 125 0
INSERM 2 85598 340 1

164 Liver Cells and Drugs. *Cellules Hépatiques et Médicaments.*
Edited by A. Guillouzo
ISBN : John Libbey Eurotext 0 86 196 128 5
INSERM 2 85598 341 X

165 Hormones and Cell Regulation (12th European Symposium). *Hormones et Régulation Cellulaire (12ᵉ Symposium Européen).*
Edited by J. Nunez, J.E. Dumont and E. Carafoli
ISBN : John Libbey Eurotext 0 86 196 133 1
INSERM 2 85598 347 9

167 Sleep Disorders and Respiration. *Les Evénements Respiratoires du Sommeil.*
Edited by P. Lévi-Valensi and D. Duron
ISBN : John Libbey Eurotext 0 86196 127 7
INSERM 2 85598 344 4

171 Structure and Functions of the Cytoskeleton. *La Structure et les Fonctions du Cytosquelette.*
Edited by B.A.F. Rousset
ISBN : John Libbey Eurotext 0 86 196 149 8
INSERM 2 85598 351 7

172 The Langerhans Cell. *La Cellule de Langerhans.*
Edited by J. Thivolet and D. Schmitt
ISBN : John Libbey Eurotext 0 86 196 181 1
INSERM 2 85598 352 5